"Dr. LaLonde presents a deeply creative and interdisciplinary path for clinicians, artists, humanists, and trauma survivors to develop novel ways of thinking about and healing from traumatic experiences. Her ideas and explorations of the relationship between trauma, resilience, and literature will deeply touch anyone who has found solace in immersing themselves in the literary world."

Dr. Alix Rivière, *Childhood Trauma Research and Policy Analyst at the Office of the Child Advocate of Massachusetts*

"Humanizing and transformative! Dr. LaLonde provides a unique perspective on trauma and posttraumatic growth, applying a humanities and literature lens supported by anecdotical data, narratives, and her own experiences working in academia and classroom settings. While discussing the main contributions of neurologists, psychiatrists, psychoanalysts, medical anthropologists and other relevant disciplines, the author takes the audience on a historical journey from the beginnings of how trauma has been conceptualized over time and further discusses the significance of resilience and post-traumatic growth. A wonderful book for current and future professionals and practitioners working in the field of trauma and resilience to develop an interdisciplinary perspective."

Dr. Elizabeth Trejos-Castillo, *Professor and Traumatologist at Texas Tech University*

Trauma, Posttraumatic Growth, and World Literature

Pandemics, global climate chaos, worldwide migration crises? These phenomena are provoking traumatic experiences in unprecedented ways and numbers. This book is targeted for clinicians, scientists, cultural theorists, and other scholars and students of trauma studies interested in cultivating interdisciplinary understandings of trauma and posttraumatic conditions, especially resistance, resilience, and posttraumatic growth. Following clinicians' invitation for trauma survivors to wear a philosopher's hat, to engage in creative activities, and to employ cognitive exercises to combat psychic constriction, the author introduces the concept of a Literary Arts Praxis. The Praxis is built on clinical research and literature seeped in existential, phenomenological, and aesthetic themes. She argues that an educational training in a Praxis might help trauma survivors to get at trauma, as they engage in: imaginative escapades, interpretative exercises, and creative writing endeavors, which include turning testimonies into imaginative stories.

Suzanne LaLonde holds a PhD in French Language and Literature, has served as an Associate Professor of Cultural Studies at the University of Texas-Rio Grande Valley, and serves currently as a Humanities Instructor in the Honors College at Texas Tech University. Her areas of research have centered on French and Francophone Literature, World Literature, Trauma Studies, Psychoanalysis, and Ecocriticism. In her book *Paris and Its Revolutionary Ideas* (2021), she invites readers to reconsider the concept of revolutions, which take place in minds and hearts, through an exposure to the arts populating the Parisian landscape. Her teaching record and interests center on French Culture, European Art History, Humanities Driven STEM courses, and Medical Humanities classes, including "Narratives of Illness and Reflective Writing" and "World Literature and Global Health."

Literary Criticism and Cultural Theory

Trans(in)fusion
Reflections for Critical Thinking
Ranjan Ghosh

Ghostly Encounters
Cultural and Imaginary Representations of the Spectral from the
Nineteenth Century to the Present
Edited by Stefano Cracolici and Mark Sandy

Gender and Memory in the Postmillennial Novels of Almudena Grandes
Lorraine Ryan

Recycling Virginia Woolf in Contemporary Art and Literature
Edited by Monica Latham, Caroline Marie and Anne-Laure Rigeade

Lu Xun's Affirmative Biopolitics
Nothingness and the Power of Self-Transcendence
Wenjin Cui

Queer Women in Modern Spanish Literature
Activism, Sexuality, and the Otherness of the 'Chicas Raras'
Edited by Ana I. Simón-Alegre and Lou Charnon-Deutsch

Telling Details
Chinese Fiction, World Literature
Jiwei Xiao

Erich Auerbach and the Secular World
Literary Criticism, Historiography, Post-Colonial Theory and Beyond
Jon Nixon

Living with Monsters
A Study of the Art of Characterization in Aldous Huxley's Novels
Indrani Deb

Trauma, Posttraumatic Growth, and World Literature
Metamorphoses and a Literary Arts Praxis
Suzanne LaLonde

For more information about this series, please visit: https://www.routledge.com/
Literary-Criticism-and-Cultural-Theory/book-series/LITCRITANDCULT.

Trauma, Posttraumatic Growth, and World Literature

Metamorphoses and a Literary
Arts Praxis

Suzanne LaLonde

Routledge
Taylor & Francis Group

NEW YORK AND LONDON

First published 2022
by Routledge
605 Third Avenue, New York, NY 10158

and by Routledge
4 Park Square, Milton Park, Abingdon, Oxon OX14 4RN

Routledge is an imprint of the Taylor & Francis Group, an informa business

© 2022 Suzanne LaLonde

Library of Congress Cataloging-in-Publication Data
A catalog record for this title has been requested

ISBN: 9781032256887 (hbk)
ISBN: 9781032257099 (pbk)
ISBN: 9781003284642 (ebk)

DOI: 10.4324/9781003284642

Typeset in Sabon
by Taylor & Francis Books

In loving memory of my brother, Robert J. LaLonde

Contents

Acknowledgments

This text has undergone its own metamorphoses thanks to the constant support of my colleagues, editors, friends, family, and students. I would like to thank the initial invaluable feedback I received from Dr. Eve Golden. She was instrumental in helping me to define interdisciplinary links between the sciences, medicine, and the humanities and to render abstract discussions on literature and art more concrete for a scientific community of readers. I am also indebted to my colleagues Luis Rodriguez-Abad, Bill Yaworsky, and Joe Hodes who have read various iterations of my writing and poured over them with a fine-tooth comb. Special thanks are in order to my former graduate students Maria González and Erin Knobloch who assisted me with foundational research and engaged in stimulating conversations about trauma and resilience. My gratitude extends to my editors at Routledge, Mitchell Manners, Michelle Salyga, and Cherry Allen, and copy-editor Hamish Ironside, whose assistance and professional input were unwavering. This book would not have come to fruition without the constant moral support of my family. During the pandemic especially, our Zoom calls provided sustenance in the form of witty and warm exchanges. Special thanks especially to Joe, Marc, Mimi, and Alex for cultivating a sense of direction and continued passion for this book project. Most importantly, I wish to acknowledge the debt I owe to my former undergraduate students at UT-RGV who taught me about courageous and creative acts of resistance, resilience, and growth to combat the devastating effects of trauma. Your lives are inspirational testaments of determined drives to flourish emotionally and intellectually. Finally, grateful acknowledgement is made to Johns Hopkins University Press and Kent State University Press for granting me permission to use parts of previously published material in my chapters on Jean-Marie Gustave Le Clézio's *Desert* and Albert Camus's *The Plague*.

Introduction

Trauma, Posttraumatic Growth, and Pedagogy

The seeds of this book on trauma, posttraumatic growth, and world literature were planted in classrooms where I learned about the traumatic
experiences of my students. By traumatic experiences, I am referring to both
trauma and traumatism.[1] Trauma can refer to physical or psychic wounds
caused by either a physical or psychic event or events that are "extraordinary, not because they occur rarely, but rather because they overwhelm
the ordinary human adaptations to life."[2] Traumatism includes subsequent
states, ranging from posttraumatic stress disorder (PTSD), "with its intrusive and fixed remembrances or its opposite, resilience."[3] Posttraumatic
states also include resistance and growth, and even recovery, cure, and
healing.

My interest in these topics started in my course on French intimate
literature, which I taught at the University of Texas–Rio Grande Valley
(UT-RGV). Many of my students were Mexican, crossing the border from
the neighboring state of Tamaulipas to Brownsville to attend classes.[4] We
read chronicles, essays, reveries, diaries, journals, memoirs, and letters in
French. We spent the semester in the company of Victor Hugo to Simone de
Beauvoir. And yet, I also spent time in my students' heads. I asked them to
keep a diary in French. This was an advanced undergraduate course, and my
students possessed advanced college French skills owing to their native
Spanish. Their journal entries did not simply amount to enumerations of
daily activities. Students also dialogued with the philosopher Jean-Jacques
Rousseau about inequalities and with the psychiatrist and philosopher
Frantz Fanon about oppression and violence. The Renaissance philosopher
Michel de Montaigne turned to writing essays in response to the despair he
felt during the French Wars of Religion, whereas the existentialist philosopher and writer Jean-Paul Sartre took up his pen during World War II to
make sense of the role of the arts amidst evil. For my students, course
readings appeared to translate the untranslatable, while journaling seemed
to provoke new ways of contemplating what defied contemplation. This led
me to ponder: How are psychic trauma and posttraumatic experiences related to the literary arts, including storytelling, decoding stories and literature, and creative writing?

DOI: 10.4324/9781003284642-1

This question was predicated not only on my students' experiences but on my own confrontation with the prevalence of trauma in the community. I had been contacted earlier in my teaching career at UT-RGV by law-enforcement officials to serve as a translator for a case involving the murder of a young woman. She had been kidnapped by a Mexican cartel and brought to the United States, where she was exploited as a sex slave, brutally tortured, and eventually killed. Her enslavement and murder were recorded in confiscated letters exchanged among cartel leaders, including those from a French cartel. Thus, the reason for the letters in French and Spanish. While I thought I knew what to expect, I failed to imagine the extent of the brutality. I returned the packet of letters to an officer, refusing the job. "Fine," replied the agent with a misplaced grin, "but you know … the cartels are like cockroaches." Confused, I asked the agent why he was cautioning me. "They're everywhere, underneath the woodwork, up on the rafters. You'll come across them when you turn on the lights at night." With images of cockroaches and the young woman's murder haunting me, I struggled to return to my teaching and research duties. The struggle intensified as I wrestled with the thought of my students' welfare. It was not a question of whether they had been exposed to such traumatic experiences. It was a question of how many.

The first assignment in my French intimate literature course confirmed my worst fears. Students were asked to record their weekend activities and whether they found Montaigne's description of hypocrisy in his essay "Of Cannibals" relevant today. My student Luz-María's diary entry was shocking.[5] She described how her fiancé had been kidnapped that weekend. Her family was forced to pay some $20,000 for his release. How was she able to write about this in French, no less in her native tongue? In short simple sentences, she outlined how "they" (cartel members) stormed in on the family-owned recycling business, held her fiancé at gunpoint, blind-folded him, and swept him off in a car that sped into dusty fields outside Matamoros, the Mexican city on the other side of the Rio Grande River. Once the ransom was delivered, her fiancé was returned, and Luz-María and he spent the evening locked in each other's arms. As for Montaigne's "Of Cannibals"? "They're still eating us," she wrote, finishing the sentence with blank pages. When I returned her journal, I asked if I could speak to her after class. She seemed stuck in a shaken state, but also somehow resolute. "This is a way of life for us," she explained firmly in English. "The cartel seeks businesses for revenue. They kidnapped my fiancé to cement the 'partnership'. They keep us 'safe,' we finance them." "Even a recycling business?" I asked naively. "It's the copper they're after. Anything that generates money." "But are you OK?" I pressed on. "That's why I'm here," she responded with a smirk to hint at the double entendre of her words.

I did not learn directly about Juan-Carlos's traumatic experiences in his diary. Details arose only subtly. His family had owned a cell-phone store in Matamoros until cartel members ransacked and took it over. Hints of this traumatic event found their way into his journal in response to Albert Camus's essay "The Myth of Sisyphus." "The cartel leaders are the gods; we are Sisyphus," he wrote. "We have no freedom going up the mountain. But we do on the way down. We can swear at those monsters and defy them in subtle ways. Sisyphus is my hero." After class, I told Juan-Carlos how moved I was by his writing. He followed me back to my office and spurted out in English: "I could have been killed." "Killed?" I managed to formulate. "Yes, killed. I was only twelve. I had been under the store counter organizing merchandise in the cabinets of my father's shop. I heard the brass bells on the door ringing wildly. A man started screaming at my uncle about my father. 'Where is he?' Where is he?' I heard gunshots. My uncle fell to the ground behind the counter. A stream of blood spilled on the floor." How was I supposed to react? I managed to say, "*Lo siento mucho*" and added, "I'm very sorry." He dodged my condolences by explaining that the cartel kidnapped his father to "help" with their illegal telecommunication services. Fleeing for their lives, Juan-Carlos and his mother crossed the border without papers to start a new life. He was majoring in psychology. He aspired to become a social worker to help migrant families.

Certainly not all my students shared their stories. Or if they did, were their experiences as traumatic. However, whether it was in my "French Intimate Literature" class or in "Narratives of Illness and Reflective Writing," it became obvious that I was working with a unique group of students. There were others like Luz-María and Juan-Carlos, to be sure, but also the undocumented and DACA students.[6] As they asked me to write letters of recommendations for scholarships or for DACA applications, I learned more about traumatic experiences of migration, not least those of family members separated and deported back to cartel-ridden Central America. How was I to process these narratives? My training in French and Spanish languages and literatures did not seem immediately applicable. Besides, was I somehow stepping outside my job responsibilities by listening so intently to their stories? Or was I perhaps serving as a witness to their traumatic experiences? What was clear was the humanitarian crisis along the US–Mexican border and throughout Central America, and it just did not seem right to remain inured or silent about it.

At the time I wrestled with this reality, I had not yet acquainted myself with scientific trauma theories—developed by psychiatrists, neurologists, psychoanalysts, psychologists, clinicians, anthropologists, and sociologists. Nor had I been exposed formally to trauma studies, an interdisciplinary domain of research (from psychiatry to sociology to the arts) that investigates traumatic experiences and posttraumatic conditions and treatments. Nor with cultural trauma studies cultivated by historians, philosophers, and literary theorists (notably, deconstructionists, feminists, post-colonialists, and eco-critics). Nonetheless, my training in French literature and specifically existentialism and aesthetics had introduced me to the philosopher Theodor Adorno. I heard his dialectical discourse on aesthetics ringing in my ears. He is known for his much-quoted statement that "it is barbaric to continue to write poetry after Auschwitz."[7] This intimates that the arts can never do justice to experiences of horrific suffering. By attempting to make sense of horrific suffering, the arts diminish and betray it. Adorno insisted nonetheless that he was not targeting exclusively poetry or the arts. The arts are not the problem; they are a symptom of a greater problem. Life itself is void of meaning, whereas the arts appear to have meaning, after all. "The darkening of the world makes the irrationality of art rational: radically darkened art."[8] Though the arts might dwell in darkness, this state transmits messages of the disaster of suffering. In this repressed form, art "takes into itself the disaster, the principle of repression, rather than merely protesting hopelessly against it."[9] The arts become therefore a place of hidden and repressed suffering. Is this what my students had experienced while reading intimate literature and journaling? By writing about their own experiences in response to Montaigne's and Camus's literature, they seemed to silence and yet voice their suffering. Cannibals were cartel members; Sisyphus became a victim-hero. And by writing in a foreign language, my students appeared to silence the voice of suffering in their mother tongue and to give it a voice in another language. These tentative observations and interpretations based on Adorno's work prompted me to ponder more specifically: How might the literary arts reach trauma survivors in meaningful ways?

The research of literary theorist Shoshana Felman also came to mind in my early research on trauma. I was familiar with her work on Camus's *The Plague* (1947) in her co-authored *Testimony* (1991) with psychiatrist Dori Laub. When I revisited her book, I was pleased to discover how she framed her project: "Is there a relation between trauma and pedagogy?" and "Can trauma instruct pedagogy and can pedagogy shed light on the mystery of trauma?"[10] In some respects, her questions reflected my own. One of her findings was that her students experienced an "encounter with the real" in her course.[11] By studying literature and viewing autobiographical videotapes of Holocaust survivors, her class found itself "entirely at a loss, uprooted and disoriented, and profoundly shaken in its anchoring world views and its commonly held life-perspectives."[12] Uprooted? Disoriented? Profoundly shaken in one's anchoring world views and commonly held-life perspectives? This vocabulary echoed my students' and yet sounded foreign. True, my students appeared shaken when they elaborated on their traumatic experiences in more detail outside the classroom. And true, I felt deeply disoriented when I realized just how prevalent trauma permeated the community and marked my students. Still, traumatic experiences in everyday life had already uprooted, disoriented, and disrupted their lives. The classroom on the other hand served as a haven. Tossed about in rough waters every day, they seemed to arrive at a calm port where they could anchor their being. Course readings and writing exercises appeared to help them reorient themselves. They rewrote stories, when stories failed, and communicated in a language removed from the original trauma. Between discovering my students' stories of trauma and learning about resistance, resilience, and growth from them and from scientific literature, I sensed that posttraumatic recovery might be caught up with pedagogy. That is, pedagogy rich in the literary arts did not seem to disrupt, but to bolster and build a mind suffering from traumatic experiences. Thus, I rephrased Felman's question about "a relation between trauma and pedagogy" to: How is posttraumatic growth (PTG) and other states, such as resistance and resilience, related to pedagogy?

I did not contemplate this question lightly. In the back of my mind rang the arguments of psychiatrist Peter D. Kramer about literature and mental illness. In his *Moments of Engagement* (1994), he writes about his fraught search for meaning in his early career as a therapist: "My collapse came," he confesses, "during the hospital stay of an affable, unflinchingly suicidal young man—let us call him Alex—who had decided on the basis of reading Kurt Vonnegut and Albert Camus that 'pain in the world' made living illogical."[13] Subsequent to his encounter with Alex, Kramer learned to detect neurological disorders in college students when he heard them talk passionately about the German writer Rainer Maria Rilke.[14] One need not be a professor of literature to find it disturbing that the names of Vonnegut, Camus, and Rilke could serve as dog whistles for neurological disorders.

Kramer builds on this alarming idea by maintaining that a near-obsessive devotion to literature is a sign of psychopathology. (This insinuates that most literary theorists are walking neurotics.) He confesses that he too was "under the influences of the beauty and intricacy of literature" when he underwent his own personal psychoanalysis.[15] His use of the term "under the influences" obviously connotes an addiction. There was something pathological about his devotion to literature. Though he explores the relationship between psychotherapy and literature and though he concludes that psychotherapy is both an art and technique designed to create a fiction by the analyst and patient, Kramer certainly casts a dark shadow on the consumption of literature. To his mind, an attachment to literature is a symptom of mental turmoil, whereas psychotherapy mimics the art of literature by producing new narratives. How should we reconcile this dissonance? Could reading and interpreting literature, keeping diaries, and storytelling be therapeutic precursors or companions to psychotherapy? And furthermore, could they not be important artifacts of trauma?

It bears stressing that I am not arguing that my course was therapeutic or that the literary arts can heal directly. Nonetheless, the students in my intimate literature course did teach me about trauma and traumatism and provoked a series of questions leading to this book. Since I could not study my students quantitatively or qualitatively, I turned to what I knew best—literature and literary theory—and embarked on a heuristic research project. And in tribute to my students who had exhibited creative resources to live through their traumatic experiences, I focused on the topics of resistance, resilience, and growth rather than on the psychopathological effects of trauma. True, traumatic events can impact the body, brain, and mind leading to depression, PTSD, and other physical and mental disorders. Still, "most individuals do not develop such illnesses after experiencing stressful life events and are thus thought to be resilient."[16]

While venturing down this research path, I anticipated raised eyebrows. Whereas the terms resilience and resistance have become buzzwords in the twenty-first century, many in the field of cultural trauma studies employ them sparingly.[17] Moreover, many cultural theorists fixate on trauma. Literary theorists, not least those cut from a deconstruction fabric, might also look askance at any attempt to find meaning in literature and more specifically connections between the literary arts, trauma, and posttraumatic growth. After all, for many deconstructionists, literature, language, and literary theory are ipso facto defined by gaps, silences, and dead ends. Even if connections exist, they should remain mysterious, some might add. These topics will be amplified in Chapters 4 and 6. Suffice it to say for now that though cognizant of these possible misgivings, I have also been unduly aware of some students, who after attending literature classes replete with postmodernist obscurantism and nihilism, have felt overwhelmed by doubts about careers in the humanities, not to mention about the use of studying the arts. Most importantly, I have come to appreciate the prevalence not only of trauma, but also of posttraumatic resistance, resilience, and growth and that individuals and communities deserve our devotion to imaginative research about these topics.

I turned therefore to research from applied and pure sciences and the humanities to respond to the fundamental questions outlined in this introduction. I tapped into scientific trauma theories from neurologists, psychiatrists, psychoanalysts, and psychologists, such as Pierre Briquet, Jean-Martin Charcot, Pierre Janet, Sigmund Freud, Abram Kardiner, Paul Chodoff, Frantz Fanon, Donald Winnicott, Otto Rank, Judith Herman, Boris Cyrulnik, Barbara Shapiro, Bessel van der Kolk, Peter Levine, Robert Scaer, Sophia Richman, Aaron Beck, Judith Beck, Edna Foa, Richard Tedeschi, Lawrence Calhoun, George Bonanno, and Marylene Cloitre.[18] From the field of narrative medicine, I relied on the research of medical anthropologists Arthur Kleinman and Allan Young, physician and literary theorist Rita Charon, and sociologist Arthur Frank. Finally, from cultural trauma studies, I dialogued with Geoffrey Hartman, Shoshana Felman, Cathy Caruth, Dominick LaCapra, Roger Luckhurst, and Ruth Leys and postcolonial theorists such as Stef Craps, Michael Rothberg, Roger Kurtz, and Irene Vissier. In addition to my students who have inspired me to embark on this research journey, these mentors have guided me along the way.

Organization, Arguments, and Goals

This text relies on the metaphor of a metamorphosis to convey its main arguments about trauma, posttraumatic conditions, and world literature. The metaphor refers to not only a possible metamorphosis of the mind but also changes to a historical narrative about trauma studies and to the field of trauma studies itself.

The book is divided into four parts where attempts are made to cultivate these metamorphoses. Part I (Chapters 1–2) offers a synthesis of embryonic concepts of trauma and traumatism from Cuneiform clay tablets to Ovid's *Metamorphoses* to Enlightenment philosophy. By locating artifacts of these notions, I thus put pressure on Allan Young's argument that prior to the nineteenth century writers of literature could not refer to traumatic memory or to PTSD.[19] I also put forward that Enlightenment philosophers helped to transform Western society's understanding of human suffering and provoked in turn the eventual development of the concept of psychological trauma in the mid-nineteenth century. In Chapter 2, I further enlarge our understanding of the development of the notions of psychological trauma and PTSD by locating quasi-medical terms that pre-date the birth of these concepts. In addition, I expand the historical narrative of trauma studies by underscoring research from Briquet, Charcot, Janet, Kardiner, Chodoff, and Fanon that provide an integrated and contextual understanding of trauma and recovery mechanisms. This more expansive perspective aims to cultivate a metamorphosis of the historical narrative of trauma studies, while responding to several physicians' concerns about biologically focused research on human emotions.[20]

In Part II (Chapters 3–4), I seek to provide a synthesis of contemporary trauma theories from the perspectives of medicine, the biological sciences, and the humanities. In Chapter 3, I paint a landscape of current scientific trauma theories, while in Chapter 4, I sketch a portrait of cultural trauma studies. These syntheses are designed to respond to a dearth of pluri-disciplinary research on posttraumatic growth that, according to psychologist Richard Tedeschi and his colleagues, characterizes trauma studies.[21] Literary theorist Roger Luckhurst echoes this reading by referring to a need to regard: "trauma as a complex knot that binds together multiple strands of knowledge and which can be best understood through plural, multi-disciplinary perspectives."[22] While providing examples of transdisciplinary research projects, I also seek to offer a wide horizon where an inter-disciplinary project and a metamorphosis of the field of trauma studies might come to fruition in the other parts of this book.

In Part III (Chapters 5–6), I provide a synthesis of recognized clinical treatments for trauma survivors and then propose the creative and critical concept of this book: a Literary Arts Praxis. The Praxis refers to an educational training in the literary arts (telling and interpreting stories; reading and decoding literature rich in philosophical content from existentialism, phenomenology, and aesthetics; and creative writing, such as journaling). It is buttressed by clinical trauma theories on the importance of engaging in cognitive exercises (Janet, Beck, Foa, Tedeschi, Calhoun, and Cloitre) and the importance of engaging in imaginative or creative activities (Winnicott, Rank, Herman, Levine, Cyrulnik, Bonanno, and Richman).[23] Combining this clinical research with theories from the social sciences and literary studies, I address the main question of this research project: how a Literary Arts Praxis might "somehow get at trauma."[24] Though I do acknowledge researchers' attempts to describe this relationship, I propose several new theories from disperse fields. A Literary Arts Praxis seeks to provide therefore a bridge between the humanities, neuroscience, and clinical medicine to stimulate new research projects.

Part IV (Chapters 7–9) offers illustrations of a Literary Arts Praxis. Before engaging in a close reading of characters from world literature who engage in such a Praxis, I begin with a general discussion of world literature, which seems well positioned to morph our understanding of traumatic and posttraumatic conditions. Like existential conundrums, traumatic and posttraumatic experiences can be universal themes that world literature portrays in familiar and foreign ways. By contemplating these portrayals, familiar stories may very well seem foreign, while the foreign might appear familiar and stir the pot of our received ideas. Works to be analyzed include *Don Quixote* by the Spaniard Miguel de Cervantes (1547–1616); *The Plague* from the Franco-Algerian Albert Camus (1913–1960); and *Desert* by the Franco-Mauritian Jean-Marie Gustave Le Clézio (1940). Their pieces, though dense with other meaning, are a contemplation and dramatization of trauma and posttraumatic states. From youth to the autumn of life, the human condition can be riddled with trauma and a powerful drive often prevails to transform traumatic experiences and memories into positive conditions through creative mechanisms.

My analyses and creative concept of a Literary Arts Praxis neither claim to be empirical nor propose prescriptive clinical methods. Further, nothing that I propose in this text should be construed as trivializing traumatic suffering. Nor should my interpretations on the relationship between trauma and the literary arts be interpreted as excessively practical. I do wish to stress however that the literary arts can illuminate the dynamics of resistance, resilience, and posttraumatic growth and hence merit our careful critical and creative attention. Amplifying Herman's position that political movements provoked advances in trauma theories, this book argues that the humanities (literature, philosophy, and the arts) have also changed minds and fostered the development of a more nuanced and humane understanding of traumatic experiences.

Finally, three principal research gaps in trauma studies call for such a pluri-disciplinary project. Scientists and clinicians have insisted that there is a relationship between trauma and narratives, but they fail to explore in detail that connection. Still others encourage trauma survivors to become philosophers and/or creative storytellers and yet neglect to imagine how one can assume these roles. Third, cultural trauma theorists tend to fixate on trauma, as opposed to the topics of growth or recovery, whereas clinicians have begun to move in these research directions. A Literary Arts Praxis aims to address these three gaps, while engaging in theoretical discussions and textual analyses of fiction.

Projected Audience and Engaging with this Text

This text is targeted for clinicians, scientists, cultural theorists, and students of trauma studies. How might scholars and students from such disperse fields engage in this book? The evolutionary biologist E.O. Wilson suggested that the connections between the arts and sciences are strengthened when contemplating the issue of complexity. "The love of complexity without reductionism makes art; the love of complexity with reductionism makes science."[25] Wilson's description can be applied to the field of trauma studies. Traumatologists from clinical and basic sciences (i.e., neurology) often lean towards biological reductionism, whereas scholars from the humanities may luxuriate in the unknown nature of human experiences. This research project invites traumatologists from both ends of the spectrum to engage in new ideas about trauma and posttraumatic conditions and in turn cultivate new understandings of and treatments for trauma survivors.

The prevalence of trauma and PTSD is another reason why scholars from a wide audience might be interested in this text. Since the 1980s the topics of trauma and PTSD have consumed us. The American Psychiatric Association estimates that 60% of all Americans have undergone a traumatizing experience in their lifetime.[26] Whereas the backdrop of this research project has been the trauma defining my students' lives, the foreground is COVID-19. Much of this book has been written during the pandemic when millions have lost their jobs, fallen ill, suffered, and died. To add to this immeasurable suffering, great swaths of healthcare and front-line workers worldwide remain emotionally and physically depleted caring for the critically ill. Their and many others' traumatic experiences will persist beyond the pandemic. Along with COVID's legacy of trauma, the entire globe struggles to adjust to migrant and environmental crises. In fact, an editorial appearing (September 2021) in more than 200 medical journals—from *The Lancet* to *The New England Journal of Medicine*—stresses that the world cannot wait for COVID to pass before addressing climate change, the "greatest threat" to public health.[27] The future defined in these terms brings us back to the beginning of this introduction. The displaced are not just youngsters fleeing cartel violence from Latin America. Many of us will be among the displaced. Our life's journey will bring us to stormy waters where we are apt to experience trauma. Now more than ever, scholars from medicine, science, and the humanities are beckoned to engage in creative research on treatment methods for trauma survivors, and this book serves as an invitation to take a voyage where metamorphoses of the mind might just take place.

Notes

1 Psychiatrist Boris Cyrulnik makes the distinction between "trauma" and "traumatism" as in the difference between the original event and the follow-up psychological conditions ranging from PTSD to resilience. See Cyrulnik "Children," 24.
2 Herman, *Trauma*, 33.
3 Cyrulnik, "Children," 24.
4 Students from Mexican states along the US–Mexican border enjoy in-state status for tuition and fees at the University of Texas-Rio Grande Valley, which means that many Mexican middle-class families can afford to send their children to UT-RGV and other UT institutions on the border.
5 My students' names and circumstances have been changed to protect their privacy.
6 DACA refers to the "Deferred Action for Childhood Arrivals," an American governmental program that defers the removal of some undocumented immigrants who were brought to the United States as children and have been law abiding, stayed in school, and/or enlisted in the armed forces.
7 Adorno, *Notes*, 358.
8 Adorno, *Aesthetic*, loc. 1409.
9 Ibid., loc. 900.
10 Felman and Laub, *Testimony*, loc. 232.
11 Ibid., loc. 150.
12 Ibid., loc. 151.
13 Kramer, *Moments*, 44.
14 Ibid., 60.
15 Ibid., 224.
16 Wu et al., "Understanding," 1; we will define the terms of resilience, resistance, and posttraumatic growth in Chapter 5.
17 Currently, the term "resilience" is applied most notably when referring to the natural environment and its ability to endure and recover from human abuse.
18 Since I am neither a clinician nor a scientist, I made sure to rely on rich and diverse research, especially meta-analyses from the Cochrane and PubMed websites.
19 See Young, *Harmony*, loc. 28–30.
20 I am referring to Judith Herman's and Raymond Tallis's concerns, which we shall explore in Chapter 2.
21 See Tedeschi et al., *Posttraumatic*, 9.
22 Luckhurst, *Trauma*, 214.
23 I lean heavily on the idea that resilience is linked to regenerative experiences, such as "engaging in new creative activities"; see Bonanno, "Resilience," 136.
24 LaCapra, *Writing*, 183; we shall discuss this term in more detail in Chapter 6.
25 Wilson, *Consilience*, 59.
26 US Department, "How common."
27 Sommer, "Climate."

Part I

An Evolution of Key Concepts and Terms

1   Embryonic Concepts of Trauma and Traumatism from the Humanities

"All that the historian or ethnographer can do and all that we can expect of either of them is to enlarge a specific experience to the dimensions of a more general one, which thereby becomes accessible as experience to men of another country or another epoch."[1] Such is the advice of the anthropologist Claude Lévi-Strauss. His recommendation prods us to enlarge the "standard" history of trauma studies to make it more accessible to traumatologists from dispersed fields.[2] As pointed out in this book's introduction, trauma studies is an interdisciplinary domain of research (from psychiatry to sociology to the arts) that investigates trauma and traumatism (posttraumatic conditions from PTSD to growth).[3]

The "standard" history of the field begins with the etymology of the term "trauma." It hails from Greek and refers to a physical wound. This fact is followed by an announcement that the related term "traumatic neurosis" was first used during the industrial revolution to refer to something more than a physical wound. It described psychic disturbances caused by railroad accidents. What typically ensues is a short list of discoveries in the nineteenth and twentieth centuries from Western psychiatrists, neurologists, and psychologists. A most notable discovery was the concept of "psychogenic trauma," which refers to psychic wounds having a psychological rather than physical origin. The narrative crescendos with the American Psychiatric Association's recognition of posttraumatic stress disorder (PTSD) in 1980. An epilogue containing contributions beginning in the mid-1980s from cultural theorists (social scientists, historians, and literary theorists) follows as well as an enumeration of scientific and clinical research, both quantitative and qualitative in nature. Following Lévi-Strauss's advice, I aim to enlarge this historical narrative of trauma studies by highlighting contributions from the humanities, as embryonic as they might be. After all, the past is a foreign land where fresh ideas can be harvested for future heuristic and transdisciplinary investigations.

I explore first notions of trauma and posttraumatic conditions in early writing.[4] I consider illustrations of war trauma found in Cuneiform clay tablets and in the work of Greek historian Herodotus (fifth century BCE) and the Roman poet Lucretius (first century BCE); rape and physical abuse

DOI: 10.4324/9781003284642-3

trauma in the myths brought to life by the Roman poet Ovid (first century CE) and the Roman philosopher Apuleius (second century CE); and catastrophic and collective trauma traced by the Spanish missionary and writer Bartolomé de las Casas (1484–1566) and the French philosopher Michel de Montaigne (1533–1592). I also pay close attention to illustrations of what today we would call PTSD, resistance, resilience, and growth in these texts. Although these writers do not employ the terms "trauma" and "PTSD," they describe kindred concepts through moving prose and vivid metaphors.

After examining these early concepts, I make another main adjustment to a standard history of trauma studies. I put forward that eighteenth-century philosophers Voltaire, Jean-Jacques Rousseau, and Denis Diderot provoked a psycho-philosophical revolution that would lead to an adjustment of the term "trauma" in the nineteenth century.[5] They prepared the terrain for the term to be nuanced by planting new notions of extreme suffering; offering visceral descriptions of the suffering of others; and spurring readers' emotions. Their ideas were then harnessed to the Romantic movement before the term evoked psychic suffering caused by accidents. This brings us to the industrial revolution and to the major catastrophic events and social injustices of the nineteenth and twentieth centuries and to their relationship to trauma theories, a history to explore in Chapter 2.[6]

The Framework behind an Examination of Embryonic Concepts

The framework of my examination of embryonic concepts of trauma and traumatism is sustained by several pillars consisting of common sense, etymology, and previous related research. While the origin of the term "trauma" (to refer to psychological wounds) comes from industrial accidents, it defies common sense to imagine that only these accidents played a role in the term's birth. These accidents might have provoked an adjustment to the word, but the development of the concept and kindred ones are another story. What about previous pandemics, wars, pogroms, genocides, witch hunts, barbaric punishments, not to mention natural disasters that had plagued human communities prior to the nineteenth century? Weren't they considered traumatic? Didn't they cause deleterious posttraumatic conditions? Were humans previously *übermensch*? These rhetorical questions invite us to recognize that there must have been related concepts to trauma that existed prior to the nineteenth century.

The framework of my examination is also buttressed by the etymology and history of another important term in the history of ideas, "*teologia*" (theology). The twelfth-century philosopher Abélard coined the Latin word to refer to the study of the nature of God and religious belief. The Church objected to his dialectical analyses of God and threw his books on the bonfire.[7] Just because Abélard was responsible for the coinage of the term does not mean that the concept or embryonic concepts did not exist prior. Early Church fathers Ambrose and Augustine (from the fourth and fifth centuries

CE) practiced theology. Scholars even refer to them as theologians.[8] The concept of theology predates the coinage of the term, even if these early Church fathers' concepts were different (less provocative) than Abélard's. Similarly, the concepts of trauma and traumatism predate the coinage of these terms, even if writers from Mesopotamia to revolutionary France spoke of them differently. And if Ambrose and Augustine were called "theologians" before the word "theology" existed, early writers from the cradle of human civilization to the Romantic movement could be called traumatologists.

This attempt to propose a new narrative about the history of trauma studies is built additionally on the foundation of anthropologist Allan Young's arguments. In his *The Harmony of Illusions* (1995), he proposes three divergent interpretations from the standard history of the concepts of psychogenic trauma and PTSD. To his mind, it makes little sense to imagine that the concepts of traumatic memory and PTSD are timeless. They are found neither in Shakespeare's or Samuel Pepys's writings nor in the *Epic of Gilgamesh*, he asserts. Second, these works could not refer to psychogenic trauma because this type of traumatic memory was previously "unavailable."[9] It was not until the nineteenth century, Young claims, that a new concept of memory developed. Namely, the mind could torment the mind, producing memories that were concealed in automatic and repetitive behavior that defied conscious control.[10] Third, the anthropologist maintains that the concept of PTSD is not characterized by some built-in order. "Rather, it is glued together by the practices, technologies, and narratives with which it is diagnosed, studied, treated, and represented and by the various interests, institutions, and moral arguments that mobilized these efforts and resources."[11] Whereas I share Young's opinion that the concepts of psychogenic trauma and PTSD did not formally exist until the nineteenth and twentieth centuries respectively, I part company with him by stressing that embryonic forms of these notions did. I also put pressure on his position that the conceptualization of traumatic memory was unavailable to people prior to the nineteenth century. I not only locate hints of traumatic memory, as seen in Montaigne's work, but also argue that Enlightenment philosophers helped to raise conscious awareness about psychic and psychogenic suffering. By painting portraits of human suffering, philosophers from Voltaire, Rousseau, and Diderot put the topic on the map, paving the way for Romantics to take up the Enlightenment torch.

My more expansive approach to understanding the roots of the concepts of trauma and traumatism is also founded on an alarming perspective that psychiatrist Judith Herman raises in the 1997 afterword to her *Trauma and Recovery*. She writes: "The very strength of the recent biological findings in PTSD may foster a narrowed, predominantly biological focus of research."[12] Clinical neuroscientist and physician Raymond Tallis echoes this position and has coined the term "neuromania" to refer to a current obsession to understand emotional experiences from a neurobiological perspective, as evidenced in the terms "neurotheology" and "neuroaesthetics."[13] In more general terms, "the rise of neurobiology is leading to a kind of reductionism in which mental states are reduced to brain states ... and the key dimensions of our humanness—language, culture, history—are ignored."[14] In light of this biological reductionism, I search the humanities for artifacts of trauma and posttraumatic conditions. From earliest civilizations in Mesopotamia to the Renaissance and the Enlightenment, humanity has endured trauma and left traces of its experiences. Seen from another perspective, before there were scientific theories about trauma and traumatism, there were stories and art.

Furthermore, recent research findings and trends call for a wide-angle lens when considering the history of the concepts of trauma and PTSD. Contemporary scientific investigations have taught us several important lessons. There is a wide variety of traumatic experiences from wars, genocides, and natural disasters to complex and prolonged traumatic experiences, such as childhood neglect and abuse, clinically known as Adverse Childhood Experiences (ACE). The subjective nature of trauma renders it even more complex. The depth, width, and variety of traumatic experiences demand a more enlarged historical narrative of the field, since pivotal related information from the humanities may be discovered in the strata of time.

A history of trauma studies could benefit from an addition from the humanities for another reason. The current historical narrative remains misaligned with important contemporary trends in the field. Post-colonial theorists and anthropologists have added novel theories from non-Western sources, topics to be discussed in Chapter 4. The field has also undertaken research on resistance, resilience, and growth, rather than focusing on trauma and PTSD.[15] Still, cultural trauma studies scholars, save for post-colonialists, have not followed suit. Psychologist Richard Tedeschi and his colleagues complained in 2018 that "there has been almost no study of PTG [posttraumatic growth] in the humanities other than references to the concept of growth ..."[16] While scholars from the humanities are invited to investigate PTG going forward, all researchers might look back on the arts, which might offer a trove of findings.

Artifacts of War Trauma from Pre-history and Classical Antiquity

If our species is referred to as "Homo Narrans," it seems logical for records of traumatic or kindred experiences to exist since the beginning of writing. Portraits of traumatic and posttraumatic conditions are found in Cuneiform, the earliest form of writing developed by the Sumerians in Mesopotamian (*c.* 3500–3000 BCE). One might even say that the birth of writing came from the labor pains of trauma. This may seem like an exaggeration, for early writing consisted principally of simple notations of commercial exchanges on clay tablets. From records of bushels of wheat and chickens arose notes on traumatic events endured by farmers. Cuneiform medical records kept track of war wounds.[17] They "describe posttraumatic stress disorders as mental health manifestations of severe mental and/or physical (traumatic) stress that does not usually cause the death of the patient."[18] The fact that medicine of the times could do little to heal serious physical wounds meant that the specter of death was ever looming. There were psychic wounds, too. Tablets refer to nightmares, flashbacks, insomnia, and a sense of depression plaguing soldiers.[19] For the Mesopotamians, these symptoms were caused by a "spirit affliction."[20] The spirits of those whom the soldier had killed provoked subsequent psychic disturbances.

The ancient Greek historian Herodotus refers to a psychic condition that resembles posttraumatic stress disorder in his account of the Battle of Marathon (490 BCE) of the Greco-Persian Wars. The soldier Epizêlus "was stricken with blindness, without blow of sword or dart."[21] This sounds like a psychosomatic disorder or in metaphorical terms, a heavy blanket of fear placed a shadow on the soldier's eyes. If Herodotus speaks about a psychosomatic disorder caused by fear, the Roman poet Lucretius refers to battle dreams in which "High commanders take the field and lead troops into battle/, Sailors keep on dueling it out with the winds, their sworn foe."[22] The image of sailors fighting the winds suggests madness. Lucretius makes a generalization in fact about the nature of the human mind: "men often physically collapse beneath the sway/ Of mental dread."[23] In trauma theory parlance, the traumatic event lives on in the mind, thus rendering the term "posttraumatic" misleading.

Traces of Rape and Physical Abuse Trauma in Mythology

Ovid's narrator of the *Metamorphoses* (8 CE) seems to be obsessed with the topics of trauma and metamorphoses, as the title intimates. Countless mortals undergo traumatic experiences and metamorphoses in his epic poem. A target of the lustful eye of Apollo in Book I, Daphne, the nymph (a term referring to an insect that undergoes an incomplete metamorphosis as well as a minor female nature deity) tries to fend off her rapist by escaping into the woods. She turns to her father, the river god Peneus, and beseeches him to change her into a laurel tree. Fixed to the ground, her branches grow, leaves sprout, and flowers bud. Ovid saw to it that the nymph's protective state would not rest completely dormant. Daphne escapes the traumatic rape and the experience of being broken and defiled. But the haunting memory of her turmoil is lodged in her roots, while her divine blossoming is undermined. As for the mortal Arachne in Book VI, her traumatic experience defies interpretative flexibility. Famed for an ability to weave fine tapestries, Arachne engages Minerva (goddess of war, wisdom, and crafts) in a competition. Inflamed with jealousy after finding no flaw in her competitor's tapestry, Minerva hits Arachne, which drives the mortal to hang herself. Sprinkling a poisonous liquid onto her, the goddess changes her into a spider destined to weave the same senseless tapestry for eternity. With no way to escape her punishment, there is no posttraumatic condition for Arachne. Trauma becomes eternal. Period. The metamorphosis is defined by death, not new life.

Similarly, the second-century CE Latin author Apuleius spins tales of trauma and transformations in his *Metamorphoses*, known also as *The Golden Ass*. Akin to Ovid's Minerva, the goddess Venus feels jealous of the beautiful mortal Psyche. If Minerva turns Arachne into a spider, Venus orders her son Cupid to inspire Psyche to fall in love with the most wretched of men. Beauty does not fall for the beast. Cupid hides her in a remote place where the two commune in the dark until she, moved by importunate curiosity, shines a lamp upon Cupid's face, forcing him to flee. She falls into the hands of Venus who punishes her. Moved by the mortal's suffering, Cupid rescues Psyche. And thanks to the god Jupiter, she is transformed into an immortal.

Like Daphne and Arachne, Psyche is traumatized by an immortal. But unlike Daphne's and Arachne's enduring posttraumatic state, she escapes the immortal's punishment. Her metamorphosis into a goddess is often interpreted as an allegory of the power of love to edify. Even if Cupid plays a role in her transformation, the couple is still dependent upon Jupiter for the metamorphosis. The Greek word "*psychē*" means soul, breathe, and butterfly. This etymology indicates that Psyche's posttraumatic experience had built into it a liberating metamorphosis.

Vestiges of the Trauma of Colonialism and Civilian Trauma from the Renaissance

The Renaissance is reputed to be one of the most magnificent eras of human history. Dürer's self-portraits, Leonardo's *Mona Lisa*, Michelangelo's *David*, Brunelleschi's Dome, Dante's *Divine Comedy*, Petrarch's poems, and Copernicus's, Kepler's, and Galileo's celestial discoveries. Clearly, a bountiful human flourishing. And if Renaissance historian Giorgi Vasari sings the praises of achievements such as these, the nineteenth-century historian Jules Michelet sums up the era as "the discovery of the world, the discovery of man."[24] However, while Vasari was writing about frescoes, paintings, and sculptures in Florence and Rome, missionary and writer Bartolomé de las Casas focused on the discovery of another world and another people. His *Tears of the Indians* (first published in 1552 as *Brévisima relación de la destrucción de las Indias*) describes the flow not only of tears but also of blood from the Americas in the sixteenth century. While his work is a diatribe against the hypocrisies and cruelty of the Spanish crown and colonizers, it also offers a raw depiction of the traumatic experiences of Native Americans in the early colonial period.[25]

Kindred to previous writers discussed, de las Casas does not employ the term "trauma." But he does imply the concept in more ways than one. Descriptions of Spanish atrocities against the Indigenous fill the pages of his book. He employs various tools to convey the genocide and reach his readers. Metaphors and similes render his message clear. Native Americans are "quiet lambs," whereas the Spaniards are "like most cuel [*sic*] Tygres, Wolves, and Lions, enrag'd with a sharp and tedious hunger ..."[26] Vivid imagery also renders his writing uncomfortably raw. The Spaniards considered the Indigenous "as if they had been but the dung and filth of the earth."[27] In addition, in several chapter introductions, de las Casas invites readers to contemplate for themselves Spanish barbarity and to feel the suffering of Native Americans: "Two or three of their most hainous crimes I will rehearse, whereby the reader may judge of the wickedness of those which remain untold."[28] While this invitation may be interpreted as an insult to contemporary readers' intelligence or moral fabric, it bears stressing that when the *Tears of the Indians* was first published, its content was considered staggering. It was one thing for de las Casas to criticize vehemently the Spanish crown, it was still another to run to the defense of a people who were considered "dung and filth of the earth" by writing a biography on their suffering. De las Casas's history on the trauma of colonialism awkwardly kept company with Renaissance books on great artists and great architects. If the dominant book of the Middle Ages was the Bible, the Renaissance not only welcomed books about refined Culture from the Ancient Greeks to Raphael, but it also made room for narratives of human suffering. These were neither stories of Christ's calvary nor of the bitter wine he tasted on the cross. They depicted instead the suffering of those deemed less valuable by hegemonic European cultures.

Another important book in the Renaissance collection was philosopher Michel de Montaigne's three-volume *Essays* (first published as *Les Essais* in 1580, 1588, and 1595). The French word "*essai*" comes from the verb "*essayer*," which means "to try." The Renaissance writer tries to make sense of suffering intrinsic to life, such as diseases. He also tries to grasp the moral depravity that allows humans to inflict pain on others. And he tries to wrap his head around his own suffering. Even if he does not employ the term "trauma" in his *Essays*, he describes experiences and conditions akin to trauma and PTSD. He explores the suffering of the sick and dying; soldiers in battle; and the subjugation of the colonized and civilians in wartime, including his own. And yet, his work serves not only as an ethnography of trauma, but also as a treatise on something kindred to posttraumatic growth.

These topics come into clear relief gradually as the essayist attempts to convince readers that he is painting above all a self-portrait. We learn for example how his bowls function and how he likes to make love. Despite these traces of self-indulging humor, his *Essays* are wrapped in a shroud. Death is constantly on his mind. In his essay "Of Experience," he writes:

> Death is more abject, more languishing and troublesome, in bed than in a fight: fevers and catarrhs as painful and mortal as a musket-shot.

> Whoever has fortified himself valiantly to bear the accidents of common life need not raise his courage to be a soldier ...[29]

Montaigne's novel perspective about suffering endured in bed, as opposed to suffering on the battlefield, seems to stem from his having witnessed first-hand the death of his dear friend Étienne de la Boétie.

Beyond contemplating suffering intrinsic to life, the essayist comprehended firsthand the traumatic experiences of war. His life was tainted by the French Wars of Religion (1562–1598) and the Saint Bartholomew's Day Massacre (August 24, 1572), the very day he began his *Essays*. The massacre touched the philosopher personally. It took place on the wedding day of his Protestant friend Henri de Navarre to the Catholic Margarite de Valois. The French Catholic Regent Catherine of Medici supported the union to forge peace between the factions. Her hopes were dashed when Catholics butchered Protestant guests at the Louvre where they had been housed for the festivities. The Seine turned red as the corpses of 3,000 Protestants were thrown into the river.

Rather than provide explicit descriptions of the Wars of Religion, the essayist relies on mentors such as Herodotus and Virgil to retell stories of wars fought by the Ancient Greeks, Persians, Romans, and Turks. Why did he call upon them? Montaigne had to worry about the Catholic Church's Index of Prohibited Books.[30] Furthermore, battle stories from Antiquity could convey what should remain masked not only from the Church's point of view, but also from a psychological one. He might not have been emotionally ready to create a narrative of the brutal acts he witnessed. He might have been so traumatized that he struggled to express that which defied expression. Fully aware of human moral depravity, he might have found comfort in these mentors. The works of Herodotus and Virgil might have served as an antidote to his sense of despair about humanity. There can be no doubt that Montaigne looked up to his mentors, literally. On the ceiling beams of his castle library in Bordeaux, he engraved the maxims of great writers from Antiquity to keep him company.

It is not simply a matter of conjecture that the essayist was convinced of human moral depravity. He states in his essay "Of Cruelty" that cruel souls "would hack and lop off the limbs of others; sharpen their wits to invent unusual torments and new kinds of death, without hatred, without profit, and for no other end but only to enjoy the pleasant spectacle of ... the lamentable groans and cries of a man dying in anguish ..."[31] This constitutes the most extreme form of cruelty, the essayist contends, and yet it occurs every day. As much as this cruelty is frequent, it is widespread. In "Of Cannibals," he refers to cruel forms of punishment among both Native Americans and the Portuguese in South America. But the latter are more barbaric, as they remain "blind" to their barbarity.[32]

Another form of cruel suffering is mental angst. The essayist describes the psychic trauma, including his own, experienced by civilians during the war. In "Of Vanity," he confesses to going to bed nervous, afraid that he will be butchered in the night. A civil war is the worst kind of war, he adds, for you become a sentinel forever guarding your own home.[33] These confessions are significant, as they suggest that the essayist was suffering from a type of PTSD and that he tried to paint a rich and subtle portrait of this complex condition in his *Essays*.

Does Montaigne paint more than a self-portrait and a landscape of suffering? In his final essay "Of Experience," he calls upon Plato to sum up his final position. Speaking about pleasure and pain, he states that the Greek philosopher couples them together. They are two fountains from which one can draw nourishment. In the case of pain, one can learn to cultivate fortitude. As for pleasure, one can perfect self-control. The essayist sums up his attempt to make the most of pain and pleasure by confessing, "I am a great lover of fish, and consequently make my fasts feasts and feasts fasts ..."[34] By this metaphor, he makes it clear that in addition to the suffering he witnessed and experienced himself, he could turn famines into feasts, especially as the writings of his mentors nourished him. It is in this way that Montaigne's *Essays* are not only an ethnography of trauma, but also an account on a form of posttraumatic growth.

Roots of the Concept of Trauma and Posttraumatic Growth in the Enlightenment

Enlightenment philosophers wrote profusely about the topic of human suffering and hence provoked a psycho-philosophical revolution. This revolution of the mind helped in turn to give birth to the modified concept of trauma and related concepts in the nineteenth century. This perspective is built on the history of ideas from the eighteenth century as well as from Enlightenment literature.

Let us first sketch a history of the revolutionary period in France before unfolding these ideas. There were many causes of the French Revolution of 1789, including droughts and famines that plagued France during the 1770s.[35] However, a more subtle cause was the psycho-philosophical revolution predating the actual political revolution. This revolution was triggered by the formation of the Republic of Letters during the eighteenth century. The Republic revolved around books and especially those by Enlightenment philosophers, such as Voltaire, Rousseau, and Diderot. Men and women of different classes would gather in salons to exchange conversations and philosophic and scientific texts, as well as literature and pamphlets (*libelles*) containing provocative content.[36] Philosophical essays and stories fostered conscious awareness of human suffering and individual rights. Incendiary pamphlets provoked critical thinking, rather than a docile acceptance of the power of the status quo. Scientific texts cultivated a method of thinking based on logic and empiricism. Moreover, the scientific method endorsed by Enlightenment thinkers was not applied solely to the natural world. Humans and human communities could be studied and manipulated. They were not etched in stone by a divine hand. Between the Enlightenment's insistence on the malleability of humans and human societies and its emphasis on logic, empiricism, critical thinking, and conscious awareness about others' conditions, the movement provoked a revolution of the mind leading to a political one in 1789.

In a similar vein, Voltaire, Rousseau, and Diderot spurred a psycho-philosophical revolution that helped to promote the modification of the term "trauma" in the nineteenth century. Before supporting this claim by textual analyses, let us break down this argument into two parts. First, by probing the topic of extreme human suffering, these philosophers prepared the mental terrain for the term to be altered. Voltaire, Rousseau, and Diderot highlighted that not all suffering was created equal. Natural disasters and physical infirmities lead to extreme suffering. Atrocities caused by humans also provoke extreme suffering. Still, while earthquakes could not be prevented, unjust punishments and slavery could. This distinction promoted a critical analysis of the origin of extreme suffering. It was not a fact of life. One could no longer simply blame human suffering on neurotic gods and goddesses or on the will of an omniscient God.

These comments harken us back to our discussion on the philosopher and theologian Abélard in this chapter. Recall that just because he was responsible for the term "theology," does not mean that embryonic concepts of it failed to exist previously. Recall as well that the Church objected to his dialectical analyses of God. What was there to analyze? God was God. End of the discussion. But for Abélard, God was not just God. There was more to God than what doctrine taught. There was no end to the discussion about God. Similarly, Voltaire, Rousseau, and Diderot brought the discussion of human induced sufferings to the table for discussion. Human suffering was not just human suffering. There was more to suffering than what religion and the powers-that-be upheld. There was an endless discussion about human suffering about to unfold.

Secondly, the philosophers helped readers to become not only consciously aware of extreme suffering but also emotionally involved with scenes of suffering. The philosophers' novellas, novels, plays, essays, historical writings, and intimate literature prodded readers to establish emotional connections with those depicted in their writings, a trial run for connections with others in everyday life.

To support these interpretations, we turn to Voltaire's testimonies, which include a portrait of what appears to be his own traumatic and posttraumatic experiences and those endured by others during colonization and war. He understood painfully well the topic of cruel punishments. He was held under house arrest, imprisoned in the Bastille, and forced into exile on several occasions. Voltaire's first crime committed in 1717 consisted of writing a tragedy *Oedipus* in which he accused the French Regent of incest. After his second imprisonment in 1726, which lasted eleven months, he was placed under house arrest at his father's estate. From there, he fled to England. Voltaire's letter from October 26, 1726, the day he arrived on the island, gives us a clear impression of his condition: "I was without a penny, sick to death of a violent fever, a stranger, alone, helpless, in the midst of a city, wherein I was known to no body ... I could not make bold to see our ambassador in so wretched a condition. I had never undergone such distress ..."[37] Though the French monarchy tried to repress his voice, he continued to use his pen as a sword to fight against injustices, hypocrisies, and human suffering. Under the heading "Religion" in his *Philosophical Dictionary* and thanks to the interventions of an imaginary genie, readers learn about "abominable monuments to barbarism and fanaticism."[38] The genie refers to an "inquisition" in the Americas and a "massacre" and estimates that 12 million Indigenous people had been killed all because they had not been baptized. In his *Age of Louis XIV*, the philosopher neither hides behind a genie nor minces his word about human barbarity that provokes traumatic experiences: "The Americans, from whom we have wrested their continent after having dyed it with their blood, look upon us as the foes of humankind, who came from the farthest part of the globe to butcher them, and afterward to destroy one another."[39] Again, he puts extreme suffering on the map and blames humans for it, implying that it can be abolished provided the West reset its moral compass.[40]

Even if Voltaire repeatedly portrays the issue of human-induced suffering, even if he makes readers aware of the topic, does it matter? Can such portraits have revolutionary effects? While his *Candide* might leave us with the impression that suffering caused by others is simply part of the human condition, his *Zadig* gives us the opposite impression. The main character Zadig, the Minister of Justice of King Moabdar of Babylon, is an instructor of emotions. The mantra he follows is: "When you feed, feed the dogs also, even though they bite you."[41] Motivated by compassion, he runs to the defense of an Egyptian woman who was accosted by her lover; helps abolish the tradition of burning widows; and gives alms to the destitute. To erase these forms of suffering requires an emotional connection with others and a resolve to act on these connections. He teaches these lessons to his elite guests who come to his home to watch "tragedies produced which excited tears, and comedies which provoked laughter."[42] Whether it is Zadig who provokes emotions in his guests or Voltaire who makes his readers shudder with disgust or bellow with laughter, the philosopher's intent is unequivocal. He wants us to feel and to feel the pain of others who are victims of social injustices.

Following Voltaire's example, Rousseau paints landscapes of human-induced suffering and spurs readers to feel the pain of others. In his *Discourse on the Origin of Inequality*, he stresses that there are different types of inequalities that cause suffering. There are those that occur naturally and those cultivated by societies. His social contract, an agreement between individuals to respect each other's rights and needs, is an attempt to abate human-induced suffering. Rousseau clarifies his position: "All power comes from God, I admit; but so does all sickness: does that mean that we are forbidden to call in the doctor?"[43] The philosopher invites readers to reconsider human suffering stoked by social inequalities. Differences in resources are not etched in stone. They can be abolished through human connections and agreements.

Like a doctor who prescribes a regimen to patients, Rousseau prescribes both a social contract and a particular form of education to abate human-induced suffering. The stimulation of emotions, especially empathy, is key to achieve this goal. In his *Confessions* and *Reveries of the Solitary Walker*, the philosopher discloses his love affairs and life's regrets, thus encouraging readers to contemplate themselves. And by stimulating conscious awareness of our own emotions, we may have prepared ourselves to imagine those of others. Rousseau's treatise on education *Emile* is a blueprint for emotional intelligence. He advocates a curriculum based on observing, gathering data, questioning, doubting, forming opinions, and growing aware of one's opinions. But, just as this scientific method is key, so too is the cultivation of emotions and senses. One cannot be consciously aware of the world (including other humans), without being connected with it emotionally and physically (phenomenologically). And for Rousseau, humans must be trained to cultivate these intellectual, emotional, and physical connections in societies.

Diderot also believed in his pen's power to cultivate emotional connections among humans. In his *Encyclopedia* (1751–1780), he writes under the entry "encyclopedia": "To entertain and please, when one can instruct and move, is to miss the mark."[44] The philosopher does not miss the mark, as he privileges both teaching and stirring emotions in his political writings, often plumed anonymously. He employs powerful writing devices for instance to spread abolitionist and anti-imperialist messages. In his *Supplement to the Voyage of Bougainville* (1796), he creates an imaginative soliloquy from a Tahitian man: "If someday a Tahitian landed on your shores and engraved on one of your stones or the bark of one of your trees: This land belongs to the inhabitants of Tahiti, what would you think?"[45] The philosopher is not simply stating a position about how colonialism and enslavement are wrong. The Tahitian's question gives us the impression that he is speaking directly to readers. Prodded to imagine how it would feel to watch Tahitians engraving their names on the hardwood trees of European forests, readers feel the suffering pain of the colonized. In his *History of Two Indies* (*Histoire de Deux Indes*, 1770), co-authored with Abby Guillaume Thomas Raynal, Diderot pleads with his fellow Europeans:

> You have not even any rights over the lifeless and insensible productions of the land you have arrived in, and yet you claim one over your fellow man. Instead of recognizing this man as a brother, you see in him

only a slave, a beast of burden. This is the way that you think, this is the way that you behave, oh fellow Europeans, and yet you have notions of justice, a code of morals and a sacred religion, you share a common mother with those you treat so cruelly.[46]

The philosopher does not mince his words. He refers to colonialism as "lifeless and insensible productions." He reproaches his fellow European for treating natives as "slaves and beasts of burden." And he calls out European hypocrisy of upholding justice, a moral code, and religion while treating natives so cruelly. By speaking directly with readers and allowing an imaginary Tahitian to voice his complaints, Diderot publicizes the suffering of others as well as encourages readers to feel connected with others and to act upon those connections. He was an unapologetic moralist when it came to slavery and colonization and paved the way for others, such as the Haitian revolutionary and abolitionist Toussaint Louverture and the French revolutionary and abolitionist Abbé Grégoire, to spearhead political movements that established a greater recognition of human rights.[47]

The Enlightenment's emphasis on human-induced suffering caused by injustices and inequalities; atrocities caused by humans; and an understanding of others' emotions were grist for the mill to alter the West's notion of psychic suffering. Philosophical texts and stories cultivated conscious awareness of human suffering and individual rights. Provocative pamphlets triggered critical thinking. Scientific writings fostered a method of thinking based on logic and empiricism. And on a related note, the scientific method advocated by Enlightenment philosophers was applied to individuals and communities, which could be analyzed and molded. Voltaire, Rousseau, and Diderot underscored that societies in part determine human destinations, and once it became clear that not all were destined for hell on earth, the concept of psychological trauma could be teased out of the false notion that it was automatically part of life. Trauma up until this time was the problem without a name because it was seen as simply part of the human condition and hence immutable. In sum, the Enlightenment created a psycho-philosophical environment where the notions of "trauma" and "PTSD" could eventually develop in the nineteenth and twentieth centuries. This argument finds resonance with Judith Herman's position that collective awareness of psychological trauma grew thanks in part to associations with political movements. She maintains that the first concept of hysteria emerged from "the anticlerical political movement of the late nineteenth century in France."[48] While I do share her position about the importance of political movements, I argue instead that the Enlightenment first prepared minds and hearts to recognize eventually psychic and psychogenic trauma.

Roots of the Concepts of Trauma and Posttraumatic Growth in Romanticism

Many Romantic writers dipped their plumes into Voltaire's, Rousseau's, and Diderot's inkpots. Though they might have objected to the scientific method prevalent in Enlightenment literature, they did gravitate toward an equally important emphasis on affect. Voltaire's and Rousseau's intimate literature provided the Western world with a blueprint for writing about emotions and psychic experiences, including those that resemble trauma and posttraumatic conditions, as argued above. The Romantics followed this tradition, recording the voices of trauma survivors. Though poems and novels obviously do not provide quantitative research, they do offer records of personal trauma made public by writers such as William Blake, Samuel Taylor Coleridge, William Wordsworth, Wolfgang von Goethe, Heinrich Heine, Germaine de Staël, François-René de Chateaubriand, and Victor Hugo. Literary theorists (such as Paul de Man, Geoffrey Hartman, and Cathy Caruth) have investigated the relationships between trauma theories and Romanticism. While I will not summarize their scholarship, I will highlight Hartman's research because it serves as a segue into the mind–body issue dominating trauma theories. Hartman considers Romantic literature as a testimony and transmission. William Wordsworth's poetry serves as a testimony of trauma while transmitting it "into personal and cultural memory."[49] Part of this transmission consists of impasses. Romantic poetry, Hartman maintains, is punctuated with gaps and dimness. Yet, these gaps are filled, and dimness fades through the intervention of the human imagination and body. Hartman finds that Samuel Coleridge's "The Rime of the Ancient Mariner" is a "remarkable externalization of an internal state."[50] When reading the poem, the imagination gets to work, making us feel physically the images produced by words on the page and in our gray matter. The abstract becomes concrete in the form of somatic feelings. This leads Hartman to conclude that "Perhaps the only way to overcome a traumatic severance of body and mind is to come back to mind through the body."[51] This conjecture suggests that Romantic poetry might have already served as a balm to traumatized minds well before the formal scientific therapies of hypnosis and psychoanalysis developed at the end of the nineteenth century, topics to be analyzed in the next chapter. Hartman's ideas about the stimulation of the imagination and somatic feelings obviously do not apply exclusively to poetry. Nor does his conjecture that one can return to the mind through the body occur solely when reading Romantic literature. Romantic writers had been inspired by Rousseau's character Emile, who taught us about the importance of experiencing the world through the body.[52] And as we shall encounter in Part IV of this book, Miguel de Cervantes (1547–1616) situates the topic of the stimulation of emotions at the very center of *Don Quixote*.

Conclusions: Future Interdisciplinary and Symbiotic Research

What pivotal information from this enlarged historical narrative of trauma studies have we gained? From clay tablets to Herodotus's historical narratives and Ovid's and Apuleius's *Metamorphoses*. From Montaigne's *Essays* to de las Casas's *The Tears of Indians*. From Voltaire's philosophical essays to Rousseau's intimate literature and Diderot's *Encyclopedia*. The message is unequivocal. Authors of imaginative writing have spoken about the unspeakable and provoked somatic feelings in readers well before the Romanticists penned verse and clinicians and scientists developed the term "trauma" and described different states of traumatism in the nineteenth and twentieth centuries.

As far as specific lessons about their notions of psychological trauma, two cogent topics appear. From the Mesopotamians, we learned that symptoms, such as insomnia and nightmares, were triggered by a "spirit affliction" or the spirits of those whom soldiers had killed. This concept underscores that the trauma and traumatism experienced by combat soldiers and perpetrators of violence are complicated by issues of regret, self-reproach, shame, and guilt. The recovery process may therefore need to involve opportunities to acknowledge personally and publicly these burdensome feelings. This may include apologies, acts of contrition, including self-forgiveness, and cathartic processes. While these notions may be widespread among clinicians, they certainly do not populate the research work of cultural theorists. As for the Renaissance writers Montaigne and de las Casas, their narratives on Native Americans highlight traumatic-like experiences associated with racism, slavery, and colonialism in clear and visceral language. The Enlightenment philosophers Voltaire, Rousseau, and Diderot followed suit. Their writings were an honest assessment of European hypocrisy and moral depravity. They stirred Europeans to look themselves in the mirror where they could observe their racism, feel the pain of the colonized and enslaved, and move towards abolishing slavery and eventually colonialism. In brief, the trauma and traumatism associated with these abominations were written in between the lines of their prose.

Readers might object that these lessons are not new to the contemporary world. Post-colonial researchers have devoted reems to these themes. We should pause nevertheless to consider that the *DSM-5* (the manual that defines and classifies mental disorders with the aim of improving research, diagnoses, and treatments) has multiple nuanced entries on trauma, but does not include the trauma of racism or impoverishment. It is almost as if culture does not cause trauma, or better yet, it only causes certain types. By reading literary texts such as these (or contemporary works) on the traumatic experiences of prejudice and poverty, clinicians may develop a keener awareness and feeling of these widespread forms of trauma.

As far as discovering a trove of findings about resistance, resilience, growth, and recovery, we should recall the clever and subtle methods characters and writers have employed to transcend their traumatic suffering. Ovid relies on the river god, Peneus, to transform Daphne into a laurel tree, lest she be raped by Apollo. The metaphor is powerful. It intimates that even if the traumatic experience has deeply altered Daphne, it has not impeded her growth altogether. She has resisted and can grow, although she might not be able to recover fully. Even if the anxiety of the rape is rooted in her being, she still flourishes somehow as branches grow, leaves sprout, and flowers bud. Similarly, Apuleius's Psyche is not stuck in an eternal traumatic situation. Cupid rescues her from his mother's punishments, while Jupiter transforms her into an immortal. Even if Cupid and Jupiter play a role in her transformation, the Greek word "*psychē*" means soul, breathe, and butterfly. That is, Psyche's posttraumatic experience had built into it a liberating metamorphosis. This may be a very uplifting message for trauma survivors. For Montaigne, finding solace posttraumatic experience is work. It consists of trying to make sense of suffering. Beyond the trauma he experienced and witnessed, he was able to turn famines into feasts, as he nourished himself with the writings of his mentors. He quotes Plato, Aristotle, Cicero, and Lucretius to express what he fails to express and calls upon them to keep him company by engraving their sayings on the beams of his library. Montaigne's reliance on these writers brings to mind what psychiatrist Peter D. Kramer wrote about his patients who were extremely devoted to literary authors. As reviewed in this book's Introduction, Kramer found that such devotion to literature was a dog whistle for neurological disorders. Montaigne's work and life story imply that such a devotion may very well be a dog whistle for coping mechanisms, such as cultivating resistance, resilience, and a desire to learn and to grow.

Our findings from these textual analyses remind us that the humanities held a privileged position in society for millennia until the explosion of empirical science in the late nineteenth century. Enlightenment thinkers coupled the scientific method with the humanities as seen in the writings of Voltaire and Diderot. Far from remaining on the cultural fringe, as they might today, members of the humanities produced research on psychic suffering. By advancing an alternative history that relies on the literary arts, history, and philosophy, this research project moves beyond a reductive trend in trauma studies to "medicalize" human emotions and experiences of suffering. Indeed, the Enlightenment's duo emphasis on both the humanities and the sciences could serve as an excellent template for the future of scientific trauma theories and cultural trauma studies.

Notes

1 Lévi-Strauss, *Myth*, 40.
2 When I employ the expression "standard" history of trauma, I am referring to the historical narratives proposed by key theorists from science to cultural studies, such as Judith Herman, Ruth Leys, and Cathy Caruth, among others. Herman's

epilogue to *Trauma and Recovery* (2015) makes important additions to the "standard" historical narrative, whereas I attempt to make others. For a summary of the "standard" history, consult Young, *Harmony*, loc. 57–65.

3 Recall that psychiatrist Boris Cyrulnik makes the distinction between "trauma" and "traumatism" as in the difference between the original event and the follow-up psychological conditions ranging from PTSD to resilience. See the Introduction for a discussion of this distinction.

4 This raises the parenthetical issue that primitive societies might have used similar terms that we can only conjecture about in the absence of written records.

5 By emphasizing the contributions from philosophers and the importance of a psycho-philosophical movement, I thus divert from Herman's argument that, "Without the context of a political movement, it has never been possible to advance the study of psychological trauma. The fate of this field of knowledge depends upon the fate of the same political movement that has inspired and sustained it over the last century." Herman, *Trauma*, 32.

6 In contrast with this narrative, Allan Young argues that William Shakespeare and Samuel Pepys "could not have been referring to the thing we call traumatic memory, for this memory was unavailable to them." See Young, *Harmony*, 4.

7 See Abélard, *Letters*, 13.

8 See Chadwick, "Introduction," xxi–xxii.

9 Young, *Harmony*, loc. 40.

10 Ibid., loc. 50.

11 Ibid., loc. 66.

12 Herman, *Trauma*, 240.

13 See Tallis, *Aping*, 60.

14 Rose and Abi-Rached, *Neuro*, 20–21.

15 See Blum, "Resilience," 173.

16 Tedeschi et al., *Posttraumatic*, 9.

17 Scurlock and Andersen, *Diagnoses*, 345.

18 Abdul-Hamid and Hughes, "Nothing," 6.

19 Ibid., 2.

20 Ibid., 1.

21 Herodotus, *Histories*, 347.

22 Lucretius, *Nature*, 159.

23 Ibid., 98.

24 Michelet, *Histoire*, 51.

25 To be sure, de las Casas viewed the Spanish with contempt and sought to paint an arresting portrait of them. He writes, "This I will also add, that from the beginning to this day, the Spaniards were never any more mindful to spread the Gospel among them, then as if they had been dogs …" De las Casas, *Tears*, loc. 2008.

26 Ibid., 3.

27 Ibid., 6.

28 Ibid., 77.

29 Montaigne, *Essays*, loc. 20939.

30 Montaigne's *Essays* were placed on the Catholic Church's index of forbidden books in 1676.

31 Montaigne, *Essays*, loc. 8577.

32 See ibid., loc. 4450.

33 See ibid., loc. 18602.

34 Ibid., loc. 21064.

35 See LaLonde, *Paris*, 42–47.

36 The historian Roger Chartier maintains that literacy rates in France by the end of the eighteenth century had reached 47% for men and 27% for women, increasing

from 29% and 14% respectively from the end of the seventeenth century. Before the French Revolution of 1789, bookstores and libraries were few. All texts were reviewed by the *Librairie*, the French monarchy's official censuring body, and their decisions were enforced by the book police. Chartier's research reveals, all the same, that presses in Switzerland and Holland were busy printing and shipping material covertly to France. The book smuggling business became prominent as readers sought revolutionary literature. Of the approximately 1,500 titles published in France in 1764 (and still available today) only 40% had been approved by the official censuring body. See Chartier, *Origines*, 106–111.

37 Voltaire, *Lettres*, 72.
38 Voltaire, *Philosophical*, "Religion."
39 Voltaire, *Age*, 261.
40 It is important to point out that Voltaire did not always practice a sense of empathy for others. He was anti-religious, anti-Semitic, Islamophobic, and a misogynist. See LaLonde, *Paris*, 45 and 59.
41 Voltaire, *Zadig*, loc. 280.
42 Ibid., loc. 550.
43 Rousseau, "Discourse," chap. 3.
44 Diderot, "Encyclopedia."
45 Diderot, *Supplément*, 188. My translation; the original reads: "*Si un Tahitien débarquait un jour sur vos côtes, et qu'il gravât sur une de vos pierres ou sur l'écorce d'un de vos arbres: Ce pays est aux habitants de Tahiti, qu'en penserais-tu?*"
46 Raynal, *History*, 112–113.
47 A most moving testimony of the complete disregard for the rights of enslaved colonial subjects can be gleaned from Abbé Grégoire's "Letter to the Citizens of Color and Free Negroes of Saint Domingue" (1791). See Müller, *Crossroads*, 39.
48 Herman, *Trauma*, 9.
49 Hartman, "Traumatic," 552.
50 Ibid., 541.
51 Ibid.
52 These comments also draw upon Hartman's comment that "the poets were there before Freud." See ibid., 551.

2 The Birth of the Terms Trauma and Posttraumatic Stress Disorder

According to the psychiatrist Judith Herman, there have been three times between the late nineteenth and twentieth centuries when a collective awareness of psychological trauma has flourished. Hysteria, a mental malady afflicting women with so-called defective wombs, was the first form of trauma that was recognized collectively. The concept emerged from "the anticlerical political movement of the late nineteenth century in France."[1] The second form was shell shock or combat neurosis. It was somewhat studied during World War I and became a topic of interest during the Vietnam War. "Its political context was the collapse of a cult of war and the growth of an antiwar movement."[2] The last and most recent forms of trauma to enter collective awareness are sexual and domestic violence. "Its political context is the feminist movement in Western Europe and North America."[3] It should be clear that Herman emphasizes political movements that promoted the development of these three separate forms of trauma investigation.

While I do not dispute the importance of these developments triggered by political movements, I consider other phenomena that might have expanded the West's concepts of trauma and posttraumatic conditions during the nineteenth and twentieth centuries in this chapter. For instance, rather than focus on railroad accidents as *the* reason for the coinage of the word "trauma" to refer to mental disturbances, I uncover a series of previous and simultaneous terms that publicly legitimized psychic suffering. This more enlarged reading is thus a continuation of the previous chapter in which I delineated embryonic forms of these concepts in literary texts and argued moreover that the Enlightenment prepared the mental and emotional terrain for the notion of psychic trauma to come to fruition in the mid-nineteenth century. I propose this enlarged history to respond once again to current biologically oriented research on emotional experiences, especially trauma.[4]

We shall enlarge and thus adjust the standard history of trauma studies in several ways. French doctors and generals were already alluding to a type of posttraumatic stress disorder (PTSD) at the end of the eighteenth and early nineteenth centuries. We also pause to consider overlooked notions about the social causes of hysteria from the middle of the nineteenth century. With piercing insight, the French physician Pierre Briquet identified the

DOI: 10.4324/9781003284642-4

relationship between poverty, child abuse, sexual abuse, and rape and hysteria. We then pause to consider "irritable heart syndrome," a term coined by the cardiologist Jacob Mendes Da Costa, who treated veterans from the American Civil War. Returning to Paris, we visit the investigative theater of neurologist Jean-Martin Charcot, who studied women suffering from hysteria. Of equal interest was his interdisciplinary research in the humanities, not to mention his mentorship of two leading traumatologists, psychologist Pierre Janet and neurologist Sigmund Freud. Both developed novel concepts from "fixed ideas" to "dissociation," not to mention talk therapy. Though these contributions have been monumental, they have stirred controversy meriting attention.

This brings us to a discussion of World War I and to the birth of the expression "shell shock." Even though the prevalence of traumatized minds could not be denied during and after the war, much of the medical field neglected to develop compassionate treatments for combat veterans, while Freud expressed doubts about their recovery. In contrast to Freud's pessimism, the American psychiatrist Abram Kardiner created an encyclopedia, as it were, on combat-veteran posttraumatic conditions ("war neurosis" and "combat fatigue") from both world wars. Simultaneously, psychiatrists William Niederland, Paul Chodoff, Leo Eitinger, and Henry Krystal researched Holocaust survivors and catastrophic and collective trauma, stimulating interest in extreme and collective forms of trauma. This leads us to the topics of other forms of extreme and collective trauma (racism and colonialism) and to the research of psychiatrist and philosopher Frantz Fanon. From the topic of decolonization follows the related topics of the Vietnam War, sexism, and sexual abuse. Thanks to both the anti-Vietnam War and women's liberation movements and the research contributions mentioned above, the term "posttraumatic stress disorder" was coined in 1980.

Whereas this history of scientific trauma studies seeks to stretch the field of investigation to include quasi-medical and related-medical terms, it stresses above all that the study of psychological trauma also rests on the humanities. In other words, it was not just political movements, like French Republicanism and the pacifist and feminist movements, that sparked interest in and collective awareness of psychic suffering. Writers, artists, and clinicians trained in the humanities also provoked an acknowledgement of a unique form of collective repression. Humanity had denied the prevalence and complexity of trauma, and it took not only scientific research but also exposure to literature and art to cultivate a greater awareness of it.

Combat Psychic Suffering, Hysteria, and "Irritable Heart Syndrome"

Prior to and during the early part of the nineteenth century, there was an attempt to recognize medically the existence of mental turmoil in soldiers engaged in the French Revolutionary Wars (1792–1802). Doctor René-Nicolas Desgenettes describes soldiers suffering from psychic disturbances in his

Histoire Medicale (1802). He refers to an emotional aberration (*aberration*) of a soldier who upon seeing a friend killed in battle fell into a state of shock (*stupeur*); wailing (*gémissements*); and fury (*fureur*).[5] In addition, there was a quasi-medical precursor term "the symptom of the cannon-ball wind" (*le symptom du vent du boulet*) to describe mental disturbances during the Napoleonic Wars (1804–1815). General Baron de Marbot employs the expression in his Napoleonic war memoirs (1807).[6] The term refers to mental wounds of combat soldiers. Even though they were not hit directly by cannon balls, they had appeared to be struck by a great gust of wind. Marbot also describes his own traumatic experiences, including how he was nearly killed in a hand-to-hand bayonet combat with a Russian officer. The general relates his emotional shock. He was crushed (*anéanti*) during the horrific battle but regained his mental faculties (*facultés mentales*).[7] Referring to the Napoleonic Wars, the Romantic writer René de Chateaubriand elaborates on these experiences in his *Memoirs from Beyond the Tomb* (1849–1850). "Never, it must be admitted," he insists, "have men been put to so great a test and suffered such agonizing torment."[8] These testimonies from Desgenettes, Marbot, and Chateaubriand are remarkable for three main reasons. They offer a novel perspective about combat mental turmoil. According to the physician Emmanuel Régis (1855–1918), it was believed that an antidote to psychic suffering was to engage in revolutions.[9] By prescribing more violence and terror, there was a dismissal of veterans' psychological wounds, whereas Desgenettes, Marbot, and Chateaubriand highlighted them. Further, these testimonies may very well have helped to raise awareness of psychic suffering of combat soldiers, just as Enlightenment literature provoked conscious awareness about the topic of human induced suffering. And today, these works offer evidence of other embryonic expressions and concepts related to trauma and PTSD that pre-date the coinage of the term "trauma" during the Industrial Revolution.

By the middle of the century, physician Pierre Briquet had contributed significantly to understanding mental suffering by elaborating on hysteria prevalent in different segments of society.[10] This may seem trivial to contemporary minds who consider hysteria a non-scientific concept, not to mention, a sexist one. Nonetheless, Briquet's enlarged notion of hysteria leaves us with the impression that he, like the authors studied above, was referring to trauma without using the word trauma. This leads us to conjecture that his understanding of hysteria played an important role in the birth of the concept of psychic trauma, especially for Jean-Martin Charcot. One might even say that his modified notion of hysteria was the mid-wife that helped give birth to the new concept of trauma later in the century, at least in France.

Briquet was a taxonomist of the mind. Visiting thousands of patients in the Children's Hospital and Hospital of Charité in Paris, he would observe patients, record and categorize information, and draw conclusions about those who suffered from mental disturbances, including hysteria. What were his main contributions? I will mention only four from his untranslated seven-hundred-page *Traité Clinique et thérapeutique de la hystérie* (1859). First, he applied the term "hysteria" to both men and women, boys and girls. The word comes from the Greek "*hyster*," which means uterus. It had been used from the time of Hippocrates (460–375 BCE) to refer to pathological conditions allegedly unique to women.[11] Briquet along with other doctors from the early and mid-nineteenth century argued that hysteria was not an illness caused by a defective womb.[12] He observed convulsions, paralysis, speech impediments and other conditions common in hysteria in men and boys.[13] His nuanced understanding of hysteria signals a general acknowledgment that men and boys could suffer from mental disturbances as well. This finding should be of special interest, as both Janet Oppenheim and Elaine Showalter have argued that Anglo-American physicians did not widely accept the idea that both men and women could experience hysteria until World War I.[14] Briquet's finding also contrasts sharply with the policy of "prescribing" revolution to soldiers who suffered from mental disturbances, as discussed previously. Second, he emphasized that hysteria was not fundamentally biological. It was a "neurosis of the brain" (*névrose d'encéphale*).[15] By employing the terms "neurosis of the brain," the physician puts into sharp relief that the condition is not caused by an organic disease, but rather by the reactions of the mind to events. More specifically, it is caused by perturbed "affects and passions" to events.[16] Third, Briquet contributed a long list of other "predispositions" to hysteria, including social circumstances and emotional sensibility.[17] Contrary to a widely held opinion at the time, he argued that the poor were more apt to suffer from hysteria than the rich.[18] This finding is particularly significant, because many were convinced that the poor were "accustomed" (*habitués*) to hardships and were not susceptible to hysteria.[19] Fourth, and equally as remarkable, he observed correlations between child abuse, sexual abuse, and rape and hysteria.[20] It should be stressed finally that he included a hundred-page discussion of the different types of treatments he employed to treat hysteria.

An acknowledgement of psychic suffering in men and boys? An emphasis on affects and passions, as opposed to diseased wombs? A long list of predispositions for nervous disorders? An acknowledgement of social conditions, such as poverty and exposure to abuse and rape? These are significant contributions to understanding psychopathologies. Curiously, though, Briquet's name seldom appears in narratives of the history of trauma studies.[21] Unfortunately, his interest in mental disturbances triggered by poverty, rape, sexual abuse, and child abuse has not always been shared. Other researchers from this period focused on physical accidents, rather than societal aberrations, that could cause mental disturbances. Still, Briquet's pluri-disciplinary research on hysteria paved the way for other clinicians to study and care for those suffering from traumatism from different perspectives.

On the other side of the Atlantic appeared noteworthy trauma research by the American cardiologist Jacob Mendes Da Costa. After having treated veterans during and after the American Civil War, he coined the term "irritable heart syndrome."[22] The cardiologist recorded the following symptoms: attacks of acute heart palpitations during both exercise and rest, especially at nighttime, headaches, and dizziness, while pain is constant but either dull or piercing. He describes it as a "curious cardiac malady of which we saw so many examples in soldiers."[23] Why curious? Though he did not explicitly state that the syndromes were psychosomatic, he stressed that he failed to find the malady's physical etiology.[24] Mendes Da Costa was on to something. Today, "irritable heart syndrome" is called neurocirculatory asthenia and is indeed considered an anxiety disorder.[25]

The Birth of the Word "Trauma" and Erichsen's and Oppenheim's Contributions

Simultaneous to Briquet's research on hysteria caused by social factors, other clinicians investigated how industrial accidents could provoke a host of physical and psychological ailments and some even with no obvious somatic origin. In 1866, British physician John Erichsen identified a "trauma syndrome" in survivors of railway accidents, which he called "railway brain" or "railway spine."[26] Railway or other serious accidents, such as falling from a carriage, could damage the spinal cord. The spine, like the brain, could suffer a concussion that led to "molecular changes" that provoked subjective symptoms, he maintained.[27] Railway spine could cause memory loss, confused thoughts, perturbed sleep, impaired sense of hearing and touch, sexual impotence, changes to gait, loss of motor skills, loss of sense of the limbs, among other symptoms.[28] His conviction that these symptoms were due to a somatic injury, rather than a psychological one, was strengthened by his observation that both men and women experienced railway spine. In a twisted form of reasoning tainted with sexism, he could not imagine that a male survivor of a railroad accident could be so vulnerable to his mental reactions (affects, including anxiety) to the accident. His symptoms must have been caused by a physical disruption of the spine, the psychiatrist reasoned. He asked rhetorically, "Is it reasonable to say that a man has suddenly become 'hysterical' like a lovesick girl?"[29] Had Erichsen read Briquet's work, then he might have been convinced that men could suffer from hysteria and that purely psychical causes, such as fright, could account for nervous states and physical disorders. In fact, the British physician writes that "Hysteria, whether in its emotional or its local form, is a disease of women rather than of men, of the younger rather than of the middle-aged and old..."[30] He supports this claim by indicating that he has never seen or read about a middle-aged hysterical man.[31]

The German neurologist Hermann Oppenheim endorsed a more subtle understanding of psychic trauma. In 1886, he delivered a lecture entitled "The meaning of fright for the diseases of the nervous system."[32] He then coined the expression "*traumatischen Neurosen*" (traumatic neurosis).[33]

Between this term and the title of his lecture, it becomes apparent that Oppenheim stresses the psychic dimension of trauma, rather than a physical one, as in the case of Erichsen's conviction of a damaged spinal cord that led to symptoms. Not only did Oppenheim intimate that neurological diseases could be caused by psychic conditions, namely fear, he nuanced this position by referring to "another somatic mediating force."[34] More specifically, "(hysterical) paralysis resulted from the loss of memory pictures, i.e. ideas of the movement, in the brain (Oppenheim, 1889)."[35] Thus, he defined the underlying issue of traumatic neurosis as neurological or quasi-neurological, resulting in muscle cramps, tremors, and paralysis, among other symptoms.

Charcot's Interdisciplinary Research

If Erichsen attributed the condition of "trauma syndrome" to physical injuries to the spinal cord and Oppenheim connected "traumatic neurosis" to psychic causes with an accompanying physical mediating force, Jean-Martin Charcot stressed psychic causes for the origin of "traumatic hysteria." He went so far as to argue that the actual traumatic experience played less of a role in posttraumatic conditions than hereditary dispositions for nervous disorders.[36] Seen from another perspective, traumatic experiences served as the catalyst ("*agent provocateur*") for a nervous disorder such as hysteria that already existed in some form.[37] Confirming Briquet's position, Charcot concluded that hysteria occurred in both men and women and presented itself in the form of cataleptic, lethargic, and sleepwalking symptoms.[38]

The neurologist would demonstrate these symptoms in real time. He transformed the Salpêtrière hospital in Paris into a refuge for those suffering from mental disturbances. From the streets came the homeless, prostitutes, and the so-called insane. Weekly, the hospital would become a "theater" where medical doctors, writers, and artists would observe the neurologist engage his patients (principally women suffering from hysteria) in hypnosis. (Charcot himself was an amateur artist and loved going to the theater.) The idea behind hypnotism was to create psychopathological states to be analyzed in controlled settings. Herman contends that "Though Charcot paid minute attention to the symptoms of his hysterical patients, he had no interest whatsoever in their inner lives. He viewed their emotions as symptoms to be cataloged."[39] No interest whatsoever? This seems to be an unfair assessment. Granted it is easy to object to the sexist connotations of displaying women suffering from mental turmoil to a public, as if they were circus animals. Granted he did not devote himself to listening to his patients the way his students Pierre Janet and Sigmund Freud did.[40] Be that as it may, let us not forget that Charcot was a neurologist not a psychiatrist, psychologist, or psychoanalyst, a vocation that did not even exist at the time of his early career. The point is that neurologists typically do not rely on talk therapy to diagnose pathologies the way psychoanalysts do. It might be more accurate to state therefore that he was interested in the inner lives of those suffering from hysteria in general but not in individual suffering. He pursued nomothetic research, seeking general patterns, as opposed to idiographic research based on individual cases.

Charcot broadened his understanding of hysterical neuroses by turning to art. His co-authored and untranslated *Les Démoniaques dans l'art* (1887) is a collection of art showcasing religious versions of hysterical individuals. He included reproductions of ivory carvings, mosaics, and drawings of the "possessed" and those being healed. Until the scientific method was employed to study and treat neuroses, the clergy "diagnosed" and "treated" them. An individual suffering from hysteria was referred to as "a perversion of the soul,"[41] which allegedly demons had caused. It is paradoxical that "demons" were seen as the cause of a "perversion of the soul" when in many cases sexual assaults committed by men provoked hysteria, a conclusion that Freud drew but tragically later renounced, as we shall discover.

From his study of hysterics or "*démoniaques*" depicted in art, Charcot concluded that the condition was not a by-product of modern society. Its presence was extensive in the Middle Ages, as art from the period documented. The neurologist included artistic depictions of hysterics from artwork perhaps to gain elucidation that his scientific lens failed to provide. Charcot refers to a multiprong approach to studying hysteria. His research consisted of embarking on voyages to other countries to speak with colleagues, visit museums and private collections, and study photographs and sculptures.[42] The field of investigation was not just the examining room at the hospital; it extended to the Louvre. His tools of study were not simply hypnosis. They consisted of paintings, sculptures, and photography. His colleagues were not exclusively medical doctors. The writer Émile Zola frequented the neurologist's theater, as did artists such as André Brouillet. And they came from far and wide, while Charcot traveled across Europe exchanging ideas on the condition of hysteria. To illustrate even more the multidisciplinary nature of his research, one need consider that the neurologist even wrote a text on religious healings of those suffering from hysteria.[43] In short, Charcot was deeply committed to pluri-disciplinary research about traumatic neurosis. This provides evidence of his devotion not only to his patients but also to his students Janet and Freud, who established the more interdisciplinary fields of psychological-analysis and psychoanalysis, respectively.

Janet's, Freud's, and Breuer's Key Theories of Trauma

Janet and Freud lasered in on causes of symptoms and embarked on an investigation of their patients' inner lives. Janet employed the terms traumatic neurosis (*névrose traumatique*) and traumatism (*traumatisme*) to refer to psychological disturbances subsequent to traumatic choc, accidents (*choc et accident traumatiques*), and more generally, hysterical trauma (*hystérie traumatique*).[44] Following Charcot's lead, he also employed the term hysteria to refer to the psychopathological condition of patients subjected to traumatic experiences.

While Janet left a formidable corpus of research, three of his contributions to the field of trauma studies merit special attention. He defined hysteria as (a) a form of mental depression characterized by a constriction of conscious awareness and a tendency to both (b) experience dissociation and (c) create fixed ideas.[45] Rather than focusing on the traumatic event itself, Janet targeted emotional reactions (*emotion-choc*) that undermine conscious awareness. Why this focus? Patients often feel ill-prepared to process their emotional reactions, according to Janet. Rage, sorrow, fear, and compromised cognitive processes may feel overwhelming. This emotional load may in turn produce a maladaptive strategy of constricting awareness of one's experiences and surroundings. Related to this constriction is the tendency to engage in dissociation (*dissociation*), another maladaptive strategy to endure posttraumatic experiences. Dissociation is a constricted mental state. It occurs when a trauma survivor is so exhausted psychologically that she fails to view herself and her experiences from an overarching perspective. There is thus neither a synthesis nor a meta-analysis of her existence. This constricted state facilitates the formation of fixed ideas (*idées fixes*), which are rigid and thus distorted memories.[46] Memories are cemented, deformed, and off limits, as a patient fails to integrate them into her conscious realm. Nevertheless, fixed ideas can appear in sleepwalking and "brain fugues" or memory lapses. They can also make themselves known through behavior. Janet describes patients who would imagine themselves to be in hell among demons or transported to heaven.[47] One of his patients, Louise Lateau, would even reenact scenes of Christ's crucifixion.

On a related note, Janet argued that fixed ideas can manifest themselves in physical ailments in the stomach or intestines. He maintained in fact that all maladaptive modifications of the body triggered by representations (ideas) indicate hysteria.[48] Recalling Charcot's lessons, he sums up the power of the mind to torment the mind and body as: "It is not necessary that the carriage wheel should really have passed over the patient; it is enough if he has the idea that the wheel passed over his legs."[49] This implies that the patient's traumatic affects are reactivated and aggravated during the posttraumatic experience. The posttraumatic experience is defined by the emotional fall out. While Janet's findings highlighted above shed light on posttraumatic conditions, they are not universally accepted today. His concepts of fixed ideas, rigid and distorted memories, and dissociation are controversial. They have provoked bitter controversies among psychiatrists, psychologists, and cultural theorists and will be examined in Chapter 6.[50]

Freud and his colleague Joseph Breuer also focused on the issue of memory in traumatic neuroses. They were convinced that "hysterics suffer from reminiscences."[51] As innocuous as this may sound, it points to the hard-to-grasp nature of traumatic memories, which are out of reach to the conscious mind and buried in unconscious psychic space. Freud also considered traumatic neuroses "grounded in a fixation upon the moment of the traumatic disaster."[52] Related to fixation, is Freud's notion of trauma as "economic." "For the expression 'traumatic' has no other than an economic meaning, and the disturbance permanently attacks the management of available energy."[53] The traumatic experience is so intense that its assimilation and eventual elaboration cannot be achieved by normal mental mechanisms. If one follows Freud's metaphor of trauma as "economic," one can conclude that a pronounced assimilation and elaboration is required to match a pronounced traumatic experience.

This led the psychoanalyst to draw the conclusion that "the disturbance permanently attacks the management of available energy."[54] Nightmares are examples of mental stimulation tormenting the mind. Repeated dreams might allow the patient to relive and perhaps even work through the trauma. Similarly, survivors might benefit from the stimulation of memories. Though he did employ hypnosis to stimulate memories, Freud moved on to develop psychoanalysis. Traumatic reminiscences are excavated from the strata of the unconscious through talk therapy. The survivor freely associates, exposing memories by sharing whatever comes to mind. The patient is invited to "abreact"—to explore phobias, daydreams, and desires particularly sexual ones.

Despite sounding encouraging, Freud's theories contained a heavy dose of pessimism about traumatic neuroses. Even though his psychoanalytic therapies were designed to work through traumatic experiences, the psychoanalyst maintained that his patients were "unable to free themselves therefrom and have therefore come to be completely estranged from the present and the future."[55] His vocabulary "unable to free themselves" and "completely estranged" insinuates that recovery from traumatic experiences is unlikely.[56] To strengthen this interpretation, it bears mentioning that Freud contended that unconscious wishes were "indestructible" and that "nothing can be brought to an end in the unconscious; nothing can cease or be forgotten."[57] Again, his choice of superlative words ("indestructible," "nothing can be brought to an end," "nothing can cease or be forgotten") underscores his sense of pessimism about successfully treating traumatic neuroses. Psychoanalyst and Freudian disciple Karen Horney elaborates: "Freud's pessimism as regards neuroses and their treatment arose from the depths of his disbelief in human goodness and human growth. Man, he postulated, is doomed to suffer or to destroy."[58] Between Freud's own writings and Horney's reading of her mentor, it is obvious that one must accept his theories with a grain of salt, as they are shrouded in darkness. This warning applies especially to "First Wave" cultural trauma theorists who remain devoted to the father of psychoanalysis. Besides his pessimism, Freud undermined his own research. He discovered a relationship between hysteria and childhood sexual abuse. The prevalence of hysteria led him to conclude that pedophilia was "endemic, not only among the proletariat of Paris, where he had first studied hysteria, but also among the respectable bourgeois families of Vienna, where he had established his practice. This idea was simply unacceptable,"[59] at least to Freud. After making this discovery and in an act of treason against his patients, science, and humanity, he swept his theory of the traumatic origins of hysteria under the rug.

World War I and Shell Shock

From the concepts of the symptom of the cannonball wind, hysteria, irritable heart syndrome, railway brain, traumatic neurosis, neurosis in the brain, fixed ideas, traumatic memories, and reminiscences came "shell shock," a consequence of the trauma of traumas, World War I. If railroad and industrial accidents had traumatized the body and mind in unprecedented ways and frequency in the 1800s, the machinery of the Great War assumed this dubious honor in the 1900s. The term "shell shock" first appeared in an article in the *Lancet* journal in 1915 by the British physician David Forsyth. Sharing case studies of soldiers suffering from "traumatic neuroses" (also called hysteria, neurasthenia, and soldier's heart), Forsyth nuances the term by asking: "Why do some men exposed to a psychical trauma develop neuroses, others under the same strain escaping, little if at all affect?"[60] It is not so much the circumstances or the intensity of the trauma, but rather the psychological profile of the patient. He delineates a patient's psychological history that could determine psychopathic tendencies, "such as previous nervous breakdown, sexual impotence, a habit of worrying in a morbid degree over the ordinary affairs of life, or of drug-taking."[61] Forsyth's article is a medical *J'accuse* (the article Zola wrote to denounce the French Third Republic's anti-Semitism made obvious in the Dreyfus Affair). The British doctor's article on "nerve-shock" was a diatribe against sending broken soldiers back to the front.

Meanwhile on the other side of the English Channel, Janet's colleague Georges Dumas observed a relationship between war engagement and mental turmoil, a type of hysteria, without trace of physical harm. Though this may seem self-evident today, many in the past doubted that wars and revolutions could provoke mental illnesses. Recall that some even argued that they cured mental illnesses rather than caused them.[62] The rude reality of World War I debunked this position. While it became increasingly clear that the "traumatic shock" (*choc traumatique*) of war caused shell shock ("*choc de l'obus*" or "*hypnose des batailles*"), the etiology of the condition remained unclear. Was it caused by inherited personality traits, the environment, or the result of previous physical pathologies? Was it the war itself that triggered the mental disorder? And was the pathology neurological, physiological, psychological, or a combination of all three?[63] Dumas and other doctors posed these questions as they struggled to treat a complex condition that seemed just as much psychological as physical in nature.[64]

With a limited understanding of shell shock after World War I came a "psychiatry of war." Previous and new treatments were employed—such as hypnosis, psychoanalysis, sedatives, narco-analysis, and electrical current (faradization). Patients were eventually given short shrift as the medical field turned its attention to other mysteries of the mind and investigations of the brain. Perhaps clinicians, who had treated so many traumatized soldiers, were suffering from their own form of trauma and hence split off this topic from their cognitions and focused on other topics. One notable exception to that tendency was André Breton, a World War I medic and surrealist writer who developed artistic and literary activities designed to break the silence of traumatic experiences. His automatic psychic exercises, including doodling and collaging, provided keys to unlock the unconscious realm.[65] Art spoke when speech was arrested. This is a staggering statement for several reasons. It points obviously to a therapeutic effect of art and calls into question Freud's pessimism about his ability to treat veterans, a topic to unfold in Chapter 5 in our discussions of treatments for survivors of trauma.

The American psychiatrist and psychoanalyst Abram Kardiner believed that Freud had failed to address the traumatic neuroses of war.[66] In his eyes, the Freudian theory of the libido and ego were inadequate to understand wartime cases of neurosis. In his published *The Traumatic Neuroses of War* (1941) (later revised as *War, Stress, and Neurotic Illness*), he presents his research on US World War I veterans. One of Kardiner's most important contributions is his piercing complaint against the capricious research on traumatic neuroses. He complains that "the public does not sustain its interest, which was very great after World War I, and neither does psychiatry."[67] As a consequence of this whimsical attention to the topic of war neuroses, research was conducted only periodically, owing to the declining reputation of veterans, according to Kardiner. In response to this neglect, he endorsed psychoanalysis and other forms of dynamic psychotherapy to treat traumatic war neuroses. "Traumatic neuroses," would be categorized today as posttraumatic stress disorder—PTSD. And of special interest is his summary of the condition: "The nucleus of the neurosis is a physio-neurosis."[68] This intimates that the body lodges and responds to the original traumatic event. It is not only psychological, but also physiological.

World War II, Kardiner's Trauma "Encyclopedia," and the Use of "Truth Serum"

During World War II, Kardiner continued to develop trauma theories, a symptomatology guide, and treatments. A chief contribution was his detailed descriptions of symptoms related to acute war stress and chronic neurotic illnesses. The most prominent symptom in the acute phase of war stress is an unconscious state with eyes closed and flaccid limbs. The face is pale, the pulse is slow, and respiration is superficial. The patient is "impervious to external stimuli and insensitive to pain..."[69] The chronic phase includes hypochondriasis, schizophrenia, transference, defensive ceremonials and tics, autonomic disturbances, psychosomatic disorders, sensory-motor disorders, acute shock psychosis, and an epileptic symptom complex. This enumeration is meant to convey his detailed research. One might say that he created the first encyclopedia on trauma. As far as actual treatment findings are concerned, Kardiner along with psychiatrist Herbert Spiegel stressed that the best way to protect against debilitating anxiety from warfare was to establish bonds among soldiers. Simultaneously, British and American psychiatrists William Sargant, John Spiegel, Roy Grinker, and others treated World War II veterans suffering from "combat fatigue" with barbiturates. Often in catatonic states, returning soldiers were administered sodium amytal ("the truth serum") to trigger the brain's principal inhibitory system, like alcohol or *vino veritas*. Uninhibited, veterans would accept food and drink and express themselves more freely. This loosening of the tongue would allow patients to access and relive their traumatic memories. Such a cathartic experience was considered key for bringing traumatic memories into conscious awareness and for forming a narrative of the traumatic experience. Historian Ruth Leys points out nevertheless that Sargant's position on the motives for employing drug catharsis was mixed. On the one hand, he considered it a mechanism to reproduce the original traumatic event. It was a re-enactment as well as a mental encounter. On the other, he felt that "the cure depended on an intense, mimetically or hypnotically induced discharge of emotional scenes that might be authentic copies of the original but were frequently fictional in character."[70] Drug catharsis might produce not so much exact memories but rather a liquidation of feelings associated with those past experiences. The issue of truth seemed therefore secondary to affect.

The Holocaust and Collective and Catastrophic Trauma

After World War II, the term "war neurosis" continued to be employed in the United States and Great Britain to refer to posttraumatic conditions. Nonetheless, humanity seemed to have suffered from a case of collective amnesia about war neurosis. This fact has moved Leys to write: "Not even the independent psychoanalytic studies of the long-term effects of trauma on survivors of the Holocaust ... succeeded in arousing widespread interest in trauma."[71] Her comment alludes to both a dearth of interest in the topic of war neurosis and conversely, the presence of research on Holocaust survivors. In the late 1950s and early 1960s research began to be published in different countries about personality disorders and psychiatric illnesses still present in many concentration camp survivors.[72] But how can one compose a terse summary of this research? The psychiatrist-psychoanalyst and Holocaust survivor Henry Krystal cautions: "the very attempt to generalize about Holocaust survivors is bound to introduce much error. It is not possible to achieve either a uniform, singular diagnosis or an all-inclusive view of this population, or even of their shared experiences."[73] I shall thus delineate the main contributions of four psychiatrists who devoted a lifetime studying and treating Holocaust survivors. Their research highlights both an inability to treat survivors and the very possibility of resistance, resilience, and growth.

In the late 1950s, the clinical neuro-psychiatrist William Niederland, a refugee himself of Nazi Germany, found that the Holocaust survivors he examined all continued in some respects to dwell in concentration camps.[74] This fact "deserves our attention," he writes and asks: "How can it be explained in clinical and psychodynamic terms?"[75] He explored the mental disturbances of survivors not only out of an urge to address this clinical question and a moral urge to serve his patients' needs, but also out of a literal calling. In 1961, he was named the principal consultant by the German government to diagnose Holocaust survivor claimants. Interviewing close to 2,000 survivors, he cultivated a nuanced understanding of their traumatization. A chief finding was that they suffered from "survivor guilt," "a continuing painful state of tension and unrest"[76] as one contrasts one's survival with the murder of so many others. One clinical consequence of this state was chronic depression, typically accompanied by somatic manifestations. The other was a tormenting sense of being persecuted, endangered, or attacked. He also noted that "survivor guilt... remains for the most part repressed, and tends to manifest itself clinically in the depressive, persecutory, psychosomatic, and neurovegetative symptoms of the patient, or, very rarely, in complete denial."[77] Expanding on these findings, Niederland developed the term "survivor syndrome" as a distinct condition, "which persists as a chronic state of tension, vigilance, irritability, depression, unrest and fear, usually accompanied by sleep disturbances, anxiety dreams and nightmares."[78] This term was later employed in reference to other catastrophic and collective trauma, including the genocide in Bosnia. Moreover, it helped spur the formal recognition of posttraumatic stress disorder in the *Diagnostic and Statistical Manual III (DSM-III)* (1980).[79]

Niederland maintained that psychotherapy was the preferred treatment method for Holocaust survivors. He contends that "ego strength" seems to contribute to survival. "Looking, hearing, observing, constant vigilance employed in the sense of hunted animals in the jungle were of paramount."[80] He points out nonetheless that somatic symptoms, tendencies for apathy and isolation, and the guilt and grief overwhelming survivors rendered psychotherapy challenging. Even though he contended that the "full therapeutic result" appeared "rarely possible," his therapeutic aim was to "help the patient gradually out of his anxiety-ridden, guilty and benumbed existence."[81] Thus, the goal of treatment might not have been full recovery, but rather rendering existence less of a living hell.

The psychiatrist Leo Eitinger, a concentration-camp survivor, refers to the saying that, "one year of campaigning ages a man twice as much as two years in barracks, and one year in concentration camp ages a man as much as three years of campaigning."[82] To his mind, systematic research to support this idea were few. He set out to investigate whether the severe physical and psychic stress humans were subjected to in Nazi concentration camps had psychological consequences and could be considered decisive for observed morbid conditions. He discovered that "concentration camp syndrome" correlated with the duration and severity of the camp experiences and was not related to the survivor's premorbid personality.[83] "A certain amount of mental stress ... does not break down the personality, does not blunt the ability to feel with others and can, to a certain extent, develop the personality in a positive direction, such as an increased wish to help others, and the like."[84] Conversely, a stress that goes beyond an individual's endurance and/or her values and social norms can cause profound alterations to her personality that in many incidents are irreversible.[85] This conclusion leads to the reaffirmation of the presence of a concentration camp syndrome, which occurred most often in survivors who had been subjected to "head injuries and/or encephalitis, and/or spotted fever, and/or a captivity lasting longer than three years and/or a loss of weight down to the 'living corpse' stage."[86] These findings contradicted a prevalent emphasis on premorbid personality traits leading to subsequent chronic psychiatric disorders.[87] Further, Eitinger's findings helped to define posttraumatic stress syndrome. The World Health Organization included in its *ICD-10*, a new classification category: "'Enduring personality change after catastrophic experience,' a diagnostic concept based on the work of Eitinger."[88] This (along with Niederland's contributions) indicates that it was not only the political movements (anti-Vietnam War and women's liberation) that spurred the formal recognition of posttraumatic stress disorder, as Herman contends, but also the research findings of psychiatrists treating Holocaust survivors.

Basing his 1963 report on an examination of over 200 Holocaust survivors who sought German government reparations, psychiatrist Paul Chodoff writes: "Obsessive preoccupation with recollections of the persecutory experiences was characteristic, so much so that in my interviews with some survivors I was sometimes left with the uncanny sensation of being transported in time back to the gray inferno of Auschwitz ..."[89] This echoes Niederland's impression of survivors dwelling endlessly in concentration camps and underscores how the mind can become a prison of mental torture. Chodoff's findings also mirror Niederland's regarding the presence of survival guilt. And instead of referring to a "survival syndrome," Chodoff employed the term "concentration camp syndrome" (akin to Eitinger), which consisted of severe anxiety, marked by apprehension, hypervigilance, sleep disturbances, and depression.[90] Of keen interest is Chodoff's multidisciplinary research focus. Though he might not have always provided quantitative data, he shared qualitative data about psychic suffering, especially in Jewish children who were in concentration camps, the ghettos, or shipped around to foster families during the war.[91] He compares the traumatic experiences of these children with those of children living in slums in the United States in the 1960s, and concludes, "whether they originate in malevolence as in the concentration camps or in neglect as in our urban slums, crushing forces have crushing effects and the adaptive resilience of the young human organism, though very great, is not illimitable."[92] Chodoff's comment was a warning call to American societies during the war on poverty to improve the condition of children living in abject misery in American ghettos, physical conditions kindred to those in the Warsaw ghetto.

Henry Krystal, a Holocaust survivor himself, based his findings on studies of over 2,000 Holocaust survivors over forty years. (Like Niederland and Chodoff, he diagnosed survivor claimants for the German government.) There are three contributions from Krystal's research I wish to highlight here, while others will appear throughout this book. First, he introduced the term "alexithymia" to a wider public. "Alexithymia is the single most common cause of poor outcome or outright failure of psychoanalysis and psychoanalytic psychotherapy."[93] It consists of a constriction of cognitive functions such as memory, judgment, and problem solving. Alexithymia also refers to a psychic constriction characterized by a cool indifference to the original traumatic experience, resulting in an inability not only to express emotions but also to feel them. Krystal drew attention furthermore to "anhedonia," a condition prevalent in survivors of extreme forms of trauma and describes an inability to take pleasure in life.[94] If survivors of catastrophic traumatization have lost all motivation to find pleasure in life, including looking forward to the future, if they suffer from constricted thoughts and feelings, if their verbalization has been compromised, if they are unable to interpret their emotions, then psychotherapy seems to be thwarted, a conclusion that Niederland had drawn. Thirdly, Krystal elaborated on the issue of memories in trauma survivors. In his eyes, memories and their interpretations are not inflexible, but flexible. "We now know," he informs us, "that survivors of the Holocaust have to keep reviewing and changing their perspectives and recollections of the stressful era."[95] Unacceptable memories may need to be reinterpreted or edited. "We can understand, then, the need for some Holocaust survivors and their children to keep creating new interpretations, even mythologies, that make the images of the past more bearable."[96] This becomes a mission with both positive and negative values, including a preoccupation to somehow endure a traumatic past. Working with other psychiatrists and traumatologists (such as Dori Laub whose research will be discussed in Chapters 4–6) from Yale University's Fortunoff Video Archive for Holocaust Testimonies, Krystal helped to encourage survivors to share their narratives of trauma to render the unbearable, bearable.

The findings of Niederland, Eitinger, Chodoff, and Krystal elucidate some of the psychological and physical consequences of the Holocaust on survivors. Again, responding to observations of thousands of survivors, these psychiatrists developed the terms "survivor guilt," "survivor syndrome," and "concentration camp syndrome" and elaborated on these conditions. Other contributions include insight into obsessive ruminations (Niederland and Chodoff), flexible memories (Krystal), and physical injuries and psychic suffering (Eitinger). On a more global scale, these and other findings helped to spur the formal recognition of PTSD (Niederland and Eitinger). Perhaps, more importantly, their research may very well have served as a source of inspiration to counterbalance the sense of despair felt as one grasped the extent of human evil made painfully manifest in the Holocaust. If Niederland and Krystal highlighted the difficulty of treating survivors, some have objected to the way in which Holocaust survivors are seen as "emotionally handicapped."[97] By treating survivors and sharing survivor stories, these four researchers remained true to the reality of human depravity and cruelty, while celebrating human resistance, resilience, and growth. This statement carries greater weight if one contemplates that both Krystal and Eitinger were Holocaust survivors. Their published research serves as the very symbol of resistance, resilience, and growth. As Barel et al. conclude in their meta-analysis, "Our investigation suggests that Holocaust survivors demonstrate remarkable resilience in adapting to their personal, social, and communal life. This finding is consistent with the new realm of research during the past two decades."[98] Psychiatrist Boris Cyrulnik has focused attention on the resilience of Holocaust survivors, namely those who were not necessarily in camps, but displaced and on the run from the Nazis and French authorities, just as he was as a Jewish child in France.[99] Indeed, rather than focus exclusively on trauma, as many researchers do in the fields of cultural trauma studies, this book builds on Holocaust survivor research to explore examples of "remarkable resilience" in the context of the literary arts.

The Trauma of Colonialism and Racism

Colonialism, slavery, and racism are other contexts of extreme and collective trauma meriting our attention. Of course, philosophers (Montaigne, Voltaire, and Diderot) and abolitionists (Toussaint L'Ouverture and Abbé Henri Grégoire) explored these issues and helped fuel movements against racism, colonialization, the slave trade, and slavery. There were thus both philosophical and political forces that provoked liberating changes for traumatized communities before the twentieth century's decolonization revolutions.[100] Though self-evident, this statement assumes a subtler hue when placed once again against the backdrop of Herman's more one-sided argument that "the systematic study of psychological trauma therefore depends on the support of a political movement."[101] The systematic study also depends on philosophy, literature, and art, as Frantz Fanon's work makes abundantly clear.

Fanon was a psychiatrist and philosopher and as expected, offers an interdisciplinary (philosophical, political, artistic, and medical) understanding of psychic trauma caused by racism and colonialism.[102] Born in Martinique under French colonial rule, he was trained in psychiatry in France and administered a psychiatric hospital in Algeria from 1953 to 1956 during the Algerian War of Independence (1954–1962). His work has been largely ignored by trauma theorists (except by anthropologists and post-colonialists). This is paradoxical since racism, colonialism, and slavery seem to encapsulate the very definition of traumatic experiences. Is this an illustration of repression and denial among scientific and cultural trauma theorists? These topics are the elephants in the research room that few have called out and examined, and hence the reason to add them to a historical narrative of trauma studies.[103]

Fanon's research centers on creative and critical adjustments to previous theories. He breaks with Freud's explanation of sexual fantasies as the cause of neuroses. At the same time, he repairs (to a certain degree) the harm that Freud committed by readjusting the concept of "first traumas" (child sexual assault and incest). Traumas associated with racism and slavery are kindred to first traumas. They involve the subjugation of one individual or group by a more powerful individual or group. Fanon begins his *Black Skin, White Masks* (1952) asking how Freud's and Alfred Adler's theories are applicable to black people's understanding of the world. Reminding readers that their theories focus on the family, he writes: "A normal black child, having grown up with a normal family, will become abnormal at the slightest contact with the white world."[104] It is not so much the family that is the source of psychopathologies, but the world itself for a black person. Fanon elaborates further on the traumatic experiences of living in a white world. "The black problem is not just about Blacks living among Whites, but about the black man exploited, enslaved, and despised by a colonialist and capitalist society that happens to be white."[105] These degrading experiences are accompanied by a complete sense of alienation. For Fanon, the colonial mother is protecting her children from themselves, from their egos, physiology, biology, and ontological misfortune. Thus, colonial subjects and the colonizers become totally alienated from themselves, and from each other, and suffer dissociation on a massive scale.[106] The dehumanization of populations of people of color festers in a white dominated human family. If there is any doubt about how traumatic this alienating experience might be, we can consider that Fanon likens colonialism to Nazism to stress this psychopathology. He writes: "The African people must likewise remember that they have had to face a form of Nazism, a form of exploitation of man, of physical and spiritual liquidation."[107] Fanon's analogy is no exaggeration. He contemplates how the colonized, like Holocaust victims, are completely depersonalized. Identity is reduced to a deplorable profile crafted by the colonizers for their own advantage. Without an authentic identity, colonized subjects wear a white mask, thus assuming a false, dissociated-like, and repressed identity divorced from their own culture and race.

Besides these creative and critical adjustments to Freudian trauma theories from the perspective of victims of racism and colonialism, Fanon addresses therapeutic treatments. He examines the topic of cure from a dialectical perspective. On the one hand, one could seek violent retaliation. How else is one to respond? One cannot employ words. They are nothing more than double-talk. How can one communicate with others who are constantly speaking a language devoid of authentic meaning? What is one translating? The words? Or their masked meaning? If they are weapons to manipulate minds, it makes more sense to respond with weapons that pierce bodies. It is difficult to erase moreover the physical and mental memories of violence. It leaves its traces in the tissues of the body and brain. Even though Fanon understands intellectually why the urge for violent revenge would overwhelm a traumatized survivor, he cautions against violence. He could not be any clearer: "What aberration of the mind drives these famished, enfeebled men lacking technology and organizational resources to think that only violence can liberate them … ? How can they hope to triumph?"[108] The psychiatrist need not state explicitly that violence fails to heal the mind. He writes about his devastated patients who engage in violence. An Algerian man suffers from acute anxiety after he kills a French mother in retaliation for the French murdering his mother. He is mentally tormented by the image of the French woman seeking to destroy him. Imprisoned in the mind, the memory of violent acts torments him further.

On the other hand, one could seek to purge and heal the mind and body. For Fanon, a cure cannot occur unless hidden psychopathologies are analyzed and treated first on individual and collective levels. Both colonizers and the colonized must purge themselves of disingenuous and degrading roles and assume a more authentic identity. Like existential heroes, they both must remove the masks that bind them and pursue a more authentic identity. Even though colonizers teach the colonized to distrust their own "inferior" culture, there exist modes of healing.[109] The psychiatrist stresses that prior to colonization, people used to find constructive outlets for their repressed emotions. Anger, frustration, and fear were acted out in the community. Listening to myths and dancing purged the mind and body of negative emotions and the physical residue of traumatic experiences.[110] The dance symbolizes a well spring of ablutions and purification. It also erupts like a volcano, spewing forth violent urges.

A well spring? An active volcano? Fanon's images put Hamlet's "To be or not to be" in the contexts of colonialism and decolonization. Does one attempt to heal through purification mechanisms from the traumatic experiences of colonialism and racism? Or does one harbor violence that serves as the fuel to slash the colonizer from the colonized? In other words, by engaging in healing processes, does one not perhaps betray the original trauma? What is more unethical, acting violently or failing to acknowledge the original traumatic event through reprisal? How does one define reprisal? Does it have to be violent? Can it not consist of "benevolent retaliation"?[111] Couldn't one perform incredible acts of kindness and pursue exquisite aesthetic pursuits in defiance of malevolence and evil? These are some of the questions that flow from the erupting volcano of Fanon's own writings. In addition to teaching us about the power of body-centered therapies, he brings to the forefront of our minds the ethical challenges associated with healing from trauma. In a day and age when the deleterious effects of racism still dominate communities, Fanon provides scientific and cultural trauma theorists a wellspring of research. Though his work might guide post-colonialists, it is paradoxical that it remains practically unknown among body-centered trauma theorists and therapists.

The Vietnam War, the Feminist Movement, and PTSD

Alongside the decolonization revolutions of the 1950s–1970s came anti-war movements. Significant additions and changes to the concept of trauma and posttraumatic conditions came as the Vietnam War unfolded. Veterans formed and fueled an anti-war coalition to voice their suffering publicly. Noteworthy was the creation of the organization Vietnam Veterans Against the War. This was an unprecedented move for veterans to organize against the very war in which they had engaged. Joined by psychiatrists (notably, Robert Jay Lifton and Chaim Shatan), anti-war veterans developed "rap groups."[112] No longer exclusively dependent upon the Veterans' Administration for help, they assumed greater control of their care, and by the mid-1970s rap groups met throughout the country. These groups prompted the creation of Operation Outreach within the Veterans' Administration, a program founded on self-help and peer-counseling. The anti-war movements, combined with the creation of rap groups and Operation Outreach, helped to raise collective awareness of the psychic trauma endured by veterans. Consequently, the American Psychiatric Association was moved to include in *The Diagnostic and Statistical Manual of Mental Disorders* (*DSM-III*) a new concept called "posttraumatic stress disorder" in 1980. According to the manual, PTSD occurs when a "person has experienced an event that is outside the range of usual experience and that would be markedly distressing to almost anyone, e.g. serious threat to one's life or physical integrity."[113]

The *DSM-III-R* stresses that (a) the event is persistent, relived through disturbing recollections, dreams, illusions, hallucinations, flashbacks, and psychological distress on anniversaries of the original traumatic event.[114] The manual also underscores (b) numbing, which appears as an inability to remember (psychogenic amnesia) and to feel emotions about the original traumatic event. Numbing also triggers a sense of detachment or alienation from others, among other symptoms. Contrary to numbing is (c) increased arousal manifesting itself not only in hypervigilance, but also in an inability to fall or stay asleep, to concentrate, to control one's responses in the form of startle responses and anger management. The formal diagnosis and the diagnostic criteria gave legitimacy to the idea that traumatic conditions could have serious psychological repercussions, such as psychosomatic and psychological conditions, following exposure to war and other traumatic events. Although PTSD had been assigned other terms since the birth of writing, although it had been described by researchers of survivors of the

Holocaust and victims of racism, it was thanks to veterans' groups and anti-war protestors that the condition was officially recognized.

Kindred to the Vietnam veterans' and anti-war protests, the women's liberation movement of the 1960s and 1970s also raised collective awareness about trauma. Once combat veterans had legitimized the notion of post-traumatic stress disorder, it became apparent that the psychological distress of rape and incest survivors mirrored the syndromes seen in veterans. Though their research focused on traumatic sexual experiences, feminists, sociologists, and psychiatrists such as Herman (who underscored the pre-valence of child sexual abuse) contributed a more general academic and holistic treatment for posttraumatic disorders, founded on safety, narratives, and connections. The topics of traumatic sexual and combat experiences will be amplified in Chapter 5 as we unfold more recent theories and treatments for survivors.

Cultural Trauma Studies and the Unknown of Traumatic Experiences

Before painting a landscape of more recent scientific developments, it is necessary first to sketch out the early development of cultural trauma studies. Akin to feminist and post-colonial studies, the field of cultural trauma studies was inspired by the veterans' anti-war and feminist movements. The protests were moved from the streets to university classrooms. Trauma was not just a topic reserved for clinics or rap groups. It was found in books of poetry, films, and cartoons. A historical narrative of cultural trauma studies tends to begin with the early contributions of literary theorists Geoffrey Hartman, Shoshana Felman, and Cathy Caruth. It then is followed by complementary and critical analyses by anthropologist Allan Young, historians Dominick LaCapra and Ruth Leys, sociologist Jeffrey Alexander, and those by post-colonialists. A discussion of these contributions will be provided in Chapter 4. It bears pointing out for now a deep irony about the field of cultural trauma studies. If it was inspired by the political movements, as made evident in its ethical claims, it paradoxically disappeared (in part) from the streets.[115] By repeatedly advancing the unknown, the unspeakable, the gaps, and impasses of trauma, some literary theorists have secluded themselves in an ivory tower, not to mention sent a dispiriting message to trauma survivors. These claims are supported by a trend among literary trauma theorists to distance themselves from readers by writing in an obscure style. Moreover, some literary theorists seem to have put aside their original ethical claims by failing to explore resilience, resistance, and growth. While they have fixated on trauma, scientists, clinicians, and other cultural theorists, have expanded their research beyond the topic of trauma since the beginning of the twenty-first century, as we shall discover in Chapter 5. This makes us question whether a new branch of research called "resilience studies" might develop.

Conclusions: Findings and Looking Forward to What Follows in this Book

Where do trauma and PTSD come from? This question has a double meaning. It could be asking about the origins of the terms "trauma" and "PTSD." Or it could be an inquiry into the nature of trauma and PTSD themselves. This chapter has attempted to ponder the origins of the terms. Nonetheless, by investigating their etymology, we have also explored the nature of trauma and PTSD. We underscored first that doctors and generals were already alluding to a type of PTSD during the French Revolutionary and Napoleonic Wars. This finding is important because it stresses how psychic suffering was acknowledged, even if it was not formally treated, in the early nineteenth century by medical and military personnel. Briquet however made up for this neglect in the middle of the nineteenth century by researching the nature of hysteria. In a truly revolutionary way, he stressed the relationship between poverty, child abuse, sexual abuse, and rape and hysteria. Simultaneously, Erichsen and Oppenheim focused more on physical and psychic trauma caused by industrial accidents. Erichsen held that the nature of psychic trauma was caused by physical wounds, whereas Oppenheim pointed to psychic causes with an accompanying loss of memory regarding movement.[116] The topic of the underlying causes of traumatic hysteria was not as important to Charcot, even though he devoted himself to studying how hysteria manifested itself through hypnosis. Charcot's two students Janet and Freud contributed to our understanding of the nature of trauma by developing such concepts as fixed ideas and dissociation, while their talk therapy was monumental in defining treatments.

Whereas Freud stressed the difficulty to treat veterans suffering from PTSD, Breton proposed exercises in art, whereas Kardiner offered an encyclopedia on traumatic experiences of combat soldiers from both world wars and endorsed psychoanalysis and other forms of dynamic psychotherapy to treat traumatic war neuroses. While research on World War II veterans might have remained limited, investigations into the psychological and physical harm endured by Holocaust survivors occurred in response to German compensation programs. Niederland, Eitinger, Chodoff, and Krystal developed new concepts (survival guilt, survival syndrome, and concentration camp syndrome) to refer to psychopathologies of survivors. This discussion led us to another form of collective and extreme trauma that has not figured prominently in trauma studies histories, as it should. Relying on Fanon's multidisciplinary work, we summarized the nature of trauma caused by colonialism and racism. This synthesis brought us to the anti-war and feminist movements and to the birth of the term PTSD in 1980. Still, just as the pacifist and women's liberation movements helped to promote the formal recognition of PTSD, research on Holocaust survivors and victims of violent prejudice also helped pave the way for the term's adoption. And finally, this formal recognition stirred scholars from the humanities to establish the field of cultural trauma studies in the 1980s, a topic to unfold in the next chapter.

This narrative of the history of trauma studies distinguishes itself from others by enlarging the field of investigation to include quasi-medical terms and related medical terms to trauma and PTSD. And most importantly, this narrative puts forward that the study of psychological trauma also depends upon the support of the humanities. This chapter has highlighted for instance the research of medical doctors who employed multidisciplinary perspectives (Briquet, Charcot, Janet, Chodoff, and Fanon, among others). This may very well be a healthy perspective to advance. This position seems to find resonance in Caruth's opinion that "psychoanalysis and medically oriented psychiatry, sociology, history, and even literature all seem to be called upon to explain, to cure, or to show why it is that we no longer simply explain or cure."[117] I divert from her in a fundamental way. I object to her use of the word "even." It is not that "even" literature seems to be called to explain ... but rather, *especially* literature.

Notes

1 Herman, *Trauma*, 9.
2 Ibid.
3 Ibid, 10.
4 Recall from Chapter 1 that I highlighted Herman's and Tallis's concern about the mental health field's current biological focus on psychological conditions.
5 Desgenettes, *Histoire*, 93–94.
6 Marbot, *Mémoires*, 352.
7 Ibid.
8 Chateaubriand, *Memoirs*, 296.
9 See Emmanuel Régis, "*Précis*," 25.
10 My synthesis of Briquet's research adds a new take on the history of trauma studies. After all, it was not until the late-nineteenth century and the ideals of the Third Republic that interest in hysteria emerged, according to the most prominent traumatologist Judith Herman. See Herman, *Trauma*, 9.
11 In his *Diseases of Women* (*Maladies des femmes*), Hippocrates (460–375 BCE) refers to treatments for women suffering from "hysteria" (*hystérie*) (par. 151) and "hysterical suffocation" (*suffocation hystérique*) (par. 200), which refers to an inability to talk because of psychic suffering. Hippocrates, *Maladies des femmes*.
12 Briquet, *Traité*, 11.
13 Briquet devotes an entire chapter section ("*Influence du sexe*") on hysteria in men and provides examples of men and boys suffering from hysteria throughout his text. See Briquet, *Traité*, 528–530.
14 See Oppenheim, *Shattered*.
15 Briquet, *Traité*, 3.
16 Ibid., 3–4.
17 Ibid., 9–11.
18 Ibid., 108–109.
19 Ibid., 105; one might even say that Briquet's emphasis on the relationship between poverty and hysteria stands in sharp contrast with the current

DSM-5's near neglect to address the topic of a relationship between poverty and trauma, a topic to be discussed later in this chapter.

20 See Briquet, *Traité*, 184 (child abuse); 171 (rape); 171 (sexual abuse).
21 Though Herman does mention Briquet in her *Trauma and Recovery*, she fails to mention his significant contributions to the field of trauma studies. In fact, she refers to Jean-Martin Charcot as "The patriarch of the study of hysteria." Herman, *Trauma*, 10.
22 Mendes Da Costa, *Medical*, loc. 5165.
23 Ibid., loc. 5140.
24 Ibid., loc. 5157.
25 Thomas Jefferson University, "Jacob Da Mendes"; see also NCBI, "Neuro-circulatory asthenia."
26 In his letter to the *British Medical Journal* dated December 15, 1866, Erichsen underscores that it is not so much that the gravity of railway accidents was unprecedented but rather the frequency of grave railroad accidents. Erichsen, "Mr. Erichsen's," 679.
27 Erichsen, *Concussion*, 158–159.
28 See Erichsen, "Mr. Erichsen's," 678–679.
29 Erichsen, *Railway*, 93.
30 Ibid., 92.
31 See ibid., 93.
32 See Holdorff and Dening, "Fight," 466.
33 See Färber, "Hermann," 1102.
34 Holdorff and Dening, "Fight," 466.
35 Ibid.
36 Ibid.
37 Ibid.
38 As far as Charcot's conviction that men suffered from hysteria is concerned, see Charcot, *Salpêtrière*, locs. 32 and 46; concerning these three principal symptoms, consult Charcot, *Divers*, 403–404.
39 Herman, *Trauma*, 11.
40 Pierre Janet provides us with convincing proof of his dedication to his patients in his *Etat mental des hystériques* (1892) by writing about the process of listening to and recording in detail the remarks of his students. See Janet, *Etat*, 3.
41 See Charcot and Richer, *Démoniaques*, v, my translation; the original expression is: "*une perversion de l'âme*."
42 Ibid., loc. 279.
43 See Charcot, *Foi*.
44 See Janet, *Névroses*, 117, 175, and 184, respectively.
45 See Ibid., 345. The summary of Janet's three main contributions stems from a summative statement that reads: "*L'hystérie devient alors une forme de dépression mentale caractérisée par le rétrécissement du champ de la conscience personnelle et par la tendance à la dissociation et à l'émancipation des systèmes d'idées.*"
46 See Ibid., 327. Summary of material; the original reads: "*j'ai montré dans beaucoup d'observations détaillées que l'hystérie était souvent une maladie déterminée par des idées fixes. Il y a de ces sortes d'idées fixes dans les somnambulismes et dans les fugues.*"
47 Ibid., 8. Summary of material; the original reads: "*Dans d'autres cas de ce genre, les idées fixes porteront sur des faits tout à fait imaginaires comme on peut le voir chez les sujets qui se figurent être en Enfer, au milieu des démons ou qui se croient transportés dans le Ciel, ou qui jouent comme Louise Lateau la scène de la crucifixion.*"

48 Consult ibid., 328. Summary of material; the original reads: "*premier caractère de l'influence des idées sur le développement de la maladie. Moebius, Strumpell, Forel, répétaient comme Charcot: 'On peut considérer comme hystériques toutes les modifications maladives du corps qui sont causées par des representation'.*"

49 Janet, *Major*, 324.

50 Concerning the heated debate about the issues of fixed ideas, memory, dissociation, and trauma, see McNally, "Debunking," 817–822 and Krystal and Krystal, *Integration*, 220.

51 Breuer and Freud, *Studies*, Foreword.

52 Freud, *Introductory*, 186.

53 Ibid.

54 Ibid.

55 Ibid., 185.

56 This more pessimistic view of curing traumatic neuroses corresponds to Freud's overall pessimistic view of humanity. See especially chap. 5 of his *Civilization and Its Discontents*.

57 Freud, *Interpretation*, 367.

58 Horney, *Inner*, 19.

59 Herman, *Trauma*, 13–14.

60 Forsyth, "Functional," 1401.

61 Ibid.

62 See Régis's "*Précis*," 25–26. Summary of material; the original reads: "*Morel a été jusqu'à dire que les Révolutions, en fin de compte, guérissaient plus de nerveux et de déséquilibrés qu'elles n'en produisaient.*"

63 This material is gleaned from an article by Henri Wallon in "Lésions," 69–91.

64 See G. Haury's untranslated, *Les Anormaux*, chap. 7.

65 See LaLonde, *Paris*, 132–133.

66 See Leys, "Death," 46.

67 Kardiner and Spiegel, "War," 1.

68 Kardiner in van der Kolk, *Body*, 11.

69 Kardiner, *Traumatic*, 130–131.

70 Leys, *Trauma*, chap. 6.

71 Ibid., Introduction.

72 See Chodoff, "Holocaust," 153.

73 Krystal and Krystal, *Integration*, 220.

74 Niederland, "Psychiatric," 469.

75 Ibid.

76 Ibid., 470.

77 Ibid., 471.

78 Ibid., 459.

79 Stahnisch, "Niederland," 2187.

80 Niederland, "Psychiatric," 468.

81 Ibid.

82 Eitinger, *Concentration*, 180.

83 According to Eitinger (ibid., 25), the term "concentration camp syndrome" was employed already in 1954 by Hermann and Thygesen.

84 Ibid., 74; there are caveats to this finding. Premorbid deviations appear to play a role in the development and upkeep of psychoses (ibid., 115).

85 Ibid., 184.

86 Ibid., 96.

87 Ibid., 54.

88 Chelouche, "Leo Eitinger," 210.

89 Chodoff, "Holocaust," 153.

90 Chodoff, "Nazi," 30–31.
91 Eitinger makes the claim that Chodoff did not provide proper quantitative data. He writes: "Chodoff's analysis is very thorough, but the material is too small and what is more, too heterogeneous ... to be able to reach any general conclusions from it." Eitinger, *Concentration*, 29.
92 Chodoff, "Nazi," 36.
93 Krystal and Krystal, *Integration*, xi.
94 See ibid., 252–256.
95 Ibid., 220.
96 Ibid.
97 Harel et al., "Effects," 924.
98 Barel et al., "Surviving," 694.
99 See Cyrulnik, *Resilience*, chap. 3.
100 If Herman refers to the political movements associated with the traumatic phenomena of hysteria at the end of nineteenth-century France and the political movements addressing the traumatic experiences of veterans and women at the end of the twentieth century, I contend that the decolonization movements sought to publicize the traumatic conditions of colonialism, slavery, and racism.
101 Herman, *Trauma*, 9.
102 Fanon employs the term "psychic trauma" in his *Black Skin, White Masks*, 122.
103 To illustrate just how much Fanon's research on traumatic experiences associated with colonialism, slavery, and racism has been ignored, consider that neither Herman, Leys, nor Caruth discuss Fanon in their books on trauma.
104 Fanon, *Black*, 122.
105 Ibid., 178.
106 Albert Memmi describes the colonizer and colonized in these terms: "One is disfigured into an oppressor, a partial, unpatriotic and treacherous being, worrying only about his privileges and their defense; the other, into an oppressed creature, whose development is broken and who is compromised by his defeat." Memmi, *Colonizer*, 89.
107 Fanon, *Toward*, 171.
108 Fanon, *Wretched*, 33.
109 Ibid., 51.
110 Ibid., 176.
111 We shall elaborate further on the idea of "benevolent retaliation" in Chapter 9.
112 Lifton, *Witness*, 185.
113 American Psychiatric Association, *DSM-III-R*, 250.
114 This summative information is gleaned from the *DSM-III-R*, 247–250.
115 Geoffrey Hartmann makes claims about the ethical nature of literary trauma studies by writing: "In addition, both in literary studies and in the field of public health a new awareness arises which is ethical as well as clinical. There is more listening, more hearing of words within words, and a greater openness to testimony." Hartman, "Traumatic," 541.
116 It is interesting to note that the word "trauma" (with the psychological connotation) referred to railroad accidents. Why didn't physicians, such as Erichsen, rely on the term hysteria? It is obviously quite possible that sexism played a role in the birth of the term.
117 Caruth, *Trauma*, 4.

Part II
A Gallery of Trauma Studies

3 Landscapes of Contemporary Scientific Trauma Theories

To understand the contemporary landscape of scientific trauma theories, it is instructive to contemplate first artistic landscapes. While Neo-classicists in the nineteenth century painted idyllic landscapes from mental images inside workshops, the impressionists and post-impressionists went outside (*en plein air*) in the light of the day to paint the feeling of nature. They depicted landscapes from open fields, ocean shores, mountain tops, and city streets. Emotional reactions to fleeting moments in nature, made ephemeral by the moving sun, were captured with wild brush strokes and vivid colors. Conversely for abstract artists of the twentieth century, landscapes no longer mirrored recognizable geographical locations. Their canvases reflected instead the geography of their minds. As far as contemporary land artists are concerned, they work not only outside but also alongside Mother Nature. Helping to form a landscape from stones, pebbles, rocks, branches, bushes, and trees, she serves as the artist's co-creator.

If artistic landscapes, seascapes, skyscapes, and urbanscapes have served as a mirror of artists' relationships with natural settings, what do contemporary landscapes of scientific trauma theories reveal about our understanding of trauma and traumatism? Have traumatologists painted landscapes from workshops and/or *en plein air*, as it were? Are their theories abstract or more in tune with the lived experiences of the traumatized? Do they center on the workings of the brain or the cultural conditions that cause traumatic experiences?

As argued in the previous two chapters, the concepts of trauma and traumatism developed thanks to not only scientific research and to political movements (as Judith Herman contends), but also contributions from writers and clinicians who engaged in interdisciplinary research from the arts and social sciences. Before there were scientific trauma theories, there were stories and literature (Ovid, Apuleius, de las Casas, and Montaigne) about trauma and posttraumatic conditions, including states that resembled PTSD. And before doctors coined the term "trauma" to refer to psychic suffering due to accidents, Enlightenment philosophers and Romantic authors paved the way for physicians and scientists to acknowledge mental pain caused by both physical injuries and psychological turmoil, such as fear.

DOI: 10.4324/9781003284642-6

Furthermore, physicians from Pierre Briquet to Jean-Martin Charcot, Pierre Janet, Paul Chodoff, and Frantz Fanon built their trauma theories and practices on the social sciences and the arts.

Both the interventions of political movements and transdisciplinary perspectives have helped to bring the topic of trauma into wider focus. No longer was trauma seen as simply a result of accidents as it was during the industrial revolution. No longer was it simply a question of hysterical women with defective wombs as believed in the nineteenth century. Nor was it about men who lacked moral courage as contended during the world wars of the last century. Activists, trauma survivors, and researchers have made their voices heard, and three clear messages have resonated from megaphones: A traumatic event can damage both the psyche and body; nightmares and haunting memories can make that event seem eternal; and trauma is a lived experience for great swaths of people. Whether for Holocaust survivors, Vietnam veterans, minorities living in abject poverty, the colonized, or sexually assaulted women, a pandemic of trauma has plagued communities far and wide.[1] Humanity has been sailing through hurricane waters; many hands have been needed to steer the ship to calmer waters.

The sciences and the humanities took hold of the helm at the end of the twentieth century. The fields of psychiatry, neurology, psychoanalysis, psychology, sociology, anthropology, art, history, literature, literary theory, and cultural theory joined forces and contributed new notions of trauma and posttraumatic conditions. In this chapter, we paint a landscape of contemporary scientific contributions, focusing on the topics of trauma and PTSD found in the *Diagnostic and Statistical Manual of Mental Disorders* (*DSM*); new definitions, such as C-PTSD and Developmental Trauma; recent clinical and survey findings on war trauma; and neuroscience and neuroimages of traumatized brains. (To paint the most accurate landscape as possible, meta-analysis and systematic-review articles have been consulted when available.) Though there have been notable advances in scientific trauma theories, there have also been several shortcomings, including a tendency to maintain a myopic vision of what constitutes a traumatic experience. At the same time, a noteworthy conclusion based on more recent scientific discoveries is the complexity of traumatic experiences. The more clinicians probe survivors with surveys and neurologists with scans, the more apparent is the wide variety of brain reactions and human behaviors in response to trauma.

Trauma and PTSD in the *Diagnostic and Statistical Manual of Mental Disorders*

Recall that a chief contribution to the field of scientific trauma theories came in 1980 when the American Psychiatric Association's (APA) included posttraumatic stress disorder PTSD (309.89) in its third edition of *The Diagnostic and Statistical Manual of Mental Disorders-III* (*DSM-III*). This is however a knee-jerk historical narrative that demands nuances, which we will attempt to provide in this chapter. While the *DSM*'s classification (nosology) of PTSD might prove helpful to survivors, clinicians, and the greater community, the manual's related entries and the term PTSD itself is short-sighted and moreover, limits our view of posttraumatic conditions.

Expansive Views of Trauma in the DSM

At first glance, the landscape of PTSD in the APA's *DSM* seems expansive and thus might help clinicians to treat what they used to overlook. The *DSM-III-R* (1987) defines trauma as "an experience outside the range of usual human experience that would be markedly distressing to almost anyone."[2] The manual emphasizes that the traumatic event is reexperienced in the mind through persistent and disturbing memories and dreams. Conversely, the survivor may avoid feelings or thoughts associated with the traumatic event and may even suffer from psychogenic amnesia. Besides this attempt to avoid memories, survivors may enter an arousal state, struggling for example to sleep or concentrate.

This official description of PTSD has altered our understanding of trauma and its sequelae. It provided a conceptual framework to understand psychic, somatic, and psycho-somatic aftereffects of horrific events. It underscored that the etiology of the traumatic event is not caused by an inherent individual weakness but rather by the original event itself. It also highlighted that the term applies to not only veterans but also abused children, battered women, rape survivors, and other victims of other human-induced atrocities and natural disasters. Perhaps most importantly, the manual contributed "a model for correcting the decontextualized aspects of today's psychiatric nomenclature."[3] How did the *DSM-III* and eventually the revised *DSM-III-R* contextualize the experience of PTSD? It stressed that disorders can be the result of societies and interpersonal relationships, a much welcomed conclusion seeing that Briquet had pointed this out in the mid-nineteenth century.[4] The manual states explicitly that PTSD "is apparently more severe and longer lasting when the stressor is of human design."[5] It calls attention moreover to the "physiologic reactivity" prevalent in PTSD.[6] The residue of trauma lives on in the body like ripples in space and time after the collision of celestial bodies. This societal and bodily contextualization was most significant for it prodded clinicians to treat patients more holistically, in theory.

To contextualize further the experiences of PTSD, the *DSM IV* (1994) added new diagnostic criteria to address the symptoms observed in young children. The *DSM-5* (2013) stretched the definition and diagnostic criteria even more. The newest edition proposes a menu of symptoms and symptom clusters in related disorders.[7] To accentuate the interconnected nature of PTSD with other mental disorders, it categorizes PTSD as a "Trauma and Stressor-Related Disorder," rather than an anxiety disorder as indicated in the *DSM-III-R* and *DSM-IV*. PTSD is thus considered akin to other disorders, such as reactive attachment disorder, disinhibited social engagement disorder, acute stress disorder, and adjustment disorder; these are closely related to anxiety disorders, obsessive-compulsive disorders, and especially dissociative disorders.[8] Dissociation includes depersonalization, which refers to feeling detached from one's body,[9] as if one were watching oneself appear on the stage of life from a theater seat. Derealization, another form of dissociation, refers to experiences that seem dreamlike, unreal, or distorted. These additions and others pertaining to stressor criteria indicate that the *DSM-5* has sought to emphasize that "clinical presentation of PTSD varies."[10] Between posttraumatic affects and behavior such as grief, despair, insomnia, paranoia, panic or terror and/or mechanisms to shun situations in which the traumatic event might come to life again in the mind, the *DSM-5* makes clear the prevalence, complexity, and inter-related nature of trauma and stressor-related disorders.

Just as the APA expanded the reach of the *DSM-5* by highlighting the depth and breadth of mental disorders, it also internationalized the manual. Seeking to "harmonize" the newer edition with the World Health Organization's International Classification of Disorders (ICD), it lays out that psychic disturbances are defined by cultural, social, and familial norms. Conditions related to PTSD develop in individuals from different cultural backgrounds and manifest themselves in different ways. The newest edition for instance has organized culturally distinctive norms into three categories. First, a "cultural syndrome" refers to relatively prevalent symptoms in specific cultures. The syndrome may not be perceived as pathological inside the culture but may very well appear to be from the outside. *Ataque de nervios* ("nerve attack" in Spanish); *shenjing shuairuo* ("weakness of the nervous system" in Mandarin Chinese); and *khyâl cap* ("wind attacks" in Cambodian) are included as culturally specific syndromes that are kindred to PTSD.[11] Second, a "cultural idiom of distress" is a term, expression, or way of speaking about suffering among individuals from a common culture, religion, or ethnicity. *Kufungisisa* ("thinking too much" in Shona of Zimbabwe) is an illustration of an idiom of distress and refers to feeling overwhelmed with distressing thoughts and worries and again mirrors the condition of PTSD.[12] Third, a "cultural explanation or perceived cause" is a label evoking the origin of a symptom, pathology, or mental distress. *Maladi moun* ("humanly caused illness" or "sent sickness" in Haitian Creole) is an illness caused by another person who might feel jealous or envious of another.[13] The *DSM-5* does not claim that *maladi moun* is PTSD. Still, those who believe that a malicious person has caused their mental stress often appear schizophrenic with paranoid features, a symptom prevalent among individuals suffering from PTSD.[14] Whether it is the explicit message that psychic disturbances are defined by cultural, social, and familial norms or whether it is the implicit message transmitted by the addition of the terms *Ataque de nervios, kufungisisa*, or *maladi moun*, the *DSM-5* has internationalized its perspective, thus emphasizing the breadth and depth of mental disorders.

Myopic Views of Trauma in the DSM

Though the *DSM-5* accentuates a variety of symptoms and though it includes culturally specific concepts aimed to help patients, clinicians, and the greater community, the landscape of PTSD in the manual remains constricted. Three issues leave us with this impression. First, the manual does not include in its definition of trauma "ordinary" stressors, such as serious illnesses or chronic forms of trauma experienced by adults and children. Malnutrition and head injury are singled out as possible traumatic experiences because they can damage the central nervous system. However, it is incomprehensible that pandemics are not included as a stressor in the *DSM-5*. Even more difficult to comprehend is that psychic turmoil associated with the COVID-19 pandemic does not meet the criteria for a diagnosis of PTSD.[15] The explosion of posttraumatic conditions related to the pandemic (from deleterious health effects for the sick to the constant exposure to death and suffering among health-care workers) might very well provoke changes, once again, to definitions and terms of posttraumatic conditions in the *DSM-5*, including PTSD.

Secondly, the symptoms, terms, and concepts included in the *DSM-5* from other cultures do not necessarily render the manual more inclusive. The inclusion of foreign terms points to idiosyncrasies that appear in the form of questions. What about other cultural elements that cannot be translated into Western mental disorders? Aren't they relevant precisely because they present a different and hard-to-grasp perspective? Does one have to turn to the World Health Organization's *ICD-11* (2018) for further elucidation? Unlike the *DSM*'s focus on classifications of diagnoses, the *ICD-11* centers on "clinical utility with reduction of number of diagnoses."[16] Indeed, the *ICD* in general offers less of a laundry list of symptom criteria, including those culturally specific. Rather than provide a separate category or glossary of non-Western expressions, the international manual underlines the dearth of quantitative research that would allow for these terms to be added to it. Clinicians are advised therefore to use the "nearest equivalent code."[17] This leads us back to the issue of different cultural elements that remain below Western clinicians' radar screen. The *ICD* reminds readers repeatedly about how diagnoses are difficult to make when cultural differences are considered. Some diagnoses may mean very little for people from certain cultures or countries, whereas for many cultures certain symptoms are twice as common in women than men.[18] The *ICD* thus emphasizes that cultural issues should be factored into diagnoses; but it does not offer specific references to other cultures. This intimates not only that an inclusion of such "foreign" terms would go well beyond the scope of the *ICD* but also that anthropologists, artists, and writers might be just as prepared to nuance these issues, albeit from a different perspective and different medium.

Third, the landscape of PTSD in the *DSM* appears even more constricted if one considers its narrow socio-economic lens. The *DSM-5* has categorized chronic emotional abuse under the heading "Other Conditions that May Be a Focus of Clinical Attention." That chronic psychological abuse should be considered traumatic is unequivocal for many psychiatrists. According to a 2015 survey headed by Michele Black et al. at the Center for Disease Control and Prevention (CDC), more than 1 in 5 (21.3%) American women had been the victims of or an attempted rape in their lifetime, while more than a third (37%) had experienced unwanted sexual contact.[19] These figures obviously highlight the prevalence of sexual assault. The CDC's summary report emphasizes that sexual assault leads to chronic psychological and physical adverse conditions. The report also points out that violent experiences of a child or adolescent is a risk factor for subsequent victimization as an adult. Recent surveys have revealed in fact a startling landscape feature of trauma. According to the CDC, 61% of adults have experienced at least one ACE (Adverse Childhood Experience).[20] This includes emotional and physical neglect; sexual and physical abuse; and dysfunctional family settings, such as having parents who were divorced or in prison or suffered from mental illnesses. Women and ethnic and racial minorities are at greater risk for ACEs, whereas exposure to these adverse experiences leads to greater risk of health problems in adult life.[21]

The manual adds that lower socio-economic status, education deficiencies, childhood adversity (i.e., economic deprivation), and minority racial/ethnic status are "risk and prognostic factors" of PTSD.[22] If this is the case, then why isn't there greater attention devoted to descriptions of symptoms and conditions of psychic suffering among those from economically and socially disadvantaged backgrounds and for racial and ethnic minorities? The rubric "Economic Problems" instead includes a simple list of conditions, such as "low income," that disappears into the ether. Besides being unhelpful, this rings of insensitivity about the economic problems faced by large swaths of people nationally and internationally. Can abject poverty not be traumatic, too? This rhetorical question is supported by research: Among veterans who have experienced homelessness, 14.1% reported that it was their "worst" traumatic event, and was associated with five-fold greater odds of current PTSD.[23] Or perhaps the experience of economic depravity is so foreign to the chairs of the APA's diagnostic working groups and task force members who oversaw the development of the *DSM-5* that it would have been insensitive on their part to write about these issues. The absence of discussions about the relationship between PTSD and the experiences of the poor and minority groups translates into a narrow snapshot of the condition. This narrow interpretation is what psychiatrist Arthur Kleinman cautioned against in his *Illness Narratives* (1986): "the science of pain must include social science interpretations together with biomedical explanations."[24]

Kleinman's comment serves as an excellent segue into the third limited feature of the *DSM*'s landscape of PTSD. It focuses on a disorder. This may seem like a tautology. It goes without saying that the concept of PTSD should center on a disorder; that is what it is. Be that as it may, the long list of syndromes and diagnostic criteria listed in the *DSM-5*'s entries brings to mind a prescient point made by psychiatrist Bessel van der Kolk. Referring to how his colleagues at a children's hospital tended to highlight patients' "conduct disorder," "oppositional disorder," and "bipolar disorder,"[25] he felt that they were missing the forest for the trees, as it were. His colleagues were disregarding patients' traumatic experiences along with their emotional suffering. This led him to wonder: "Was their underlying trauma being obscured by this blizzard of diagnoses?"[26] In short, the automatic adoption of *DSM* diagnoses could translate into an abstract process and blind clinicians to their patients' complex and subtle realities of traumatic experiences.

These shortcomings of the concept of PTSD accentuate the complexity of posttraumatic conditions. The phenomenon of engendering complexity finds resonance in the history of the first Natural History Museums formed in Europe in the eighteenth century. Early natural scientists wore three hats: empirical scientist, field investigator, and museum curator. They would collect artifacts from nature to organize the wonders of the natural world. Their project became an endless pursuit. The more they chipped away at earth's strata, the deeper they plunged into the ocean's depths, and the higher they climbed mountain tops, the more they chanced upon novel findings that pushed the limits of their organizational schemes. While scientific trauma theorists share a drive for organization with curator-scientists, some seem to be removed, like Neo-Classical artists, from the very landscape they are trying to paint. The diagnosis is in the foreground, where actual traumatic experiences remain in a cloud (*sfumato*) in the background.

A Balanced View of Trauma Landscapes in the DSM

Even if the *DSM-5* may not include seascapes, skyscapes, and urbanscapes from other continents and neighborhoods on the other side of the tracks, the newest edition emphasizes one very important issue regarding posttraumatic disorders: the boundaries between psychopathology and normalcy vary across cultures. Different cultural, social, and familial settings have different thresh-holds of tolerance for trauma. Symptoms after a traumatic experience may be seen as pathological for one culture and yet a creative strength for another. Consider this entry from the *DSM-5*: "Culture may provide coping strategies that enhance resilience in response to illness, or suggest help seeking and options for accessing health care of various types, including alternative and complementary health systems."[27] This statement points to a heightened degree of open-mindedness about coping mechanisms and thus serves as an invitation for researchers to investigate resilience strategies from other cultures.

One would expect clinicians to be flexible about new coping strategies regardless of their cultural origin. It is nevertheless undeniable that most trauma researchers hail from the West, and especially from Anglo-American cultures, and export rather than import theories and treatments. The deleterious effects of exportation of the American concept of PTSD have been documented by anthropologist Alex Argenti-Pillen. In her research on the trauma experienced by Sri Lankans during the civil war, she stresses that Western concepts of trauma and recovery could destabilize communities. Western post-trauma coaching mechanisms perturbed local strategies of healing "terrified hearts,"[28] including cleansing rituals and avoidance of direct speech. The fact that Sri Lankans use the expression "terrified hearts," while the West has employed the terms "traumatic neurosis," "trauma," "shell shock," "battle fatigue," "operational exhaustion," and "posttraumatic stress disorder"[29] reveals the acute differences in our understanding of trauma. Argenti-Pillen's findings should foster a sense of humility, nudging us to proceed with caution clinically and theoretically and to investigate alternative concepts and models that refashion our landscape of not only PTSD, but also of other posttraumatic conditions.

New Definitions: C-PTSD and Developmental Trauma

While PTSD is a very common psychiatric diagnosis, new terms have been developed in the last twenty years to refer to other traumatic experiences and posttraumatic conditions. Thanks to the efforts of psychiatrists, such as Herman and van der Kolk, chronic psychological abuse has been labeled "Complex PTSD" (C-PTSD). (Even if the *DSM-5* did not include C-PTSD, the *ICD-11* did make a distinction between the twin disorders C-PTSD and PTSD.) C-PTSD refers to repeated and prolonged traumas, most notably those experienced by women and children. (The condition is also known as "Disorders of Extreme Stress Not Otherwise Specified," or "DESNOS.") C-PTSD often involves the use of defensive mechanisms such as dissociation, which can lead to interpersonal challenges and emotional turmoil as well as typical PTSD symptoms.

Cognizant that other diagnostic criteria were necessary to refer to and treat children exposed to interpersonal violence and disruptive caregiving, van der Kolk put forward in 2005 the establishment of a "Developmental Trauma Disorder" diagnosis. He sums up his motivation for creating the term as follows:

> Whether or not they exhibit symptoms of PTSD, children who have developed in the context of ongoing danger, maltreatment, and inadequate caregiving systems are ill-served by the current diagnostic system, as it frequently leads to no diagnosis, multiple unrelated diagnoses, an

emphasis on behavioral control without recognition of interpersonal trauma and lack of safety in the etiology of symptoms, and a lack of attention to ameliorating the developmental disruptions that underlie the symptoms.[30]

At first glance, it appears ironic that van der Kolk introduces another diagnosis category ("Developmental Trauma Disorder"), while pointing an accusatory finger above at the current diagnostic system that "ill-serves" children. His criticism begs the question: Will another diagnostic tool really help traumatized children? In the same breath of his critical remark, he hints above at recovery methods. The expressions "etiology of symptoms," "developmental disruptions," and "underlie the symptoms" point to his north star argument. That is, they hint at his attempt to get at the bottom of posttraumatic conditions. Literally. As we shall discover in Chapter 5, van der Kolk's research on trauma recovery focuses on bottom-up therapies. It centers on the body that harbors the traumatic experience in its viscera. While van der Kolk has contributed to the landscape of trauma theories by developing and publicizing the term "Developmental Trauma Disorder," he has also helped steer the conversation toward the body. The landscape has shifted to a certain degree from an emphasis on theoretical work—on diagnoses gleaned from the *DSM*—to one grounded in clinical work involving the body.

New Clinical and Survey Findings on War Trauma

Barring Abram Kardiner's investigations on veterans from the two world wars of the twentieth century and those from the psycho-historian, psychiatrist, and political activist Robert J. Lifton on Vietnam veterans, there was not extensive research on posttraumatic conditions among veterans until the wars of Iraq and Afghanistan.[31] Van der Kolk makes this historical reality woefully clear by confessing that his psychiatric training had not prepared him to address the issues he had witnessed in former combat soldiers. He confesses: "I went down to the medical library to look for books on war neurosis, shell shock, battle fatigue, or any other term or diagnosis ... To my surprise the library at the VA didn't have a single book about any of these conditions."[32]

A 2015 meta-analysis found that 23% of combat soldiers from the Iraq and Afghan wars suffered from combat-related PTSD.[33] A systematic review of the same issue revealed that only 7.5% of veterans from these conflicts suffered from PTSD.[34] More alarming is the veteran suicide rate: it has outpaced at times the annual number of soldiers killed in combat during the wars.[35] "Even among the men who had experienced the most extreme combat, however, the majority of those who developed PTSD had been able to recover over time."[36] And this was the case regardless of treatment or not.

These findings lead Herman to ponder what factors might contribute to or impede recovery. Three principal factors seem to determine veterans' posttraumatic conditions: Soldiers' childhood experiences, their human connections during combat, and their personal involvement in war crimes. "Not surprisingly," she concludes, "those who had the greatest advantages in maturity, education, and social support proved the most resilient."[37] Conversely, those exposed to childhood adversity were more apt to be psychologically scarred by combat. Childhood abuse was in fact a determining factor leading to chronic PTSD. "Young age upon entering the military, low educational level, having a family member with drug or alcohol problems, and having a family member in prison were additional prewar 'risk factors' that predicted long-term difficulties after returning from the war."[38] Beyond the issue of childhood adversity, emotional support among soldiers contributed to improved posttraumatic experiences.

Psychiatrists John Walker and James Nash discovered in their research of Vietnam veterans that many of their patients did not show marked improvement in individual psychotherapy, namely cognitive therapies or psychoanalytically oriented psychotherapy.[39] Yet, they did fare well in group therapy where they felt a greater sense of camaraderie. In short, "Rage, psychic numbing, alienation, and the inability to love and trust others are corrected as the patient finds meaning in life's experiences through group work."[40] More recently, Elizabeth Goetter et al. stress in their systematic review (2015) of investigations on Iraq and Afghan War veterans suffering from PTSD contradictory findings. They found that therapy dropout rates in individual studies varied considerably (5.0% to 78.2%) and added that, "The dropout rate differed marginally by … treatment format (group treatment had higher dropout rates than individual treatment)."[41] Though it may remain ambiguous whether group or individual therapy has a higher dropout rate, what is unambiguous is the need to curb therapy dropout.[42] Hence the reason Goetter and her team conclude that novel strategies are needed to improve treatment retention. Committing war crimes was a third predictor of traumatic stress. Herman refers to soldiers who commit war crimes as "harmers" and adds that "almost two-thirds (63 percent) developed PTSD, compared with 15 percent of the men who had never harmed noncombatants."[43] Researchers concluded that the severity of combat experiences determined most of all whether a soldier developed symptoms of PTSD.[44]

Military Sexual Trauma (MST) is another posttraumatic condition to have been added to the trauma landscape in the last twenty years. The Veteran's Administration is now mandated to screen for sexual trauma, which includes sexual harassment, assault, and rape and to provide services to military victims. Herman reports in the 2015 Epilogue to her *Trauma and Recovery* that 22 percent of female veterans and one percent of male veterans who responded to screening questions disclosed an MST experience.[45] These disturbing figures correspond to those reported by the general population. These data prompt Herman to conclude: "Though the public still tends to think of trauma mainly in connection with the armed services, in fact, most interpersonal violence occurs in civilian life, most victims are women and children, and most perpetrators are men well known to their victims."[46] This conclusion may very well provoke scientists and clinicians to focus their clinical and research attention on treatments for survivors of interpersonal traumatic experiences.

In 1989, van der Kolk and psychologist Charles Ducey led an investigation related to one of the core issues of this book: creativity in posttraumatic conditions and treatments. The researchers administered the Rorschach test to a group of veterans suffering from nightmares and PTSD. The test consists of showing a series of cards of ink-blot images to stir interpretations. The researchers discovered that when veterans were shown cards containing colors, they would relive traumatic experiences. Rather than interpreting odd shapes on cards as butterflies, the veterans reacted for example in the following manner: "These are the bowels of my friend Jim after a mortar shell ripped him open ..."[47] Though most of the veterans were disturbed when viewing the cards, others remained frozen in silence. The cards represented nothing, save for ink spilled on paper. And yet, the typical human reaction to ambiguity is to search for meaning through creative interpretations. This prompted the researchers to conclude, "We learned from these Rorschach tests that traumatized people have a tendency to superimpose their trauma on everything around them and have trouble deciphering whatever is going on around them."[48] Whether it was reading dismembered body parts or finding nothing, the interpretations were extreme and reflected the traumatic experiences that reverberated in the mind. From the study, van der Kolk and Ducey also concluded that traumatic experiences alter the imagination. Both groups lost their ability to let their minds engage in imaginative play.[49] Veterans who saw nothing more than an ink blot and those who were trapped in the gory images of the past had lost the ability to engage in imaginative exercises. This is a meaningful observation, as without imagination, one is stuck in a present colored by traumatic memories and feelings of the past. The research project also revealed that trauma survivors view the world differently from others. "A stern schoolteacher may be an intimidating presence to an average kid," explains van der Kolk, "but for a child whose stepfather beats him up, she may represent a torturer and precipitate a rage attack or a terrified cowering in the corner."[50] In other words, for the traumatized, there is a backstory that appears relentlessly as the front story. The ominous background looms large in the landscape while the foreground of the present fades into a cloud.

Though these findings provide a window into traumatized psyches, van der Kolk and Ducey's study seems to have methodological shortcomings. The sample size was small, and the control group was small too. The main arguments advanced (that traumatized veterans were either stuck in a vortex of tormenting memories or in a blackhole of emptiness and that they struggled consequently to use their imagination) spur nonetheless an important debate, especially for this book's content, about creativity among the traumatized.

Neuroscience and Neuroimages of Traumatized Brains

Pablo Picasso's *Guernica* is one of the most emotionally wrenching artistic landscapes. It depicts the 1937 Nazi bombing of the Basque city Guernica, a Republican stronghold, during the Spanish Civil War. Disfigured faces. Contorted bodies. Cut-off limbs. Gaping mouths wailing in pain. The trauma of war is stamped on figures who struggle to stay alive in shades of black and white. If ever there was a way to experience the feeling of trauma without literally experiencing it, Picasso has accomplished this task in *Guernica*, provided the viewer contemplates it profoundly. The painting conveys the physical sensation of agony and the mental turmoil of suffering, prompting viewers to enter the mind and body of the traumatized. The eternal feeling of trauma in the form of PTSD is encapsulated eternally in Picasso's mural.

Although PTSD is considered mostly a psychological phenomenon—and thus perhaps more challenging to study and treat quantitatively than a physical illness—research from the last twenty years has pulled back the curtain on the condition's biological features. Unlike other psychiatric disorders, the immediate causes of PTSD often seem more immediate and hence straightforward. This fact explains in part why biological investigations of the disorder have progressed. Neuroimaging has provided brain maps of PTSD survivors. Positron emission tomography (PET) and functional magnetic resonance imaging (fMRI) scans reveal common biomarkers, which are anatomical, biochemical, and physiological features. Even if scientists have written extensively on these biomarkers, a landscape of trauma theories in this book would be incomplete without a sketch of the principal scientific findings. Such a sketch, besides, should prove useful when considering the topics of memory and different therapies for healing, explored in later chapters.

Healthy Emotional Cerebral Responses to Trauma

There appears to be two trends in brain-imaging research on trauma survivors. Investigators either strive to delineate common brain abnormalities and/or they caution against making sweeping generalizations about these abnormalities. Van der Kolk paints a coherent picture of the main cerebral abnormalities of PTSD patients. He employs metaphors to explain these complex topics: The brain is controlled by a smoke detector and a watch tower. He starts out by describing how healthy emotional reactions unfold in the space between our ears. The smoke-detector amygdala, almond-shaped nuclei in the commonly shared mammalian limbic zone, acts as the smoke detector for danger and fear. While it does not function alone, it is critical for the feeling of fear and the related expressions, such as freezing. The amygdala works automatically and quickly with the thalamus (a relay station of information from the senses), the hippocampus (a feedback loop of information about threats and past experiences), and the prefrontal cortex (PFC).[51] Depending upon the information obtained from the thalamus, hippocampus, and PFC, the amygdala then messages the hypothalamus to release stress hormones (such as cortisol and adrenaline) and the autonomic nervous system (ANS) to ready the brain and body for fight or flight.[52] Simultaneously, the prefrontal cerebral cortex (made up of the dorsolateral, dorsomedial, and ventromedial prefrontal cortices) serves as the watch tower. Located above our eyes in some of the most evolutionarily sophisticated parts of the brain, the PFC interprets experiences and feelings less rapidly and from a wider and more nuanced perspective. By considering more calmly and objectively our feelings, emotions, and thoughts, the watchtower of our brain can regulate the automatic responses of the limbic or emotional part of the brain. The PFC for example processes the "threat-related expectations" from the hippocampus.[53] It is important to stress that the brain's watch tower and the smoke detector normally work together to produce responses to lived and emotional experiences and are involved in healthy emotional function.[54]

Cerebral and Behavioral Abnormalities Caused by Trauma

Stress, heightened arousal, and trauma alter these relationships. For instance, "PTSD appears to be mediated by the dysfunction of a PFC-hippocampus-amygdala network."[55] Stressing that this *appears* to be the case, Nathaniel Harnett and his colleagues base their hypothesis on the following logic: The PFC–hippocampus–amygdala network controls learning and memory processes; these processes are perturbed in PTSD subjects; the network therefore must be faulty. When these connections are perturbed, the mind might be challenged to regulate emotional responses. Sufferers of PTSD tend to overreact to innocuous stimuli and/or struggle to edit their overreactions when they register a non-threatening situation. There seem to be several cerebral abnormalities in PTSD subjects that cause these heightened and fixed reactions.[56] First, the amygdala hyperfunctions, thus leading to more pronounced fear associations. Second, the ventromedial PFC remains in hypoactivity, therefore failing to regulate the amygdala's responses. Third, the dorsolateral and the dorsomedial PFC appear also to be altered by traumatic experiences. While both parts of the PFC aide in the creation and expression of learned fear responses, "the dorsolateral PFC activity is attenuated in PTSD patients during anticipation of emotional stimuli."[57] Conversely, the PTSD subject shows "heightened dorsomedial PFC activity during both fear acquisition and extinction recall."[58] This leads Harnett et al. to conjecture that the hyperactivity of the dorsomedial PFC might account for the production of more pronounced and fixed fear associations.

Of special interest in their research article is a caveat: The dorsolateral and the dorsomedial PFC do not react uniformly to traumatic experiences. Cerebral abnormalities vary according to PTSD phenotypes. "For example, functional connectivity from the dorsolateral PFC to the amygdala is greater in those with the dissociative subtype of PTSD than those with typical PTSD presentations."[59] The research of Andrew Nicholson et al. provides a foundation for this conclusion. Nicholson and his team argue that the amygdala and the prefrontal cortices assume different abnormal functions depending upon whether the PTSD subject suffers from dissociation. They describe these abnormal functions as "emotional undermodulation" vs. "emotional overmodulation."[60] Non-dissociative PTSD patients tend to experience emotional undermodulation.[61] This consists of reliving traumatic experiences with related hyperarousal. How does this occur? There is a decreased activity of the PFC in general, resulting in an uninhibited amygdala and in turn a hyperactive limbic system. Conversely, dissociative PTSD subjects tend to suffer from emotional overmodulation.[62] This is characterized by emotional detachment. How does this occur? The PFC (along with the anterior cingulate cortex (ACC)) overperforms, triggering an inhibition of the amygdala.

The point of this discussion is to emphasize that although brain scans do provide valuable empirical information about the deleterious consequences of trauma, neuroimaging evidence is defined by complexity. Employing scans to investigate the brain leads to one Pandora box after another. Complexity begets complexity as Harnett's and Nicholson's research implies, and thus the reason for caution when making generalizations about posttraumatic conditions, including the issue of traumatic memory.

There are several other cerebral abnormalities among PTSD subjects. Often their Broca's area (a part of the brain responsible for producing speech) is deactivated, while the visual cortex is activated.[63] An increased activity of the visual cortex can translate into a technicolor display of images, often appearing in the form of nightmares and flashbacks, whereas when the Broca's area fails to produce language, sufferers might be stuck in silence. These discoveries are helpful because they provide physical proof of what researchers have observed clinically in trauma survivors—some struggle to narrate their traumatic experiences and are tormented by graphic flashbacks and nightmares.

Areas of the brain necessary for the storage and integration of information, such as the hippocampus can also be deactivated. If this is the case, then "the imprints of traumatic experiences are organized not as coherent logical narratives but in fragmented sensory and emotional traces: images, sounds, and physical sensations," according to van der Kolk.[64] Roger Pitman and his colleagues' meta-analysis from 2012 echoes these findings. They point out that "Diminished volumes of hippocampus and anterior cingulate cortex represent the most frequently replicated neuroanatomic findings in patients with PTSD."[65] Philip Zoladz and David Diamond's meta-analysis paints however a different landscape of the hippocampus. Their findings underscore that many studies have indeed reported reduced hippocampal volume and function in PTSD, whereas other studies have not replicated these findings.[66] Zoladz and Diamond stress that even though the hippocampus "appears to be vulnerable to the pathological effects of stress, it is also involved in the formation of traumatic memories."[67] It is important to stress the ambiguity surrounding these results, for the issue of memory—defined in part by the hippocampus—is a contentious topic, especially in the field of cultural trauma studies.[68] This ambiguity leads Zoladz and Diamond to conclude that, "PTSD illustrates our inability to pigeonhole the hippocampus into a relatively simple classification scheme, unlike the prefrontal cortex, which is impaired, and the amygdala, which appears to thrive on intense stress."[69]

In short, parts of the quartet of the amygdala, thalamus, hypothalamus, and the hippocampus either overperform or underperform, while parts of the trio PFC-hippocampus-and amygdala either underperform or overperform, while still parts of the PFC either underperform or overperform, depending upon whether one has dissociative PTSD or not. These imbalances are not trivial. According to psychiatrist Daniel Siegal and psychologist Marion Solomon, "The capacity to modulate deeper emotional responses of the amygdala, to maintain social networks of support, and to find new 'meaning' from horrific events are each under the influence of prefrontal circuitry."[70] In other words, a highway of interactions between the prefrontal cortex, anterior cingulate cortex, and the subcortical amygdala seems to be biologically important, as it allows trauma survivors to find their way out of the impasse of the traumatic event(s).

Nobody can deny the importance of discoveries of PTSD biological markers to advance treatment methods, to combat skepticism about the disorder, and encourage its widespread acceptance as a clinical diagnosis. It behooves us to consider nevertheless that these discoveries involve human minds conditioned by cultural experiences and individual psychologies. Pitman and his team sum up the complexity of studying PTSD as:

> A number of biological abnormalities have been found statistically to discriminate PTSD from non-PTSD control groups in various studies; on this basis, they may loosely be regarded as biomarkers. However, none of them possesses the specificity and sensitivity that is necessary to be used as a stand-alone diagnostic test for PTSD.[71]

While this word of caution seems to be targeted at scientists and clinicians working with PTSD patients, it could also apply to cultural trauma theorists, including myself. Between the ambiguity and complexity of data and the subjective experiences of individuals, both scientists and especially cultural theorists are encouraged to go cautiously, but creatively, into the field of trauma studies that remains elusive.[72]

Conclusion: A Collage of Landscapes

What does this chapter's collage of scientific landscapes of trauma and posttraumatic conditions suggest about our understanding of these topics? Firstly, the information on PTSD in the *DSM* indicates that the disorder is viewed from both expansive and myopic perspectives. The inclusion of terms and concepts from "foreign" cultures and an emphasis on how the boundaries between psychopathology and normalcy vary across cultures produce a wide landscape. This seems to be a much-welcomed gesture towards tolerance of other cultures. Still, the content of the *DSM* has been exported along with Western products and cultural traditions throughout the globe, whereas imports of PTSD-like concepts from other cultures remain limited.[73] How does one reconcile this inconsistency? Perhaps, the limited addition of "foreign" terms and concepts is a token gesture of inclusivity. This interpretation is in line with the *DSM-5*'s rubric "Economic Problems" and sub-rubric "low income" that trail off into silence. The manual has yet to address the relationship between poverty, minority status, trauma, and PTSD. From this analysis of the *DSM*, we can conclude that trauma theorists have painted in large part landscapes from workshops: their theories center on the workings of the brain rather than on the cultural conditions that cause traumatic experiences leading to PTSD.

Despite or perhaps better yet, because of these limitations, others (such as Herman and van der Kolk) have contributed new concepts to the trauma and traumatism landscapes. The establishment of the terms "Complex-PTSD" and "Developmental Trauma Disorder" have been monumental. They have unveiled the otherwise veiled traumatic experiences of women, children, and ethnic and racial minorities. The addition of these new terms is kindred to the developments in art in the beginning of the nineteenth century. Rather than paint pictures of perfect gods and goddesses, as encouraged by the Academy of Fine Arts, Realist artists depicted society in raw form.[74] Prostitutes, beggars, and laundresses replaced Athena, Zeus, and nymphs in the Realist paintings of Honoré Daumier and Jean-François Millet. Art was brought literally down to the street level. In a similar vein, the scientific field has expanded its understanding of traumatic experiences to include marginalized communities, but in a limited fashion.

Some of the most important additions to the scientific landscape on trauma have appeared in the last twenty years. Clinical and survey investigations have improved our understanding of the traumatic experiences of veterans from the Iraq and Afghan wars. There appear to be three principal factors that determine posttraumatic conditions: soldiers' childhood experiences, their human connections during combat, and their personal involvement in war crimes. Another chief discovery is just how prevalent MST is. It is just as prevalent as sexual traumatic experiences in the general population. Even more alarming is the fact that women in the armed forces have had to remain silent about sexual assaults ever since 1948 when they first began to serve. The prevalence of this silence brings to mind how male soldiers in the past were ordered to remain silent about their traumatic experiences on the battlefield. During the Great War, traumatized soldiers were even administered electric shock to insure their silence. Van der Kolk and Ducey's Rorschach card experiment with combat veterans finds resonance in surrealist author and artist André Breton's attempts to make trauma speak through creative mechanisms. Either the returning soldiers were stuck in violent narratives or deafening silence when they would see the Rorschach cards. Their imaginative powers were compromised during the experiment, which translated into an apparent inability to move beyond the traumatic experience.

Finally, during the last twenty years brain scans of PTSD sufferers have made key revelations. Neuroimaging indicates that trauma deactivates certain parts of the brain and activates others. The reaction of the hippocampus, which is responsible in part for memory, remains ambiguous, as meta-analyses reveal. Data also suggest that biological abnormalities differ according to whether a PTSD subject suffers from dissociation or not. These findings along with the two meta-analyses reviewed in this chapter prod us to conclude that it is difficult to generalize about the cerebral and behavioral consequences of trauma. This conclusion becomes even more poignant if one considers that not all those who experience trauma suffer from PTSD. Some use their traumatic experiences to grow and even to heal.

In addition to this complexity of drawing conclusions about posttraumatic conditions, one must consider that brain images are defined by a prominent drawback. They fail to provide a feeling of what happens to the traumatized. While scans might be able to detect abnormalities in the prefrontal cortex or hippocampus, they cannot portray the mental angst and physical turmoil the way Picasso's *Guernica* or *Weeping Woman* can. This observation leads us to conclude that the humanities, whether it is art or literature, have a vital role to play in helping clinicians and patients to understand the emotional feeling of trauma.

A poignant illustration of the relationship between trauma and the arts can be found in the work of the Italian artist Carlo Zinelli (1916–1974), who lost his mother at age two and was sent to work in the fields at age nine and later at a slaughterhouse. In 1939, he was conscripted in the Alpine Corps and sent to the front of the Spanish Civil War. After a brief engagement, he was sent home as he was showing "first signs of mental disturbances."[75] He was administered electric shock treatment and eventually sent to a psychiatric hospital. After a decade of mute suffering, he began to draw and paint prolifically, mostly thanks to the support of a multidisciplinary team of doctors and artists. Producing more than 2,000 pieces containing principally contorted images of bodies, Zinelli confirmed the rapport between trauma and artistic expression that psychoanalyst and artist Carl Jung had put forward in theory and artistic practice.[76] Today, Zinelli's artwork is considered "outsider art" (or *art brut*), an ambiguous label to describe pieces that turn mainstream art upside down. The term has been enlarged more recently to include works by artists without formal training and who have endured difficult circumstances, such as trauma. Ironically, if trauma survivors were given the opportunity to engage routinely in artistic expressions, a topic we shall explore in Chapter 5, then outsider art might not appear so obscure and might even begin to enrich histories of trauma studies and, more importantly, survivors' lives.

Notes

1 Psychiatrist Boris Cyrulnik states that 60% of the American population have suffered from a traumatizing event (50% according to the World Health Organization). Cyrulnik, "Children," 3. According to the American Psychiatric Association, "PTSD affects approximately 3.5 percent of US adults every year, and an estimated one in 11 people will be diagnosed with PTSD in their lifetime." See "What is Post-traumatic?" These figures may very well be much higher due to the COVID-19 pandemic. In fact, preliminary data suggest that this is the case. See North et al.'s "Nosological," 1–2. Although approximately 60% of the US population will experience a traumatic event within their lifetime, only a fraction of those traumatized individuals will develop PTSD. In fact, approximately 7 out of 100 people in the US will be afflicted by this debilitating condition, which intimates that "there is substantial inter-individual variability in susceptibility to PTSD." See Harnett et al., "PTSD-related" 1.
2 American Psychiatric Association, *DSM-III-R*, 250.
3 McFarlane and van der Kolk, "Long-Term," 5.
4 Recall from our discussion about the psychiatrist Pierre Briquet (1796–1881) from Chapter 2 that he too had underscored the relationship between poverty, child abuse, sexual abuse, and rape and hysteria.
5 American Psychiatric Association, *DSM-III-R*, 248.
6 Ibid., 250.
7 Friedman, "Finalizing," 550.
8 See American Psychiatric Association, *DSM-5*, 265.
9 See ibid., 272.
10 See ibid.
11 See ibid., 833.
12 See ibid., 834.
13 See ibid., 835.
14 American Psychiatric Association, *DSM-IV*, 427.
15 See North et al., "Nosological," 1; the *DSM-5* indicates that "A life-threatening illness or debilitating medical condition is not necessarily considered a traumatic event." American Psychiatric Association, *DSM-5*, 274.
16 Tyrer, "Comparison," 284.
17 World Health Organization, *ICD-10*, 19.
18 Ibid., 80.
19 Black et al., "National."
20 Ibid.
21 Ibid.
22 American Psychiatric Association, *DSM-5*, 277.
23 Tsai et al., "Homelessness" 1137.
24 Kleinman, *Illness*, 73.
25 Van der Kolk, *Body*, 108.
26 Ibid., 109.

27 American Psychiatric Association, *DSM-5*, 14.
28 Argenti-Pillen, *Masking*, 197.
29 Recall from our discussion in Chapter 2 that cardiologist Jacob Mendes Da Costa coined the expression "irritable heart syndrome," a similar term to "terrified hearts," during the American Civil War to refer to veterans who suffered from neuro-circular asthenia.
30 Van der Kolk, *Body*, 359.
31 See Herman, *Trauma*, 26.
32 Van der Kolk, *Body*, 11.
33 Fulton et al., "Prevalence," 98.
34 Goetter et al., "Systematic," 401.
35 Herman, *Trauma*, 251.
36 Ibid.
37 Ibid.
38 Ibid.
39 Walker and Nash, "Group," 383.
40 Ibid., 384.
41 Ibid.
42 See ibid., 406.
43 Herman, *Trauma*, 252.
44 Ibid., 251.
45 Ibid., 254.
46 Van der Kolk, *Body*, 254.
47 Ibid., 16.
48 Ibid.
49 Ibid.
50 Ibid.
51 See Harnett's et al., "PTSD-related," 3.
52 Van der Kolk, *Body*, 61.
53 Harnett et al., "PTSD-related," 3.
54 See ibid.
55 Ibid.
56 This synthesis has been gleaned from Harnett et al.'s review article "PTSD-related," 1–11 and Aupperle's article "Dorsolateral," 360–371.
57 Aupperle et al., "Dorsolateral," 360.
58 Harnett et al., "PTSD-related," 3.
59 Ibid.
60 Nicholson et al., "Dissociative," 2317.
61 Ibid.
62 Ibid., 2318.
63 For a discussion of this phenomenon, see van der Kolk's chapter "Posttraumatic Stress Disorder and The Nature of Trauma" in Siegal and Solomon, *Healing*, 185.
64 Van der Kolk, *Body*, 176.
65 Pitman et al., "Biological," 37.
66 Zoladz and Diamond, "Current," 881.
67 Ibid., 879.
68 Concerning the heated debate about the issue of memory and trauma, see McNally's article "Debunking," 817–822. In addition, see Rubin et al., "Memory," 1.
69 Zoladz and Diamond, "Current," 878.
70 Siegal and Solomon, *Healing*, Introduction.
71 Pitman et al., "Biological," 19.
72 Concerning the ambiguities of neuroimaging research, Israel Liberzon and James Abelson claim: "many features remain unexplained and a parsimonious model

that more fully accounts for symptoms and the core neurobiology remains elusive."
Liberzon and Abelson, "Context," 15.

73 See Watters, *Crazy*, chapters 1–4.

74 See LaLonde, *Paris*, 94–98.

75 Tansella, "Seminal," 15.

76 Even though Zinelli's life story is a powerful illustration of the relationship
between trauma and the arts, I have never come across a discussion of him in any
historical narrative of trauma studies, a reminder of the myopic view of the field;
see Jung, *Art*.

4   A Portrait of Cultural Trauma Studies

In a letter to his brother Theo, Vincent van Gogh claims not to be a land-scape artist and that human figures take instead center stage in his paintings. Though landscapes may be a background in his eyes, they still determine the "tone of the figure and the effect of the whole."[1] Figures or landscapes? The painter seeks above all to create inaccuracies on the canvas, for "those very aberrations, reworkings, transformations of reality, as may turn it into, well—a lie if you like—[are] but truer than the literal truth."[2] The artist thus renders reality unknown to make it known. Van Gogh's positions on landscapes, figures, and the aberrations and transformations of reality provide a transition from our discussion on the landscapes of scientific trauma theories to a portrait of cultural trauma theories. A landscape both provides a bigger picture ("the effect of the whole") and serves as a metaphor for the process of collecting and investigating quantitative data. Conversely, a "figure" symbolizes not only an individual but also the very process of collecting and investigating qualitative data. Artistic and literary portraits offer a type of qualitative investigation into human figures. If we draw our attention to van Gogh's self-portraits, we might notice other important trends in content and form. Several of his auto-portraits are made up of "lies" in the form of waves, swirling lines that blur the background and the foreground. The landscape transforms into the figure, while the figure transmutes into the landscape. Boundaries between them have been blended if not destroyed.

With van Gogh's notions of landscapes, figures, and self-portraits in mind, we will first paint in this chapter a portrait of cultural trauma studies from the 1980s and 1990s or during what I call the field's "First Wave." This portrait will expose the field's foundational theories of psychoanalysis, structuralism, and deconstruction. We will then focus on how First Wave theorists stressed, like van Gogh, the concept of the unknown. By claiming that trauma "resists or escapes consciousness,"[3] as Geoffrey Hartman contends, he and other literary theorists have offered a dismal view of recovery for trauma survivors. True, some psychiatrists did indeed have a bleak out-look in the 1950s and 1960s regarding Holocaust survivor recovery.[4] A trend developed all the same in the 1990s among clinicians to study the

DOI: 10.4324/9781003284642-7

"remarkable resilience" of these survivors.[5] First Wave cultural trauma theorists did not follow this trend. This is short sided, not to mention misaligned with the ethical claims they had made about being connected politically with the world.[6] Moreover, they seem to have failed to appreciate the controversial nature of the concept of unknown traumatic memories, a topic examined in this chapter. Disturbed by trends akin to these, cultural theorists from a "Second Wave" (historians and post-colonial theorists) reworked the field. While unfolding this history, we shall provide one of the motivations of this book: The canvas of cultural trauma studies could benefit from new perspectives, especially those from other fields and cultures that paint piercing portraits of posttraumatic conditions, including resistance, resilience, and growth.

First Wave Cultural Trauma Studies

Kindred to scientists and social scientists, cultural trauma theorists were inspired by the anti-war and feminist movements of the 1960s-1980s, and I would add, the research on both Holocaust survivors and to a much lesser extent, the trauma of racism and colonialism. Political movements were moved from the streets into the university. Structuralists and later post-structuralists scrutinized language and other cultural artifacts from highbrow to low. As society was marked by trauma (made manifest in wars, widespread sexual assault, refugee crises, and environmental degradation), the study of trauma figured on the agenda of scholars from the field of cultural studies. Trauma was not just a topic reserved for the clinic and the laboratory. It left its mark on books of poetry and fiction and in film. Reacting against post-modernists' rejection of an ethical agenda (in contrast to Marxist, feminist, post-colonial, and eventually queer and eco-critical theorists), cultural trauma theorists made noble claims about their research. After all, stories had always recorded psychic wounds, while literature had never shied away from, even luxuriated in, portrayals of traumatic suffering, unlike other fields.[7]

Whereas some had claimed that "The Latest Theory is that Theory Doesn't Matter," to quote a catchy 2003 headline from the *New York Times*, and while others had predicted the death of literary theory when Jacques Derrida died in 2004, it appeared that literary studies and literature could indeed make meaningful contributions. The burgeoning of trauma theories during the First Wave had appeared to create by the early 2000s an atmosphere of unity and purpose, serving as a counterforce to postmodernity's skepticism of truth and progress.

If verse and prose became the fields of investigation, what were the tools employed during the First Wave? In the 1990s, literary theorists such as Hartman, Shoshanna Felman (teaming up with psychiatrist Dori Laub), and Cathy Caruth employed psychoanalysis, structuralism, and deconstructionism to build their theories. Adding both complementary and critical analyses to these, historians from a Second Wave, such as Dominick LaCapra and Ruth Leys, tweaked cultural trauma studies as did post-colonialists Gert Buelens, Stef Craps, Michael Rothberg, Roger Kurtz, and Irene Vissier, among others. The field has therefore been defined by a background from science (psychoanalysis) and the humanities, such as deconstructionism, as well as transformations in the form of criticisms from historians and post-colonialists.[8] This turn toward multidisciplinary research has been productive in several ways, including a shift away from individuals and psychoanalysis, since trauma is tightly woven with political, social, and cultural phenomena and merits therefore a wider investigative aperture.

Psychoanalysis

Before examining how psychoanalytic theories served as a foundation for trauma studies, it is useful to explore the fundamental relationships between psychoanalysis, literature, and literary theory. These connections are based on Freud's argument that literature is a psychic artifact of the artist, just as dreams are symptoms of the dreamer. From there, some literary theorists employed psychoanalysis to explore the "unconscious" of the author, the book's content and form, and the reader, seeking often to airbrush gaps. It seems paradoxical to seek to fill them in, since the unconscious is defined by ambiguities and often made known in dreams and slips of the tongue. Or in Freud's words:

> This, then, is the keystone of the dream, the place at which it mounts into the unknown. For the dream thoughts which we come upon in the interpretation must generally remain without a termination, and merge in all directions into the net-like entanglement of our world of thoughts.[9]

Though dreams (and literature) can open a window on the unconscious realm, we confront a spider-web blocking our vision and entangling our thoughts.

The psychiatrist and psychoanalyst Jacques Lacan adjusts Freudian concepts of the unconscious. Lacan's starting point is the notion that the unconscious is structured like a language.[10] At first glance, this appears to resonate with Freud's position that psychoanalysis is a "talking cure" with speech as its tool. Lacan nuances however the language issue. In a structuralist vein, he posits that the correspondence between the signifier and the signified of language is imperfect.[11] Furthermore, speech is "empty," insomuch as the subject can never capture the essence of his/her inner instincts, drives, and desires. The clinical analyst also faces an impasse of communication. She usually interprets what she does not hear. Body language and silence communicate sometimes louder than words. Be that as it may, the analyst "has no other ears, no third or fourth ear to serve as what some have tried to describe as a direct transaudition of the unconscious by the unconscious."[12] Language is imperfect *a priori* and speech, empty? There might not be a "direct transaudition of the unconscious by the unconscious"? We need not stop at these roadblocks. Lacan's position spurs us to ponder: what about an indirect transaudition? The answer to this question might be found among the Dadaists and surrealists, whom Lacan studied with keen interest. For the Dadaists and the surrealists, the unconscious can reveal itself when one cuts up magazine images and throws them like confetti on a board to be shellacked. The surrealist writer and artist André Breton referred to this abracadabra act as "psychic automatism."[13] And what about his surrealist revolution consisting of "automatic writing" to access the unconscious realm? The idea behind such a revolution is that one can still hear the muskets fire in the dark. There are mechanisms to reach the unconscious, provided realism and empiricism face the firing squad.

Psychoanalysis and the First Wave's Fixation on the Unknowns

First Wave trauma theorists embarked on a meta-analysis, contemplating the shared links between psychoanalysis, literary theory, and literature. They built their arguments on Freud's and Lacan's concepts while constructing their own. From Freud, they relied on the notion that the unconscious makes itself known through unknown material of dreams. From Lacan, they stressed the intrinsic idiosyncrasies of language to reach the unconscious. As for traumatic memories, they are doubly defined by Freud's and Lacan's notions and thus, the intersection between knowing and not knowing. That is, memories are difficult to know, if not even impossible, just as any other unconscious material.

Hartman views psychoanalysis as distinctly pedagogical, akin to literary theory. Reception theory provides "a way of slowing reading by allowing the student's opinions, prejudices, and positions to emerge, and subduing the teacher's own rage for order."[14] Decelerating our own reading of Hartman's statement, we could replace the words "reading" with "interpreting"; "student's" by "analysand's"; "teacher's" by "analyst's." The relationship between psychoanalysis and literary theory is unequivocal. There is a shared procedure of investigating hidden meaning. By exploring dreams, slips of the tongue, memory gaps, gaffes, mislayings, misreadings, and jokes, the analysand and analyst discover the unconscious, populated by libidinal, aggressive, or anxious material. Similarly, the memories of traumatic experiences are often stored in the unconscious and require interpretative exercises, common to both psychoanalysis and literary theory. Beyond these connections between psychoanalysis and literary theory, Hartman locates links between psychoanalysis and literature. "As in literature," he argues in reference to the psychoanalytic dialogue, "we find a way of receiving the story, of listening to it, of drawing it into an interpretive conversation."[15] In such interpretive exercises, reductionism is avoided, for there is "more listening, more hearing of words, and a greater openness to testimony."[16] Words equate with psychic wounds, whereas literature undresses the wounds' bandages by employing a language that is equally as evasive as the original content of the wounds.

Felman's research builds on Hartman's notions on literature and psychoanalysis. In her eyes, "psychoanalysis and literature have come to contaminate and to enrich each other."[17] What does this shared history of contamination and enrichment look like? Both center on speech in the form of a testimony. In psychoanalysis, the patient gives a testimony; the clinician receives it. Literature mirrors this process. The writer bears witness; the reader witnesses the testimony. Further, speech is understood as a "mode of truth's realization."[18] Felman stresses that a testimony does not necessarily provide a fully baked transparent truth. It offers a mechanism to access it. She is therefore not referring to any old testimony. It is "unconscious, unintended, unintentional testimony."[19] Testimonies of the traumatic experience rely also on the listener who serves as a blank canvas upon which the experience is portrayed. Or in reader-reception jargon, the reader's mind provides a blank page where the traumatic testimony can be transcribed and assume new meaning.

Echoing and expanding upon Felman's notions, Caruth maintains that the urge to understand a traumatic event and its reverberating traumatic mental experience is no longer defined by "simple models of experience and reference."[20] What new references and experiences is she referring to? Curiously, she too stresses the concept of a testimony. (This is curious because a testimony seems to constitute precisely a "simple" model of reference, as it resembles a legal affidavit.) Following Felman's positions, Caruth maintains first that trauma narratives are a testimony of another's trauma, for "one's own trauma is tied up with the trauma of another."[21] What are the implications of having one's own testimony of trauma tied up with someone else's? A testimony of another's trauma is almost by definition shrouded in enigma and demands interpretation, just as a piece of literature craves our creative input. An individual's own trauma testimony also remains enigmatic and demands constant interpretative adjustments. Second, Caruth posits that the transmission of a traumatic experience must "be spoken in a language that is always somehow literary: a language that defies, even as it claims, our understanding."[22] That is, the transmission of a traumatic event is characterized by the yin and yang of "knowing and not knowing."[23] In either case, trauma is a story of a wound that seeks to tell a truth. "This truth," she claims, "in its delayed appearance and its belated address, cannot be linked only to what is known, but also to what remains unknown in our very actions and our language."[24] This concept can be concretized when contemplating how traumatic (and unconscious) experiences make themselves known and yet unknown in slips of the tongue, dreams, and nightmares.

These two ideas gleaned from Caruth's work should strike readers as paradoxical. (Is this perhaps what she meant when she referred to trauma narratives defying a simple model of reference?) On the one hand, trauma narratives resemble testimonies. On the other, they are like literature characterized by the knowns and the unknowns. Testimonies and literature inhabit opposite polar regions in some respects. After all, testimonies are typically seen as legal affidavits written in clear language and logical form, the very antitheses to literature. Summing up Caruth's conceptualization of trauma, literary theorist Anne Whitehead sheds some light on this paradox position: "Trauma carries the force of a literality which renders it resistant to narrative structures and linear temporalities."[25] From this we can draw three conclusions about Caruth's conceptualizations: Trauma narratives do not resemble a testimony's format. But they do rely on the concept of a testimonial witness. And they resemble the oceanic depth and breathe of literature, including the abysses of darkness. In fact, Whitehead's use of the term "resistant to narrative structures" highlights Caruth's conviction of the impossibility of narratives getting at trauma. Caruth nuances this roadblock. She evokes "The difficulty of listening and responding to traumatic stories in a way that does not lose their impact, that does not reduce them to clichés or turn them all into versions of the same story ..."[26] A memory of a traumatic event(s) might be allowed to fester in an "unknown" state, lest it become an inaccurate story. Furthermore, the unknown state of a story might also be the survivor's attempt to maintain a sense of integrity of her understanding (or lack thereof) of the original event, whose gravity might defy verbal description. The event(s) might be so encumbered with darkness that to decode it betrays somehow that evil. Although Caruth does not make the following point, the decision to "erase" the past from one's conscious awareness might translate into a sense of empowerment. By becoming "illiterate" of the traumatic memories or incapable of reading the story of the event(s), the survivor is calling the shots on her own recovery, a necessary step in the recovery process, as Judith Herman has reminded us.

Despite this positive reading of Caruth's concepts, let us return to her signature concept of the unknown nature of traumatic memories and to Whitehead's summative statement that trauma defies "narrative structures and linear temporalities." While we might be able to make sense of the twin concept of testimony and literature, it is hard to reconcile the fixation on the use of the unknowns, as it may very well have deleterious effects on trauma survivors. Another way to look at this dichotomy of testimonies and literature is to put forward that trauma survivors might rely at first on a testimony format precisely because of its straight-forward language and concision, even clichés, perhaps. It is a first line of attack to purge oneself of one's traumatic experience. Once, other stages of recovery have been reached and the mind is less tortured by stress hormones and traumatic memories, then trauma survivors can adventure into creative stories. In short, testimonies tell of trauma. Literature tells of resilience, resistance, and growth. Testimonies tell of the unknowns and knowns. Literature luxuriates in the unknowns and knowns.

Structuralist and Deconstructionist Theories

The widespread concept of the "unknowns" among First Wave cultural theorists is also built on structuralism and deconstruction. Linguist and literary theorist Roman Jakobson argued that every feeling is defined by its opposite.[27] Referring to Baroque poetry, literary theorist Gérard Genette upheld that the antithesis is its very dominant theme where despair and hope, body and spirit, god and world, hell and heaven all coexist.[28] From a structuralist emphasis on binary opposites, Roland Barthes edged his theories toward ambiguity as he claimed that "literature is intentional chicken scratch."[29] Literature is by definition ambiguous and hence does peculiar things to language. It questions the communicative nature of language; it is the site of interrogation and uncertainty that falls off the cliff of reason.

Deconstructionists drove the structuralists' duality and uncertainty of language, feeling, and literature over the precipice. Jacques Derrida ironically employs in his *Dissemination* (1969) a clear method to emphasize the unclear nature of his book. He lays the main theme out in the preface's very first line. The surrealist artist René Magritte's painting *This is Not a Pipe* becomes Derrida's: "This (therefore) will not have been a book."[30] Magritte's oeuvre (also known poignantly as the *Treachery of Images*) and Derrida's book deconstruct themselves. They both betray a fixed definition of what they are supposed to be. Derrida's act of insolence is doubly insolent. Unlike Magritte's painting that puts pressure on the image of a pipe, the post-structuralist calls into question the very tool he is employing, a book and a preface. The book's title amounts to a triple act of defiance against fixed meaning, as the term "dissemination" seeds doubt in the orderly furrows of readers' minds. The metaphor is clear, however. The dissemination of disorder might germinate a harvest of new concepts.

That said, as language and literature became known as the unknowable, it was impossible to avoid falling into a borehole. In a paradoxical act of intellectual dishonesty, the deconstructionist Paul de Man refuted not only language and literature, but also literary theory itself. The unknowable's potential to stimulate discoveries began to disappear from the map. The island of the unknowable no longer seemed to contain treasure troves. It was marked instead with crossbones. In his essay "The Resistance to Theory" (1982) de Man argues that "the main theoretical interest of literary theory consists in the impossibility of its definition."[31] This statement ironically offers a definition of literary theory (the impossibility of a definition) while claiming to reject one. By setting up this dichotomy, de Man pours scorn not only on the tools of literary theory, but also on the object of investigation, literature. Looking under the hood of literature, he finds that it is propelled by its own "autonomous potential of language."[32] It is free from referential restraints. That is, its use of language is not determined "by consideration of truth and falsehood, good and evil, beauty and ugliness, and pleasure and pain."[33] It is defined instead by a linguistic free-for-all, which casts a shadow on the "reliability of linguistic utterance."[34]

Echoing de Man's doubt on the "reliability" of language, Caruth writes: "a direct or phenomenal reference to the world means, paradoxically, the production of a fiction; or otherwise put, that reference is radically different from physical law."[35] Advancing this comparison between science and language further, she goes so far as to claim, "the only thing that was adequate to the world was, paradoxically, that which didn't refer (mathematics); and what did refer, language, could no longer describe the world."[36] By holding steadfastly to the position that language can no longer describe the world, post-structuralists have conveyed a sense that linguistic impasses are indeed valuable as they introduce the unknown. Nonetheless, don't all languages (science, mathematics, music, and art) represent intellectual and communicative impasses? And is the world unknowable as we fail to describe it in language? Aren't there other ways to communicate it as Lacan intimated when referring to the unconscious and as seen in surrealist art and literature? These rhetorical questions point to argumentative shortcomings that we shall elaborate on further below. They also point to other research directions. Historian Ruth Leys nudges us down another route (and away from the unknown) by writing: "The best practitioners have always been pragmatic in this sense, making use of whatever psychotherapeutic, medical, and other methods are available to help their patients ..."[37]

The Irony of Fixating on Unknown Traumatic Memories

Keeping Leys's comment in mind, we might put forward that Hartman's, Felman's, and Caruth's brand of psychoanalysis is not pragmatic, to say the least. "Trauma theory," explains Hartman, "introduces a psychoanalytic skepticism as well, which does not give up on knowledge but suggests the existence of a *traumatic* kind, one that cannot be made entirely conscious, in the sense of being fully retrieved or communicated without distortion."[38] Traumatic knowledge cannot be made entirely conscious? This mirrors Lacan's theories and notably his concept of accessing indirectly the unconscious through the unconscious. Traumatic knowledge escapes communication unless it is distorted? This echoes van Gogh's statement, discussed in this chapter's introduction, about creating "aberrations and transformations of reality" in order to find a truth that is "truer than the literal truth." Unlike van Gogh, Hartman neither seeks nor expects to gain knowledge. The literary theorist states in fact that, "Traumatic knowledge, then, would seem to be a contradiction in terms."[39] Thus, even if Hartman refers to a "criticism that reads the wound"[40] of trauma, he remains skeptical that this knowledge can be made conscious. Literary theory (and thus by implication, literature) covers the wound, just as much as reads it.

Felman and Caruth follow this same dialectical pattern. Felman refers to the possibility of bearing witness to a truth and yet claims that it is "essentially *not available* to its own speaker" (her italics).[41] She suggests moreover that the testimony has "an incomparable heuristic and investigative value."[42] Her vocabulary is misleading. By suggesting that a testimony can serve as an "incomparable" aid to discovery and learning, we are left with the impression that traumatized subjects might grasp the complexities of their traumatic conditions. Felman punctures this balloon of hope by adding "the speaking subject constantly bears witness to a truth that nonetheless continues to escape him, a truth that is, essentially not available to its own speaker."[43] Dori Laub, who coauthored with Felman *Testimony* (1991), echoes this position more forcefully by explaining: "Massive trauma precludes its registration; the observing and recording mechanisms of the human mind are temporarily knocked out, malfunction."[44] And although Caruth "offers the image of the voice of trauma emerging from the wound itself—a voice testifying to the role of the victim as witness,"[45] she is convinced of daunting impasses. To her mind, trauma has "an unassimilated nature" and remains "unavailable to consciousness."[46] In sum, these First Wave trauma theorists have fixated on the unknown nature of traumatic memories, which flies paradoxically in the face of psychoanalytic practices designed to cultivate many different cognitive abilities, including memory.

Second Wave Cultural Trauma Studies' Criticisms and Reworkings

During the last twenty years, a Second Wave of cultural trauma theorists have in fact reproached First Wave theorists on several accounts. The Second Wave has criticized early cultural trauma theorists for stressing the unknown and relying too heavily on psychoanalysis, which can lead to narrow perspectives, such as melancholy. It also contends that First Wave theorists suffer from Euro-American centrism and an associated fixation on trauma as opposed to resilience, resistance, and growth. As mentioned in the chapter's introduction, these idiosyncrasies provide a warrant for this book. These idiosyncrasies point to missing "figures" on the canvas of cultural trauma studies that I aim to portray in this chapter and those that follow.

Idiosyncrasies of Fixating on the Unknowns

Dominick LaCapra calls out trauma theorists (not least those cut from the fabric of de Manian deconstruction) who fixate on "the undecidable, the aporetic, the abyssal, the unnamable, the unrepresentable …"[47] Leys shares these concerns arguing that "van der Kolk and Caruth have materialized and literalized traumatic memory in ways that make it seem as if trauma stands outside all knowledge and all representation."[48] Without a critical analysis of this starting point, cultural theorists continue to fixate on the so-called "unnamable, the unrepresentable," to use LaCapra's expressions again. While his and Leys's criticisms suggest that the fixation on the unknowable is indeed a prevalent idiosyncrasy of trauma studies, this very critique may become the target of criticism, as it attempts to make the unknown of trauma studies known.[49] Irrespective of those potential criticisms, let us embark on a critical analysis of this fixation.

It is important to stress that even though Hartman, Felman, and Caruth built their arguments regarding traumatic memory on the "unknowns" of Freudian theories, structuralism, and deconstructionism, this (obviously) does not make their positions bullet proof for several reasons. A wound that escapes conscious awareness? Knowledge that is unavailable to the speaker? An experience that is unassimilated? It is one thing to employ these terms in reference to literary characters. It is still another regarding real trauma survivors tortured by a traumatic past. Upon hearing that their wounds will forever escape conscious awareness, survivors may very well respond, "If memories of my traumatic past remain unavailable or unassimilated, then why bother to strive to make sense of them? I will continue to engage in denial and dissociation to keep my memories and emotions under control." Similarly, upon learning that, "trauma is an experience that is not experienced,"[50] survivors might ask rhetorically, "Are you trying to tell me that I did not experience that rape?" A question that all too often tragically trails off into silence, while the body suffers and even recoils from the painful experience.

Further, clinical research indicates that First Wave theorists' insistence on the unknowns of traumatic memory is misguided. We should not forget firstly that among trauma survivors there is a constriction of all cognitive abilities, from memory, problem solving, judgment, discrimination, to perception, and emotional experiences. This mental shutting down seems to be an "identification with the dead."[51] And yet, Krystal points out that even though posttraumatic psychic constriction is widespread, "it varies greatly in its intensity."[52] Krystal's statement (and his findings on flexible memories reviewed in Chapter 3) suggests that trauma survivors may also feel a compelling urge to edit their stories of trauma. Herman echoes this position as well in her three-stage recovery method.[53] Second, research from psychologist Richard McNally reveals three important findings that go contrary to the First Wave's obsession with the unknowns.[54] According to McNally, memories of traumatic experiences are rarely, if ever, forgotten; they are often vivid and mutable; avoiding thoughts about traumatic experiences for an extended period is not the same as being unable to recall it. Though traumatic amnesia theorists might not agree with McNally's findings, it remains clear that the issue of traumatic memory is up for debate among psychiatrists and psychologists.[55] It should remain therefore a debatable point among scholars in the humanities. Third, current scientific research about memories (examined in Chapter 3) call into question cultural trauma theorists' starting point that knowledge of traumatic memories remains ipso facto unknown. Recall that researchers have delineated that the reaction of the hippocampus, which is responsible in part for memory, remains ambiguous in trauma survivors. Finally, the argument of the unknown of traumatic memories is on a slippery slope. It is kindred to saying that two idiopathic (without a known cause) diseases are connected because they are both idiopathic. Their shared idiopathic trait is true only because of scientific limitations. Once their etiologies are understood, they no longer share this idiopathic trait. Their link falls apart unless they share etiological and pathological characteristics. Similarly, when Hartman, Felman, and Caruth emphasize the shared element of the unknown in literature and traumatic memories, they provide only a lose link between the two.

Besides this loose link, literature or literary theory is not the only intellectual domain that is defined by the unknown. Philosophy has relished the ill-defined nature of existence.[56] Ontology and epistemology furthermore feed off the unknown.[57] The language of science (mathematics) is fundamentally ill-equipped to describe the world.[58] In this respect, we can indeed claim that language (including the language of science) cannot truly describe the world. The very fundamental nature of nature appears unknown. If critical theorists (and clinicians) are going to talk about the intrinsic deficiencies of language and the unknown nature of traumatic experiences, perhaps they should mention in the same breath that these facts govern the fields of philosophy and science and nature itself. Perhaps they should also point out that Freud stressed this in his research on the unconscious: "its inner nature is just as unknown to us as the reality of the external world, and it is just as imperfectly reported to us through the data of consciousness as is the external world through the indications of our sensory organs."[59] In short, the ambiguities of the mind are no different fundamentally from those of an expanding universe, blackholes and all. Scientists confront these impasses and yet conduct experiments and tabulate results that would make Sisyphus's charge look trivial. These phenomena in science may inspire trauma survivors as they undertake their own investigations into a traumatic past.

An Over-reliance on Psychoanalysis

Related to a fixation on the unknowable is an overreliance on psychoanalysis. How could psychoanalysis be a problematic tool for trauma research if Freud's theories grew out of and developed from early trauma investigations involving hysterical patients in Paris and shell-shocked veterans from World War I? As explored in Chapter 2, Freud was pessimistic about the possibility of healing or even growth. Moreover, Freudian psychoanalysis centers on the individual, as opposed to collectivities or cultural phenomena. Consequently, such a focus neglects the greater political and societal trends that provoke traumatic experiences. In addition, relying on Lacanian psychoanalytic theory in general might feel like attending a play in which actors appear without a script. The "blank unreadability" of trauma can lead to an impression of "unsymbolizable" reality and hence a dead end.[60] It is important to remember furthermore that the father of psycho-analysis compromised his own trauma theories. Recall from Chapter 2 that Freud discovered an unambiguous link between hysteria and childhood sexual abuse. This idea was unacceptable to the psychoanalyst, as it called out the hypocrisies of the right-thinking bourgeoisie. He thus swept his findings under the carpet. What is so paradoxical about Freud's theory regarding the etiology of hysteria is that it too remained unknown. It is as if he took his findings and sunk them below the iceberg to the ocean's abyss. To rely on his concept of the unknowable is therefore problematic for its dubious history, and it remains most curious that many trauma theorists still rely on it without second thought.[61] Finally, First Wave trauma theor-ists who rely heavily upon psychoanalysis seem to have forgotten that the field of knowledge is not simply a rhetorical device. It is also a tool to understand and alter societies, as made evident in the Frankfurt School's attempts to employ Freudian theories to comprehend and treat collective psychopathologies.[62]

A Fixation on Melancholia

Related to the obsession on the unknowable, Second-Wave theorists often find fault with the First Wave's fixation on melancholia. "To be in a frozen or suspended afterwards," writes Roger Luckhurst, "it seems to be assumed, is the only proper ethical response to trauma, displacing any other memorial relation to the past and situating memory entirely under the sign of post-traumatic melancholia."[63] Irene Visser refers to the "dictum" among early trauma theorists that "melancholy is the defining condition of trauma."[64] When paired with trauma, as in "traumatic melancholia," the term "mel-ancholia" refers to a cemented state, an inability to free oneself from the traumatic event. It amounts to holding on to a fixed memory of a traumatic experience, just as one holds onto an experience of loss in psychiatric mel-ancholic states. Moreover, an emphasis on melancholia can easily lead to a neglect of "life-affirming and activist processes," as Vissier rightfully claims.[65]

Seen from the other end of the telescope, this criticism about an emphasis on melancholia seems unfair. Melancholia after all can be a "site of crea-tivity," as Julia Kristeva reminds us.[66] She also highlights that it is the very nature of being alive, a message powerfully transmitted in Albrecht Dürer's portrait etching *Melancholia*.[67] This leads us to conclude that the issue is not so much that First Wave theorists concentrated too much on "traumatic melancholia," but rather on trauma itself as we shall discuss shortly.

Euro-American Centrism and a Failed Ethical Agenda

Besides the First Wave's overreliance on psychoanalysis and the associated concepts of the unknown and melancholia, it suffers from an acute case of cultural myopia and a failure to pursue a global ethical agenda. Originally bred in the United States and exported throughout the world, First Wave cultural trauma studies served in some respects as an uncomfortable reminder of the narrow-mindedness and hegemonic spirit dominating the West. Again, this is paradoxical, as founding members made ethical claims about their research. Hartman puts forward that the field renders "the literary object ... more connected with what goes on in a blatantly political world," thus fostering "an opening ... to public issues ... with ethical, cultural, and religious implications."[68] Caruth joins Hartman's chorus of ethical claims. Referring to the film *Hiroshima mon amour* (1959), she states that it helps spectators to develop "a new mode of seeing and of listening—a seeing and a listening from the site of trauma—is opened up to us as spectators of the film, and offered as the very possibility, in a catastrophic era, of a link between cultures."[69] This quoted segment has become almost a mantra of First Wave trauma studies. At first glance, it sounds like a goodwill message. However, this statement begs us to ask more critically, who sees whom and who listens to whom? And can our traumas truly be shared? The reality is that most fields of knowledge are shot through with Euro-American culture, and most notably Anglo-American. These dominant cultures are seen and heard, while they remain deaf and blind all too often to other cultures. It is insensitive moreover to imagine that the traumatic experiences of refugees living in squalid conditions in camps along the border could be understood by those living in privileged economic, social, and political positions. Caruth's claim above also spurs questions about resistance, resilience, and posttraumatic growth. Couldn't these experiences also be shared? Why is it just a question of shared trauma? These topics seem to have been originally off the radar screen of First Wave trauma theorists.[70]

To return to Hartman's cultivation of public issues with ethical, cultural, and religious implications, it did not exactly materialize, at least originally. Post-colonial theorists Stef Craps and Gert Buelens take this ethical claim to task:

> trauma studies' stated commitment to the promotion of cross-cultural ethical engagement is not borne out by the founding texts of the field ... which are almost exclusively concerned with traumatic experiences of white Westerners and solely employ critical methodologies emanating from a Euro-American context.[71]

Roger Kurtz also weighs in on the subject: "these built-in limitations and biases limit the ability of trauma theory to offer an effective cross-cultural ethical engagement that has global relevance."[72] Underscoring the consequences of this cultural myopia, Michael Rothberg forcefully argues: "as long as trauma studies forgoes comparative study and remains tied to a narrow Eurocentric framework, it distorts the histories it addresses (such as the Holocaust) and threatens to reproduce the very Eurocentrism that lies behind those histories."[73] If we translate Rothberg's statement into a metaphor, we could put forward that instead of the colonial master freeing the enslaved, he locks them up and throws out the key to their cerebral cell.

An Overemphasis on Trauma and an Underemphasis on Posttraumatic Growth

In addition to a tendency for Euro-American centrism, some First Wave trauma theorists overemphasize the concept of trauma. "By putting trauma at the center of a theory of representation," write post-colonial theorists Ewald Mengel and Michela Borzaga, "their melancholic vocabulary is one marked by notions of absence, holes, deferral, crises of meaning and dissociation."[74] They add that the field tends to "neglect the creativity of people in times of trauma."[75] This is an astonishing view about research on trauma and is echoed by clinicians. Psychiatrist and psychoanalyst Barbara Shapiro claims that "The psychoanalytic literature on resilience is relatively sparse."[76] Psychiatrist and psychoanalyst Boris Cyrulnik puts the point squarely: "The fact that resilience has not been studied even though clinicians have observed it says a lot about our culture …"[77] A neglect to investigate creative methods to promote agency, resistance, resilience, and growth in different cultures or even our own finds resonance in what psychiatrist Arthur Kleinman claims regarding health care: "Cultural issues are allowed to slip by, one after another in a way that would be regarded as sheer clinical incompetence if the issues were biological."[78] By integrating other cultural perspectives into the field, the ethical imperative of trauma studies, which was promised at its inception, may very well be strengthened.[79] While the medical community attempted in a very limited fashion to add other cultural perspectives to the *DSM-5* (a topic explored in Chapter 3), the Second Wave's move to decolonize trauma studies may very well provide another excellent source of multicultural perspectives of trauma and posttraumatic conditions.

The Second Wave's Efforts to Decolonize the Field

With this sketch of the idiosyncrasies of First Wave cultural trauma studies in mind, we are led to consider how post-colonial theorists have sought to decolonize cultural trauma studies. They have proposed new prerogatives and ethical claims, focusing on a non-Western trauma novel, and directing attention away from the topic of trauma to posttraumatic resistance, resilience, and growth.

New Prerogatives and New Ethical Claims

Drawing on the research of Lauren Berlant, Laura Brown, and Frantz Fanon, Craps stresses a foundational objective of the decolonization of trauma studies. This goal seeks above all to recognize toxic atmospheres of abuse and degradation as traumatic experiences. (Note that this perspective finds resonance with clinicians' attempts to define the concept of Complex-PTSD, a topic reviewed in Chapter 3.) By investigating and publicly recognizing daily toxic atmospheres, researchers might help in turn to transform their work into "a catalyst for astute political analysis and meaningful activism ..."[80] One might object that this sounds like a repeat of Hartman's ethical claims. Nonetheless, post-colonialists investigate trauma at ground zero, colonized societies and their cultural artifacts. Sonya Andermahr adds to this foundational aim by providing a summary of a decolonized trauma theory.[81] She postulates that this morphed form of trauma theory would acknowledge and make amends for the dismissal of minority and non-Western traumas; put pressure on the so-called universality of Western definitions of trauma; put forward alternate trauma aesthetics; and explore connections between developed and developing world traumas.

Pushing the Canon around: The Trauma Novel

Another way to decolonize trauma studies is to explore what should have been explored since the field's inception: post-colonial trauma novels, as opposed to British Romantic literature.[82] There has been a "decolonization" of the novel, such that post-colonial trauma fiction is enriching our understanding of literature itself. The South African writer Mothobi Mutloatse puts this attempt to decolonize literature best: "We are going to pee, spit and shit on literary convention before we are through; we are going to kick and pull and push and drag literature into the form we prefer ..."[83] What form might that be? Mutloatse's use of the terms "pee, spit, and shit" intimates that the body will be involved in the rewriting of literature. This familiar vocabulary also suggests that the "reworkings" of literature will not follow the exigencies of the establishment. His statement conveys moreover an act of colonization. Before literature can be decolonized, it must be colonized. Literature will be kicked, pulled, pushed, and dragged, just as the colonial subject was. Is this simply an act of retaliation? Mutloatse seems to be hinting at an oxymoronic process. Literature can serve as both a poison and a cure. On the one hand, literature from Balzac to Proust propagated images of bourgeois comfort and masked respectability, an "ideal" way of life for all to emulate from Paris to Abidjan. As Fanon points out, this emulation is doubly bogus. The colonized subject not only assumes a bogus mask of a white Parisian bourgeois professional, but the mask itself is bogus as only bourgeois respectability can be. On the other hand, post-colonial authors can blow up literature the way the Dadaists and surrealists did to reconfigure it. Post-colonialist subjects can denigrate Western literature by "pissing" on it and creating "a crystallization of the national consciousness" through acts of "collective catharsis."[84]

Moving Beyond Trauma: Posttraumatic Resistance, Resilience, and Growth

What about the notions of resistance, resilience, growth, and perhaps even recovery, healing, and cure in reference to decolonizing the field of trauma studies? Are these notions appropriate in the context of cultural trauma studies? Shouldn't they be reserved for the clinic? If that is the case, shouldn't trauma be a topic reserved for the clinic, as well? Are these terms even accurate? Consider the terms "recovery," "healing," and "cure." Shouldn't we harbor skepticism about employing them relative to traumatic experiences, as they seem to imply a "pathologization and depoliticization of victims of violence."[85] In effect, when we explore these latter terms, which this book has carefully avoided, we run the risk of downplaying the original traumatic event, which might have been an attack by a powerful entity on a more vulnerable community. Such an attack might stir the vulnerable to emboldened action, not to some quasi-diseased state that might eventually need to be healed or cured. It seems unwise furthermore for a specialist in literary theory and world literature to employ the words "recovery," "healing," and "cure" in a research project centering on theoretical musings and not on individuals in clinics who suffer the debilitating effects of trauma. Still, posttraumatic conditions remain all too often a lost continent. The map designating their location is marked by an "X" surrounded by images of monsters roaming the seas. Although it might be important to respect the complex and mysterious nature of these states, the literary arts often speak the same language of complexity and mystery and can serve as a source of elucidation.

Conclusions: A "Flat" Portrait of Cultural Trauma Studies and Future Visions

In his *Wretched of the Earth* (1961), Frantz Fanon describes the post-colonized painter. Rejecting the colonizers' artistic techniques, trends, and content, the post-colonized artist paints a portrait of a nation based on former national traits. His artwork is a poor rendition of the reality of the nation, according to Fanon. Colonized minds have been molded like pieces of clay in the hands of the colonizers. They have suffered from the daily traumatic conditions of racism, abuse, denigration, and alienation. The past cultural template fails to convey this reality. It represents instead kitsch and irrelevant stereotypes of yesteryear rather than relevant reflections of a cruel reality. The artist's painting turns out to be "a point-by-point representation of national reality which is flat, untroubled, motionless, reminiscent of death rather than life."[86]

Fanon's description of the post-colonized painter reflects our portrait of First Wave cultural trauma studies. Like the painter, First Wave theorists have relied on a template of the past. Harkening back to psychoanalysis, structuralism, and deconstruction, they have attempted to create a theoretical framework with an ethical cause. However, if they were inspired by the political movements of the 1960s–1980s, they removed themselves paradoxically from the reality of trauma in the streets of New York to Algiers. By stressing the "unknown" and the "unspeakable," the field created a research agenda that was "flat" in the pre-Renaissance sense that the earth's intrinsic nature was misunderstood. The catchy terms of the "unknowable" and "unspeakable" do not encompass all posttraumatic conditions. It turns out that memories of traumatic events can indeed be painfully known and communicated, as in the case of an "undermodulated" limbic zone that produces intense emotional memories, material covered in Chapter 3. Further, McNally and Krystal add varying degrees of nuanced skepticism about the notion of the unknown nature of memories. Freud has stressed moreover that the effects of trauma linger in the body.[87] It is not that traumatic experiences cannot be known or spoken, it is rather that they are made known in ways that often involve the body, as psychologist Peter Levine, psychiatrist Bessel van der Kolk, and neurologist Robert Scaer have stressed in their research, as we shall learn in the next chapter.

The terms "unknown" and "unspeakable" are also "flat" in the sense of being uninspiring, if not demoralizing. Trauma survivors may feel dispirited to learn that knowledge of the traumatic event cannot be assimilated consciously. Such a position is "reminiscent of death rather than life" to return to Fanon's statement. Why should survivors attempt to heal themselves from the psychic suffering of a traumatic experience, if the unknown will remain forever unknown? And how can they rely on the tool of language employed in psychotherapy, as well as in literature, if traumatic experiences defy language? By failing to stress or even point out that nature and human existence are also defined by the unknown and the shortcomings of language, it makes it seem as if traumatic experiences are off limits to interpretative exercises. And yet, science and philosophy engage in investigations of the unknown, precisely because it appears off-limits.

Fanon's terms "flat" and "reminiscent of death rather than life" also come to mind when considering the First Wave's heavy reliance on psychoanalysis and its associated emphasis on melancholia and trauma. The overreliance on psychoanalysis highlights a profound paradox of the field. Have First Wave theorists forgotten that psychoanalysis is not just a theory of the mind but also a practice to help treat and even cure those suffering from mental disturbances? A fixation on melancholia and trauma might also have harmful psychological effects for trauma survivors. If melancholia is not seen as a creative opportunity, trauma subjects may feel that their condition is fixed eternally in melancholic and traumatic states, even though research has shown that most recover from traumatic experiences, as clinical scientists

George Bonanno and Erica Diminich remind us.[88] From a fixation on psychoanalysis to an overemphasis on melancholia and trauma, these trends are rooted in a cultural myopia, narrowly focused on Euro-American culture and a neglect to investigate other cultural perspectives on trauma and posttraumatic conditions.

In response to this cultural myopia, Second Wave cultural trauma theorists have sought to expand the field of investigation beyond Euro-American spheres, as well as to legitimize a new canon that includes non-Western literary works. Post-colonial theorists have helped to decolonize literature. A decolonization of literature also refers to a process by which authors smash the busts of the great authors from the West and chip away at the original marble. Kicked around and spat upon, the novel encapsulates the trauma of colonization and racism. Though it may encapsulate at first a trauma novel, it often undergoes a metamorphosis. It is written anew and has something novel to say about trauma and posttraumatic conditions, especially about resistance, resilience, and growth. Since these final topics have been surprisingly neglected by both First and Second Wave cultural theorists, we shall attempt to take a brush to canvas and expand upon the portraits and landscapes of these topics in the chapters that follow.

Even more surprising about recent cultural trauma studies research is the neglect to address an important question: How does literature "somehow get at trauma"?[89] Whether it is First or Second Wave cultural trauma theorists or whether it is scientists or clinicians, they only state or hint at a relationship between literature and trauma. Another question avoided is: How do the literary arts foster posttraumatic resistance, resilience, and growth? One can imagine that the literary arts and especially the "trauma novel" may have an important role to play in posttraumatic treatments. It could invent a survivor of trauma who knows a certain degree of healing as opposed to a victim who continues to dwell in a traumatic experience. Even if post-modernists might object that it is tantamount to naivety to investigate how literature "gets at trauma" or how it might aide survivors of trauma, it comes down to an ethical imperative to examine these topics. By integrating research from both the sciences and the humanities and by blending the boundaries between the portrait of cultural trauma studies with the landscapes of scientific trauma theories, we will propose a reworking and a transformation of the field, to return to van Gogh's comments on his landscapes.

Notes

1　Van Gogh, *Letters*, loc. 3395.
2　Ibid., loc. 5449.
3　Hartman, "Words," 214. His complete comment reads: "Trauma is generally defined as an experience that is not experienced, that resists or escapes consciousness."
4　See Chapter 2 for an amplified discussion of the bleak perspective of treating survivors of the Holocaust and particularly psychiatrist William Niederland's position.
5　Barel et al., "Surviving," 694.

6 Recall from our discussion in Chapter 2 that Hartman is of the opinion that "both in literary studies and in the field of public health a new awareness arises which is ethical as well as clinical. There is more listening, more hearing of words within words, and a greater openness to testimony." Hartman, "Traumatic," 541.

7 Historian Dominick LaCapra voices a critical view of history: "The style of a widespread approach to historiography, in its quest for ready readability, entertaining anecdotes, and classical balance, may in effect take the trauma out of trauma." LaCapra, Writing, loc. 62.

8 I am not suggesting that psychoanalysis is as scientific as neuroscience. However, it is incontestable that psychoanalysis has its roots in Charcot's investigative theater in Paris and Freud's clinical work in Vienna, and hence was originally scientific in nature. Whether the field is considered a science today is obviously open to debate.

9 Freud, Interpretation, 335.

10 Lacan, Écrits, 65.

11 Lacan stresses a "resistance of signification" inherent in the connection between signifier and signified. See ibid., 181.

12 Ibid., 50.

13 Breton, Manifesto, 26.

14 Hartman, "Traumatic," 550.

15 Ibid., 541.

16 Ibid., 541.

17 Felman and Laub, Testimony, 15.

18 Ibid.

19 Ibid.

20 Caruth, Unclaimed, 11.

21 Ibid., 8.

22 Ibid., 5.

23 Ibid., 3.

24 Ibid., 4.

25 Whitehead, Trauma, 5.

26 Caruth, Trauma, vii.

27 Jakobson, Huit, 39. The original reads: "aucun sentiment n'est si pur qu'il ne soit mêlé du sentiment contraire."

28 See Genette, Figures I, loc. 610.

29 My translation. The original reads: "la littérature est une cacographie intentionnelle." The term "cacographie" refers to poor writing that is either illegible or fails to conform to basic spelling or grammar rules.

30 Derrida, Dissemination, 3.

31 De Man, "Resistance," 3.

32 Ibid., 10.

33 Ibid.

34 Ibid.

35 Caruth, Unclaimed, 76.

36 Ibid.

37 Leys, Trauma, loc. 3572.

38 Hartman, "Traumatic," 537.

39 Ibid.

40 Ibid., 549.

41 Felman and Laub, Testimony, 15.

42 Ibid.

43 Ibid.

44 Felman and Laub, Testimony, 57.

45 LaCapra, Writing, 182.

46 Caruth, *Unclaimed*, 4 and 91.

47 LaCapra, *History*, 40 and 203.

48 Leys argues: "Indeed, as I show in chapters 7 and 8, van der Kolk and Caruth have materialized and literalized traumatic memory in ways that make it seem as if trauma stands outside all knowledge and all representation." Leys, *Trauma*, loc. 1773.

49 Regarding the prevalence of Caruth's work, Tom Toremans writes: "Rather than making Caruth's work obsolete or out of fashion, however, the very fact that trauma studies is time and again forced to return to its theoretical foundations in Caruth's articulation of Freudian psychoanalysis with de Manian deconstruction is testimony to its relevance for the further development of the field." Toremans, "Deconstruction," 65.

50 Hartman, "Words," 214.

51 Krystal and Krystal, *Integration*, 160.

52 Ibid.

53 See Herman, *Trauma*, 195.

54 See McNally, "Debunking," 817–820.

55 The issue of memory is rendered even more complex by the research findings of meta-analyses on the topic. Recall from Chapter 3 that Zoladz and Diamond emphasize that even though the hippocampus seems to be affected (pathologically) by stress, it is involved in producing traumatic memories.

56 The notion of the unknowable has certainly defined metaphysics. The dialectical position of knowing and not knowing is the very alpha and omega of philosophy. In his *Republic*, Plato wishes to speak about the Good. Yet, he appreciates that humankind can never understand its intrinsic nature. He therefore represents it as the sun, thus rendering the unknowable known. In more global terms, it is the metaphor that brings the incomprehensible into an approximation of comprehensibility. For example, the classical thinker Philo of Alexandria argues that "The well is presumably the symbol of knowledge, which is in all cases hidden and hard to discover" (Philo, *De Somniis*, I.) Philo's statement puts into sharp relief not only the art of employing metaphors, but also the idea that the price of knowledge is high, as it involves gritty application.

57 In his *Time and Being*, Martin Heidegger's underscores two basic points relevant for understanding the "unknowable" of trauma and for ontological or epistemological questions. Veiling is intrinsic to unveiling, while unveiling is always veiled with a subjective covering. The communicator is the magician who veils and unveils the model, while language serves as a curtain, veiling and unveiling. This suggests that language does not describe the world as it is, but as it is perceived. Jacob Bronowski explains: "And then we invent words like 'gravitation' or 'electrons,' which are just as much inventions as the worlds 'tree' and 'love'. They are just as real, but they are also just as much something which human beings put into their interpretation of the world" (Bronowski, *Origins*, 95). This suggests that gravitation and trees are not a thing, but a think. The world is the thinking subject as well as the object being thought about. The same self-referential issue surrounds a traumatic experience. It seems unknowable since the survivor is still wrapped up in it. The question therefore is: how does one separate the subject from the object? How can the survivor of trauma resolve the conundrum of trauma if she is wrapped up in the thick of it?

58 Many scientists treat science and mathematics as a language, as mathematician Jacob Bronowski reminds us in his book on the *Origins of Knowledge and Imagination*. Furthermore, scientists and mathematics use other languages—such as English—to write articles and books that communicate their empirical results and describe the world. One seminal article written in German was by Werner Heisenberg in 1927 on the "uncertainty principle." The field of quantum mechanics (the physics of sub-atomic particles) is defined by an impossibility to measure a

physical system without perturbing it. The nature of the momentum and the position of electrons remain undefined or ill-defined by the experiment because the experiment defines the electrons. And how and when the experiment perturbed them, remains undefined. In short, all languages collapse in on themselves. They fall constantly beyond the event horizon of meaning.

59 Freud, *Dream*, 127.
60 LaCapra, *Writing*, loc. 65.
61 Besides Hartman, Felman, and Caruth who rely on the Freudian concept of the unknown, Anne Whitehead and Suzette Henke, among others, have also built their trauma theories on it.
62 I am thinking most notably of Erich Fromm's attempts to read psychoanalytically the psychopathologies of collectivities. See Fromm, *Escape from Freedom*.
63 Luckhurst, *Trauma*, 210.
64 Vissier, "Trauma," 132.
65 Vissier "Decolonizing," 11.
66 Kristeva, *Soleil*, 13.
67 Ibid., 17.
68 Hartman, "Traumatic," 543–544.
69 Caruth, *Unclaimed*, 56.
70 I stress "originally," as Caruth has given signs more recently to being drawn to the topics of resilience, growth, healing, and cure. Although she might not write about these topics per se, she has provided a platform for them to be discussed. See her book of interviews with psychiatrists, psychologists, psychoanalysts, and cultural theorists *Listening to Trauma* (2014).
71 Craps and Buelens, "Introduction," 2.
72 Kurtz, "Introduction," 9.
73 Rothberg, "Decolonizing," 227.
74 Mengel and Borzaga, *Trauma*, xiii.
75 Ibid., xiv.
76 Shapiro, "Resilience," 119.
77 Cyrulnik, *Merveilleux*, loc. 139. My translation; the original reads: "*Le fait que la résilience n'ait pas été étudiée alors que tous les praticiens l'ont constatée en dit long sur notre culture …*"
78 Kleinman, *Illness*, 135.
79 Caruth alludes to "an ethical and political paralysis" in her *Unclaimed Experience* (1996). See Caruth, *Unclaimed*, 10.
80 Craps, *Postcolonial*, loc. 2373.
81 Andermahr, *Decolonizing*, 2.
82 I am referring to Hartman's research on British Romantic poetry.
83 Mutloatse, *Forced*, 5.
84 Fanon, *Wretched*, 173; Fanon, *Black*, 123.
85 Craps and Buelens, "Introduction," 5.
86 Fanon. *Wretched*, 161.
87 Writing about his hysterical patients, Freud concludes: "I am therefore inclined to think that their appearance was not due to the same psychical process as was that of the other symptoms, but is to be attributed to a secondary extension of that unknown condition which constitutes the somatic foundation of hysterical phenomena." Breuer and Freud, *Studies*, 45. Though the origin of the hysteria might have remained unknown cognitively, it was revealed through the body, a point that serves as an invitation to nuance the issue of the unknown.
88 See Bonanno and Diminich, "Annual," 382.
89 Again, I am borrowing the term "somehow can get at trauma" from Frank LaCapra and will explore it in detail in Chapter 6. See LaCapra, *Writing*, 153.

Part III

Treatments and Educations for Trauma Survivors

5 Clinical Treatments for Trauma Survivors

"The exploration of deeply altered selves and worlds is not one that can be fully made in a consulting room or office."[1] Thus reads a summative statement by the neurologist Oliver Sacks. These words could be applied to the deeply altered world and psyche of trauma survivors. But if posttraumatic treatments might take place beyond the consulting room or office, where might they occur? And what might they consist of? Sacks's comment and these questions invite us to imagine interdisciplinary treatments based on both the subjective experiences of patients and objective empirical data.

Let us recall from our discussion in Chapter 1 that Herman casts doubt on such a convergence of perspectives. She worries about the development of a more conventional period of scientific research that evades a contextual and integrated understanding of psychological trauma. "The very strength of the recent biological findings in PTSD," she postulates, "may foster a narrowed, predominantly biological focus of research."[2] Herman is not the only one to express concern about this biological focus. Neuroscientist Raymond Tallis coined the term "neuromania" to refer to a current tendency to understand emotional experiences and to describe them from a neurobiological perspective, as evidenced in the terms "neuro-ethics," "neuroaesthetics," and even "neuro-evolutionary literary criticism."[3] Once again, this trend is summed up poignantly as, "the rise of neurobiology is leading to a kind of reductionism in which mental states are reduced to brain states ... and the key dimensions of our humanness—language, culture, history—are ignored."[4] A Literary Arts Praxis, the creative concept advanced in the next chapter and illustrated in Part IV, aims to provide a counterweight to this biological reductionism and encourage scientists and clinicians to knit the cultural skeins of languages, literature, and philosophy into their research and practice.

Before introducing the core concept of a Literary Arts Praxis and how it might "get at trauma" in Chapter 6, it is necessary to put these concepts into a wider context. This chapter therefore provides a synthesis of clinical therapies for trauma survivors.[5] There are several treatments under the umbrella of pharmacotherapy and psychotherapy. Even though the former is widely employed to treat PTSD, we will focus our attention principally on

DOI: 10.4324/9781003284642-9

non-pharmacological methods to treat trauma survivors.[6] We sketch out first foundational treatments from Pierre Janet, Sigmund Freud, and Herman. From there, we examine two current clinical trends: cognitive behavioral therapy (CBT) and somatic-centered therapies. These treatments, rich in theories and methods inherited from psychoanalysis, behavioral psychology, neuropsychiatry, and non-Western cultural sources, will prod us to examine the newest trends in psychoanalysis. This summary of clinical methods to treat trauma survivors should reveal a holistic focus on the mind and body, as opposed to a strictly biologically centered one. It should also give proof of new trends that are moving away from the concept of psychopathologies and toward resilience, resistance, and growth fostered by creative activities.

Important Definitions: Posttraumatic Growth, Resilience, Resistance, and Recovery

To understand clinical methods designed to cultivate posttraumatic growth, resilience, resistance, and recovery, let us first define these terms. Posttraumatic growth (PTG) was coined in 1995 by psychologists Richard Tedeschi and Lawrence Calhoun.[7] (I stress that the term was coined then. Before scientific theories described posttraumatic growth, there were myths, stories, religion, plays, literature, and the fine arts depicting positive changes subsequent to traumatic experiences.) PTG consists of "positive psychological changes experienced as a result of the struggle with traumatic or highly challenging life circumstances."[8] The growth experience can involve cognitive, emotional, behavioral, and physical changes, and might include alterations to one's philosophy of life, relationships with others, and self-identity.[9] This transformation boils down to ego development and self-actualization, as survivors struggle to cope with emotional distress and intrusive ruminations; develop a sense of safety through a therapeutic alliance; gravitate toward deliberate and concerted ruminations; and disclose themselves through narratives or other creative processes.[10] Engaging in these processes might engender greater self-confidence and self-reliance, which could in turn promote a steeling effect to confront subsequent stress or adversity. In sum, and as meta-analyses have shown, "PTG tends to be related to increased positive mental health, reduced negative mental health, and better subjective physical health."[11]

Though there are culturally specific characteristics of PTG and though some researchers question its prevalence, it is not an anomaly.[12] Nor is it simply a self-deceptive way to cope with highly negative circumstances.[13] If PTG consists of positive transformations resulting from mental struggles with a traumatic event, is it the opposite of PTSD? "To place PTG and PTSD at opposing ends of a continuum is simplistic, erroneous, and does not account for the complexities of human response to trauma."[14] Trauma survivors can still experience positive mental growth, such as a greater understanding of the human condition, and yet suffer from PTSD. It is also important to stress that PTG is not synonymous with positive psychology. Even though they both emphasize patients' strengths and abilities, PTG differs fundamentally from positive psychology by acknowledging the inherent distresses and suffering of life. On a related note, PTG does not necessarily represent recovery, which is characterized by a return to pre-trauma levels of psychological states after moderate to severe disruptions that decline after the course of many months.[15] Research suggests that PTG and psychopathologies can occur simultaneously, thus indicating that the former should be viewed as a process not as a cemented outcome.

PTG, resilience, and resistance seem to have synergistic relationships. Before elaborating on this idea, it is necessary to define resilience and resistance (from a scientific perspective). The American Psychological Association defines resilience as "the process of adapting well to adversity, trauma, tragedy, threats or significant sources of stress—such as family and relationships problems, serious health problems, or workplace and financial stressor."[16] The Association's definition stresses that resilience is part and parcel to life, rather than an extraordinary trait. Referring to psychiatrist Michael Rutter's research, Tedeschi et al. define resilience as "the personal attribute or ability to bounce back from difficulty, or to resist the effects of difficulties without experiencing prolonged negative effects (Rutter, 1985)."[17] Their definition insinuates that resilience and resistance are different sides of the same coin. Resilience allows survivors to bounce back, whereas resistance involves pushing back.

Still, the term resilience merits further nuance. Psychologists Christine Agaibi and John Wilson explain that "the task of predicting resiliency is further complicated because there is no universally defined concept of what constitutes resilient behavior."[18] It can be defined on the one hand by an absence of prolonged stress responses (i.e., an absence of PTSD) or maladaptive coping mechanisms.[19] On the other hand, it can be characterized by other variables, such as support from others, more positive thinking than negative, ego-enhancement, flexibility of emotional regulation, adaptive flexibility, high self-esteem, and biological traits, such as genes, neurobehavioral development, and neural-plasticity.[20] Related to these factors is the varied nature of the original traumatic event. Different forms of resilience develop following chronic adversity, such as in childhood ("emergent resilience") versus acute traumatic events ("minimal-impact resilience").[21] Contrary to the considerable biological and psychological challenges caused by chronic adversity, acute traumatic events allow for more focused coping mechanisms. Consequently, the latter leads to "little or no lasting impact on functioning and a relatively stable trajectory of continuous healthy adjustment ..."[22] Does "healthy adjustment" constitute recovery? Psychologists George Bonanno and Erica Diminich refer to a "recovery trajectory." After a traumatic experience, "normal functioning temporarily gives way to threshold or sub threshold distress and psychopathology (depressive symptoms,

PTSD) for several months before gradually returning to pre-exposure levels."[23] Recovery is thus seen as a gradual return to psychological baseline with intermittent regressive states. This intimates that recovery is contingent on regression.

Whether we are speaking about recovery or resilience, their complexity is undeniable because they cannot be measured objectively. Research from neurologist Gang Wu and his colleagues also points to genetic factors that determine resilience.[24] What remains indisputable however is that resilience is the most common outcome post stressful events.[25] Psychiatrist and psychoanalyst Barbara Shapiro sums up the relationship between psychological distress, posttraumatic growth, and resilience:

> We see many severely traumatized people who come to us plagued with problems, who with help are better able to work, love, and play, although scars persist. That person's resilience makes him or her able to use the therapeutic opportunity for reflection and growth, and the growth then makes the person more resilient.[26]

From Shapiro's remarks, it becomes clear that a treatment challenge is the cultivation of resilience leading to growth and growth leading to resilience, despite (and perhaps even thanks to) the damaged state. There are shades and nuances of growth, resilience, and resistance in posttraumatic states. Regression also accompanies these states. Another important nuance is the state of dissociation, a mental constriction consisting of banishing traumatic memories and feelings from conscious awareness. It can represent both a positive as well as negative coping mechanism. While the topic of dissociation will be included in our discussions of different clinical treatment methods for posttraumatic conditions, it is important to acknowledge for now that it has been viewed as a creative form of therapy.[27] On a related note, Bonanno, stresses that resilience is the ability to engage in creative activities.[28] This is startling, as it intimates that trauma survivors' ability to bounce back is contingent upon creative engagements. An important topic to weave in and out of the synthesis that follows is whether creativity is part of treatment methods for trauma survivors.

Janet's and Freud's Treatment Methods

While Janet and Freud valued hypnosis to reach the traumatized, they understood its limitations, too. On the one hand, hypnosis could reproduce artificially in the investigative theater similar symptoms (sleepwalking and paralysis) caused by the original traumatic experience. It was essential to observe these symptoms, just as dreams of the night make manifest unconscious fears and desires. Trauma could then, perhaps, be resolved by safely replaying the events and constructing an imaginary acceptable conclusion. On the other hand, hypnosis could not explain why symptoms were so persistent. Thus, Janet developed a multi-prong treatment method. As explored in Chapter 2, he believed that the integration of traumatic memories was the most acute challenge trauma survivors faced. He focused therefore on helping patients to recover and integrate these memories into their entire personality. He created a "psychological analysis" consisting of two principal mechanisms: a form of mental catharsis (*une décharge*) of traumatic memories and a re-education of the mind.[29]

Before outlining Janet's treatment methods, it is important to stress that he voices reservations about using the term "*psychothérapie*" to refer to his work.[30] He questions if one can call his field of research "therapy" if both the naming of psychological troubles and the diagnoses remain so arbitrary and if all too often treatment methods prove ineffective.[31] Despite casting doubt on the therapeutic nature of his research, he makes clear that his vocational goal was to teach his patients how "to augment the use of their own resources and to enrich their own minds."[32] This is Janet the professor, teacher, and mentor making a pronounced statement about how he views his role as a physician.

Writing about Jean-Martin Charcot's patients in his *L'automatisme psychologique* (1889), Janet refers to how they needed a "*longue rééducation.*"[33] What does he mean by the expression "long re-education"? He describes how in the case of one patient, "her motor education had already been under way for quite some time because she suffered from hysteria, a type of psychological instability."[34] These comments can lead us to conclude that hysteria is a pathological type of autodidacticism. It is a self-induced "re-education" of the body and mind in the form of convulsions and phobias to address the underlying fall-out of the original traumatic event(s). Janet's reliance on the term "re-education" seems to stem from another reason. He considers his traumatized patients as mentally deficient. They are not exactly demented, but they suffer from a retraction (*rétrécissement*) of conscious awareness.[35] On a related note, he portrays hysteria as a personality disorder (*maladie de la personnalité*) that requires a refashioning.[36] Another possible reason why Janet appears beholden to the concept of a re-education is found in the term's etymology. The French word "*éducation*" stems from the Latin word "*educatio,*" which first referred to raising or training animals and then to forming minds. Janet employs the term in the sense of retraining the mind by regular mental work, which today would be called "ergotherapy." Referring to Janet's form of therapy, psychiatrist Karl-Ernst Bühler and psychologist Gerhard Heime claim that its basic idea "is to train higher tendencies, to broaden the field of consciousness, and to enable it to take in several ideas simultaneously as well as to synthesize them or oppose one another."[37] Contemplating a wide horizon of ideas? Synthesizing material? Pondering antithetical ideas with the goal of promoting keener conscious awareness? These exercises imply that the process of recovery and the integration of traumatic memories is facilitated by cognitive exercises and by a discharge of emotions and memories, as we shall discover below.[38]

According to psychologists Onno van der Hart et al., Janet's treatment model is organized into three-phases designed to retrieve, explore, and modify traumatic memories gradually.[39] The first stage consists of promoting patient stabilization and symptom reduction. A simplification of lifestyle, isolation, and rest are encouraged. A therapeutic alliance based on a special and safe "rapport" between therapist and patient is simultaneously built. Though convinced of the importance of patients heeding the advice of their therapists to break the spell of hallucinations, Janet cautioned against employing suggestions to patients: "If it is possible to heal a subject through suggestion, he remains sick ..."[40] What does he mean by the term "suggestion"? Psychologist Edna Foa illuminates his use of the term by writing: "Hypnosis is a procedure generally established by an induction, during which suggestions for alterations in behavior and mental processes including sensations, perceptions, emotions, and thoughts are provided."[41] Contrary to hypnosis therapies, Janet built his treatment method on an educational method with a mentor-mentee relationship as its cornerstone. Clinicians give words of encouragement, incentives, and exercises to strengthen cognitions, such as concentrated attention and self-reflection. He summed up such procedures as: "The best methods are those that cause the assimilation of the exciting emotion, that bring the subject to comprehend ... it by reflection, to react against it correctly and to resign himself to it."[42] In Janet's playbook, reflection is a form of mental gymnastics as one stays keenly attentive, reacting against and ignoring various thoughts and emotions. Following the footsteps of his mentor Charcot, Janet also employed hypnosis in the stabilization stage to promote relaxation and to address insomnia.

In the second stage, trauma subjects are encouraged to identify, explore, and modify dissociated traumatic memories. These memories inhabit the subconscious and are often in a fixed state, emerging inadvertently as behaviors, emotional states, physical sensations, and dreams.[43] While these vestiges of traumatic events remain in the unconscious or appear in dissociated forms, the survivor's personality remains arrested.[44] However, "in uncomplicated cases, traumatic memories and the psychological charge associated with them were 'near the surface' and often available to non-trance interventions."[45] Such interventions included discussions of survivors' experiences or journaling to cultivate resolution. Another prominent feature of Janet's treatment method consisted of "discharge exercises" such as confessions, religious absolutions, reconciliations, and victories.[46] Janet stressed however that these processes of liquidating traumatic memories and the energy associated with keeping "fixed ideas" hidden should be an intense act of discharging the tension of the original trauma.[47] Once traumatic memories begin to surface, he followed up with substitution techniques, such that neutral or positive images replace traumatic memories.

In the third stage, trauma subjects seek to abate residual symptoms and prevent further ones from developing. Most importantly, they work on rehabilitating the personality, which refers to rebuilding a solid and stable sense of self through the acquisition of new psychological wisdom and engagement in social activities.[48] This translates not so much into another phase of treatment, but a new phase of life. This may very well be the moment to introduce a Literary Arts Praxis, a cognitive training to unfold in the next chapter.

As outlined previously, Freud believed at least in theory that traumatic reminiscences could be excavated from the strata of the unconscious by engaging in psychoanalysis, the talking cure. The patient freely associates, exposing memories by sharing what randomly comes to mind. The patient is also invited to abreact, to explore phobias, daydreams, fantasies, and wishes. Freud remained pessimistic however about healing traumatic neuroses. He argued that unconscious desires are "indestructible" and that "nothing can be brought to an end in the unconscious; nothing can cease or be forgotten."[49] His use of superlative words "indestructible," "nothing can be brought to an end," "nothing can cease or be forgotten" highlights both his conviction of the strength of traumatic psychopathology and his pessimism about effective treatments for trauma survivors.

Often reproached for his failure to address traumatic war experiences, Freud confessed to his inability to bring war veterans' suffering into his hypotheses.[50] What was at stake in war traumatic neuroses went well beyond his research, as this excerpt from his *Civilization and Discontents* (1930) intimates:

> No matter how much we may shrink with horror from certain situations—of a galley-slave in antiquity, of a peasant during the Thirty Years' War, of a victim of the Holy Inquisition, of a Jew awaiting a pogrom—it is nevertheless impossible for us to feel our way into such people—to divine the changes which original obtuseness of mind, a gradual stupefying process, the cessation of expectations, and cruder or more refined methods of narcotization have produced upon their receptivity to sensations of pleasure and unpleasure. Moreover, in the case of the most extreme possibility of suffering, special mental protective devices are brought into operation. It seems to me unprofitable to pursue this aspect of the problem any further.[51]

Freud is pointing to an impossibility to "feel our way into" the suffering of extreme situations of trauma, such as wars, inquisitions, and pogroms. Between the complexity of "special protective devices," such as an "obtuseness of mind" and a "cessation of expectations," he humbly relinquishes his pursuit of the issue of war traumatic neurosis. If one reflects upon his very definition of trauma, one senses this same degree of humble surrender: "The traumatic experience is one which, in a very short time, is able to increase the strength of a given stimulus so enormously that its assimilation, or rather its elaboration, can no longer be effected by normal means."[52] What does he mean by "the traumatic experience can no longer be effected by normal means"? What is normal? What is abnormal? This ambiguous definition and his failure to address traumatic war neuroses—owing to their existential and moral complexity—lead us to wonder if the father of psychoanalysis projected a deleterious message to clinicians and survivors. This question is based (in some respects) on Wu and his colleagues' research on positive emotions. They argue that optimism, an expectation for positive outcomes, "has been consistently associated with the employment of active coping strategies, subjective well-being and larger and more fulfilling social networks and connections ..."[53] While Freud's pessimism about recovery of survivors of extreme forms of trauma may be warranted in theory, it might have psychologically poisoned survivors, such that they could not employ coping strategies. Furthermore, cultural trauma theorists latched on to Freud's pessimistic viewpoint and seem to have injected the field with a toxic dose of doom.

Herman's Three-Step Recovery Process

Herman appears to rely on Janet's model as a blueprint to construct her own three-step recovery method. Her process consists of: cultivating a sense of safety; embarking on a process of remembrance, mourning, and telling one's story; and re-establishing connections with others.[54] A sense of safety is created first through a therapeutic alliance in which therapist and patient engage in the task of recovery. Aiming to reestablish trust, autonomy, competence, initiative, identity, and intimacy, the team creates a sense of safety by emphasizing care of the body. In cases of acute trauma, the survivor focuses on reducing hyperarousal and intrusive symptoms to restore biological rhythms of resting, sleeping, and eating. In cases of prolonged trauma, the subject concentrates on the integrity of the body, such as regulation of basic needs and functions (sleeping, eating, and exercising), management of symptoms, and self-destructive behaviors. These strategies seem to help the survivor cultivate a vital sense of personal jurisdiction.

Once a sense of safety is cultivated through a "therapeutic alliance" (a relationship of trust between psychotherapist and patient) and a nurtured body, the subject is encouraged to revisit the traumatic event. This is a second stage of remembrance and grieving and focuses on the survivor's narrative. "This work of reconstruction actually transforms the traumatic memory, so that it can be integrated into the survivor's life story."[55] During repeated attempts, the survivor expresses her bodily experiences, sensations, emotions, and mental images, while the psychotherapist assumes a role of an ally and witness who helps the trauma survivor to speak the unspeakable.[56] Herman stresses in fact the importance of feeling emotions while narrating a trauma story: "The recitation of facts without the accompanying emotions is a sterile exercise, without therapeutic effect."[57] Building upon emotions as the backbone of narratives, she developed a three-step narrative process of the traumatic experience.[58] The survivor first describes her dreams, relationships, and struggles before the traumatic experience. She then narrates the traumatic event in as much factual detail as possible.[59] Since the most unbearable moments might escape narration, the survivor is invited to employ nonverbal methods to communicate, such as drawing. Herman concludes that since traumatic memories are often visual, drawing appears to be the most efficient initial mechanism to capture indelible images.[60] The goal is for survivors to narrate the original event followed by an enumeration of their associated bodily sensations and imagery. Their story is not only spoken, but also felt, sensed, heard, and understood gradually by the body and mind. The survivor is then encouraged to interpret more deeply her trauma story and to act on it.[61] She might analyze moral issues of guilt and responsibility to make sense of her undeserved pain. The story process is complete, provided it is coupled with action, including grieving and public testimony. The survivor mourns the self that was tainted and even destroyed by the event(s). She makes her narrative public by providing a testimony, a private confession and/or a public political statement. "After many repetitions, the moment comes when the telling of the trauma story no longer arouses quite such intense feeling ... The story is a memory like other memories, and it begins to fade as other memories do."[62] This is an important assertion, for it calls into question the notion that memories are somehow immutable, ill-defined, and permanent. Although the reconstruction of the traumatic experience will remain incomplete, as the survivor is constantly changing, the traumatic event often ceases to be the most important part of the survivor's life and story.[63] Indeed, once the original traumatic event(s) and associated emotional experiences fade into the past, the survivor can reimagine her present life and construct her future.

This brings us to Herman's third stage of recovery, connection.[64] As the trauma begins to recede into the past, intimate connections with others can be cultivated. Venturing into wider circles and sharing her story, the survivor may connect with other survivors. New connections form as well within the subject herself. A multidimensional self has developed: the victim, the survivor, and the narrator. The subject now strives to cultivate an "ideal self." This "involves the active exercise of imagination and fantasy, capacities that have now been liberated."[65] These imaginative acts help to determine recovery, for the survivor-narrator eventually takes the place of the therapist or close friends or family members. The survivor becomes not only her own therapist, but also a philosopher, theologian, writer, and/or storyteller.[66] In short, she creates a therapeutic environment where "fantasy can be given free rein," while serving as "a testing ground for the translation of fantasy into concrete action."[67] The terms "fantasy can be given free rein," "translation of fantasy into concrete action," and "capacities for imagination and play" make clear not only Herman's endorsement of cognitive exercises, such as telling one's story imaginatively, but also that the survivor can potentially experience a marvelous expanded sense of being. Though quick to point out that no "treatment is absolute or final," she emphasizes that these creative exercises are pivotal to posttraumatic growth just as cognitive exercises and a sense of self-reliance are key to healing in Janet's educational model.[68]

Cognitive Behavioral Therapies

Cognitive behavioral therapy (CBT) has practically become a household term. The psychiatrist Aaron Beck developed cognitive therapy (the original name) in the 1970s in response to idiosyncrasies prevalent in other psychotherapies (traditional neuropsychiatry, psychoanalysis, and behavior therapy).[69] If psychoanalysis attempts to heal neuroses by excavating thoughts, fears, and desires buried in the unconscious realm; if behavior therapy seeks to alter emotional and behavioral disorders through external stimuli, including punishments and rewards; and if neuropsychiatry employs somatic therapies, such as the administration of drugs and electroconvulsive therapy to "counter-condition" behavior, then patients' attempts to use their own problem-solving mechanisms, including common sense and intuition, were undermined, according to Beck.[70] These therapies, he concludes, give patients the impression that they cannot help themselves and must rely on a professional therapist to address even everyday stressors. This is not to suggest that CBT severed itself completely from psychoanalysis, behavioral therapy, or neuropsychiatry. On the contrary, from psychoanalysis it borrowed an emphasis on insight, a cognitive process that attempts to identify hidden feelings, thoughts, and desires and their connections. From the behaviorists, it inherited a focus on learning and from neuropsychiatrists, it assumed an interest in somatic reactions, especially during a third wave of CBT centering on the body. The basic premise of CBT is that emotional disturbances develop from learned responses.[71] If they are learned, then they can be modified by exercises, at least in theory.

How does the therapist–patient alliance develop an environment where patients can learn to comprehend their emotions, thoughts, and behaviors and modify them accordingly?[72] While CBT is in some respects based on the three antecedent therapies, it distinguishes itself by stressing the development of patient problem-solving skills. It cultivates habits of the mind (similar to Janet's education model) that patients can practice without a therapist once the formal treatment is complete. The patient is therefore instructed first about CBT (psychoeducation) in preparation for her assuming the role of self-therapist. The initial exercises involve data gathering on the patient, which often means that the patient is invited off the couch, as it were, to fill out questionnaires on paper or on a white board with the therapist. The goal is for the therapist-and-patient team to pinpoint problems and objectives readily. Therapists then engage patients in exercises to foster conscious awareness of their thoughts, emotions, behaviors, and physiology. Patients are encouraged to keep a mood log, so that their thoughts, emotions, and bodily sensations become clearer. They also engage gradually in daunting behaviors while tracking their cognitive, emotional, and somatic reactions. The key is for patients to unveil the mysterious nature of their being. Or better yet, it is essential for them to understand that the nature of their emotions, thoughts, behavior, and bodily reactions can be made known and understood, provided they engage in cognitive exercises. After assuming these habits of mind, patients begin to discover their warped thinking, misunderstandings, and automatic responses that cause emotional disturbances and then concentrate on altering them.

Exposure therapy (ET) or flooding is a trauma-focused form of CBT. Building on a therapeutic alliance, the therapist and patient engage in three principal steps: psychoeducation, exposure to the traumatic event, and cognitive restructuring. Exposure therapy is designed to address defective thinking in PTSD sufferers. According to Edna Foa, their pathological cognitions take this form: "'The world is an utterly dangerous place,' and 'I am completely incompetent and unable to cope with stress.'"[73] During imagined exposure in a clinical setting, patients re-encounter the traumatic event (s) in their minds and bodies and recount (verbally) associated images, emotions, and sensations. In the case of live exposure, patients confront real stimulations, which can occur in concentrated or gradual ways. The goal of both forms of exposure therapies is to dampen the automatic emotional responses to traumatic stimuli. "By learning that nothing 'bad' will happen during a traumatic event, the patient experiences less anxiety when confronted by stimuli related to the trauma and reduces or eliminates avoidance of feared situations."[74] Several studies indicate that exposure can have a "substantial therapeutic effect on reducing intrusive and cue-related arousal symptoms in PTSD."[75] Furthermore, exposure therapy can help to address fear and anxiety but does not seem to abate guilt or other complex emotions.[76] This form of therapy presents further drawbacks. When one experiences prolonged exposure either virtually or in vivo, the body and brain can experience distress that matches the original trauma, according to neurologist Robert Scaer.[77] He warns as well that "without a concomitant and external environment that incorporates a sense of safety and empowerment, the victim may move immediately into the freeze/dissociation response."[78] Foa and her colleagues respond to this concern by addressing the issue of emotions. To their mind, the topic of emotions is the cornerstone of trauma survivor treatments. They explain: "Trauma theorists have postulated that emotional engagement with traumatic memory is a necessary condition for successful processing of the event and resultant recovery."[79] Conversely, "dissociating from awareness of the traumatic memories and emotions in the immediate aftermath of trauma can impede processing of these reactions and thereby lead to subsequent PTSD (Spiegel, 1994) ..."[80] Since the use of exposure therapy can pose risks to trauma survivors by exciting emotions, Foa and her team highlight that patients can be prepared to engage in this therapy by teaching them "skills in distress tolerance, labeling emotions, and emotion management."[81] While research findings suggest that CBT is no elixir for PTSD sufferers, they do indicate that cognitive therapies may still serve as important starting points in the challenges of posttraumatic recovery.

Psychologist Marylene Cloitre and her colleagues have developed more recently a dual cognitive-behavioral treatment for trauma survivors of chronic interpersonal trauma called STAIR/NT. The acronym stands for "Skills Training in Affective and Interpersonal Relations" and "Narrative Therapy" and is outlined in their second-edition book *Treating Survivors of Childhood Abuse and Interpersonal Trauma* (2020). STAIR focuses on the present and the cultivation of social and emotional resources, whereas NT centers on the past and the resolution of traumatic memories. The program first helps survivors to acknowledge and comprehend their trauma through exposure and cognitive reappraisal. It also includes "strategies for identifying the implicit interpersonal schemas that guide beliefs, feelings, and behaviors, and revising them through reappraisal processes and the use of role play to facilitate new learning and behavioral changes."[82]

The NT module of treatment centers on recalling traumatic memories to find meaning and to integrate experiences into a life story that aims to foster a coherent sense of self. In light of this focus, NT resembles a literature class, one might argue. "The client then identifies feelings that emerged from the telling, including what parts of the story elicited these feelings and how intense they were. Therapist and client then listen to the recording together."[83] The client interprets her story as if she were studying a piece of literature, while the clinician-professor monitors the client's interpretative reactions. This is followed by the client listening to a recorded version of her story on her own, perhaps in her home. What Cloitre and her colleagues have found from this narrative process is that "clients experience a range of reactions, many of which appear unavailable when they are engaged in the actual narration. These often include sympathy for themselves and curiosity—as if they are experiencing themselves as people with histories and with interesting stories to tell."[84] This finding is monumental, as it suggests that the trauma survivor can reach herself and her traumatic experience through an emotional and cognitive distance. The person who narrates is not the person who is the object of the narration. It is almost as if the trauma survivor needs to see herself as another—a tragic character in a story—before she can begin to gain conscious awareness about herself. Even though Cloitre and her team do not state explicitly that NT is a creative enterprise, it is obvious that it beckons creative interpretations from the trauma survivor. Curiously, they write that, "Lastly, the client's ability to 'follow their feelings' can ignite a sense of creativity and self-appreciation that may never have emerged or may have been lost a long time ago."[85] But they do not stress that the act of listening to one's life and trauma story can also be a creative enterprise. Seen in this light, this is an innovative form of therapy that could incite new imaginative treatments and trainings.

Once a narrative begins to form, the client and therapist can explore more profoundly a sense of individual identity around other themes that weigh upon survivors of interpersonal trauma: shame and betrayal, loss and grief. Shame is a particularly difficult topic to explore for survivors of chronic interpersonal trauma, because "the ensuing feelings of shame often serve as self-confirmation of their own wrongdoing, creating a vicious cycle."[86] However, that cycle may possibly be broken as the client listens to her story with her therapist or on her own and is able to reinterpret the emotions, shunning shame. In fact, the client is invited to participate in exercises in which she can practice alternative reactions. Again, she is trained to think and to feel differently (creatively) and in ways that allow her to edit her life story even more.

Levine's, van der Kolk's, and Scaer's Body-Centered Therapies

Although the somatic-centered therapies of Peter Levine, Bessel van der Kolk, and Robert Scaer borrow from Janet's, Herman's, and Beck's emphasis on establishing a sense of safety and calm, they focus principally on the storage and release of traumatic memories from the body. Another way to understand their focus is to say that Levine, van der Kolk, and Scaer are interested in implicit or procedural memories of the traumatic event. By this, I mean that they concentrate first on how our bodies react, without us being consciously aware of phenomena.

What is the logic behind a somatic-centered perspective? A most obvious answer is that emotions are not psychological reactions existing exclusively in the intercranial space between our ears. They are somatic states animating our entire being. In the field of investigation, the body of the traumatized subject appears in four possible states: hyperarousal; constriction; dissociation; and freezing (immobility) coupled with a sense of helplessness. These four reactions occur first. Other symptoms develop subsequently "if the defensive energy mobilized to respond to a traumatic event is not discharged or integrated within a few days, weeks, or months following the experience."[87] The key terms from this statement are: "if the defensive energy mobilized" and "is not discharged or integrated." The trio of body-centered scientists has explained what is at stake for trauma survivors by referring to other animals' fight–flight–freeze phenomenon. It makes sense to ponder this response, since traumatic events are based on real or perceived threats to life and are closely associated with basic survival reactions. These responses principally involve the activation of both branches of the autonomic nervous system (parasympathetic and sympathetic) and of the somatic musculature. Once a gazelle escapes a pack of lions, it will literally shake off the excess energy from the stressful event. This action resets its nervous system. Humans are anomalies. We do not automatically discharge the energy used to protect ourselves through the states of hyperarousal, constriction, dissociation, and freezing. What is the upshot? The fight–flight–

freeze messages continue to fire even once the danger has evaporated. A continued secretion of stress hormones translates into feelings of agitation and panic and in the long run wreaks havoc on both the mind and body. This phenomenon of a truncated freeze discharge "appears to be the physiological event that initiates the central nervous system changes leading to posttraumatic stress disorder."[88] In addition, this heightened physical state accompanies a mental one defined by compulsive and terrifying flashbacks, kindred to reliving the trauma. It follows therefore that since the original traumatic event reverberates in the body as excess energy, it is imperative to employ treatments to unleash that energy from the body carrying the burden of the original trauma.

Before describing the nature of body-centered treatments, let us review another argument for somatic approaches. The immediate reaction (fight–flight–freeze) to a traumatic event is not the only way the body is implicated. The body is involved in posttraumatic states that involve a unique form of memories. I am not referring here to the notion that memories of traumatic events remain unknowable or in clinical jargon, "fragmented and poorly integrated."[89] As discussed in Chapter 3, there is evidence indicating that traumatic memories can be "overly integrated."[90] I am referring instead to the fact that traumatic memories are often characterized by physical sensations and intense negative emotions such as rage, fear, shame, collapse. These responses are neurological and physiological and are difficult to alter. Because these revisited experiences feel overwhelming, subjects tend to avoid them directly. They psychologically split off or dissociate their sensations and feelings. Their bodies tighten as they fight them off. Physical sensations and emotional feelings that are not registered consciously require a formidable amount of energy to keep at bay.[91] This constitutes a form of "acting in" as opposed to "acting out."[92] That is, the trauma survivor internalizes defensive mechanisms. And yet, neglected sensations and feelings demand attention. Body treatments aim to address these pressing needs.

What are body-centered treatments and how do they function? Levine advances his own program called Somatic Experiencing®, whereas van der Kolk and Scaer provide a synthesis of body-centered therapies. In all approaches, it is a question of listening first and foremost to the body's voice by tracking inner sensations and learning new responses to them. Levine's somatic exercises zero in on a decelerated, concentrated, and mindful attention to subtle inner sensations and movements.[93] This acute sense of the self allows trauma subjects to become acquainted with their bodies' mechanisms and messages in general. Once the body's primeval sensations have emerged into consciousness, subjects can concentrate on ignored sensations—such as freezing, helplessness, and rage—and become consciously aware of them. With the help of a clinician, subjects vacillate between acceptance and resistance, exploration and fear of sensations. This process helps to cultivate a sense of agency while shedding armors that have protected against immobility, vulnerability, and fear. What is the upshot of this therapy?

> This back-and-forth switching of attention (between the fear/resistance and the unadulterated physical sensations of immobility) deepens relaxation and enhances aliveness. It is the beginning of hope and the acquiring of tools that will empower her as she begins to navigate the interoceptive (or the direct felt experiencing of viscera, joints and muscles) landscape of trauma and healing. These skills lead to a core innate transformative process: pendulation.[94]

The term "pendulation" refers to the process of gently moving in and out of accessing inner sensations and traumatic memories. The idea is that before trauma subjects can explore head on their traumatic memories, they need to build internal resources (such as confidence and compassion) that allow them to feel safe as they access bodily sensations and emotions. Thus, the treatment's goal is to become familiar with the fundamental workings of the body: not only to grow consciously aware of its pathologies and sufferings but also to learn to rely on its healing mechanisms. And finally, by developing conscious awareness of one's sensations, one can gently discharge the energy that other animals, such as the gazelle, discharge naturally.

Fundamentally related to Levine's Somatic Experiencing® method, van der Kolk's treatments consist of specific exercises that allow for better access to one's basic bodily sensations and eventually to the stored-up energy of the original traumatic event. Van der Kolk endorses a "bottom-up" therapy, as opposed to a "top-down" (cognitive) format. Bottom-up methods seek to alter the survivor's physiology and her relationship to bodily sensations. Targeting the body's viscera, the survivor is invited off the couch, so to speak, and to engage in rhythmic exercises. These include breathing exercises (pranayama), chanting, drumming, singing, dancing, and the martial arts. He refers to yoga as a "major cornerstone in our understanding that it is imperative to befriend one's bodily sensations to overcome the imprints of trauma."[95] These non-pharmacological and non-Western practices rely on rhythms and breathing to help calm somatic reactions. In brief, they help to re-educate the body and mind to feel and interpret physical sensations, so that survivors can eventually discharge the stored-up energy from the original traumatic event and prepare for future events.

Related to these rhythmic therapies, van der Kolk encourages survivors to participate in theater programs. What is the link between trauma survivors and the therapeutic potential of drama? The psychiatrist stresses that survivors are often afraid of feeling "deeply," for emotions can thwart a sense of control.[96] Theatrical performances conversely are about embodying feelings and giving them a voice. Drama exercises also encourage survivors to become rhythmically attuned with others and assume different roles, both psychologically and physically. Since drama centers so often on conflicts, survivors who perform in plays can experiment with fictional conflicts as well. This may in turn help them decipher and master their own emotions. Related to this issue of engaging in conflicts on stage, theater performances consist of exploring ways to convey truths to the audience. "This requires pushing through blockages to discover your own truth, exploring and examining your own internal experience so that it can emerge in your own voice and body on stage."[97] Finally, by taking on character roles, survivors can experience a new identity, a potential first step to shedding the constricting identity of the trauma "victim."

Similar to Levine and van der Kolk, Scaer emphasizes the importance of accessing somatic forms of traumatic procedural memories. And like his colleagues, he advocates visual, tactile, or auditory stimulation to recreate the traumatic event, while other exercises such as incantations, humming songs, or counting aloud are employed to soothe the body. Scaer endorses additionally the use of "kinesiology, a technique related to concepts of Eastern medicine, acupuncture meridians, and the flow of 'energy' within the body."[98] In 1989, psychologist Francine Shapiro developed a successful treatment method for PTSD sufferers called EMDR (eye movement desensitization and reprocessing). She discovered that moving one's eyes rapidly while contemplating an arousal-based memory dampened the anxiety associated with that memory for an extended period.[99] EMDR consists of identifying a traumatic memory and expressing a personal negative thought ("I feel ashamed"), which is then transformed into a positive one ("I am honorable"). The therapist waves her fingers before the patient's face a dozen times, while the patient follows the movement and concentrates on the traumatic memory. After each session, the therapist assesses the patient's distress level regarding the traumatic memory and the newly formed positive thoughts. The technique aims to improve the speed of processing information and the transformation of traumatic memories. To Scaer's mind, EMDR and other treatments described above serve as templates for future therapeutic models for trauma survivors, because "they represent a somatically based reflexive approach to a condition characterized by the predominantly unconscious perpetuation of conditioned neural responses that inevitably contain somatic cues."[100] Conversely, while cognitive therapies might be effective for some PTSD victims, they often do not address the underlying somatic feature of dissociation, and this might be why both CBT and psychoanalysis have added body-centered treatments to their methods.

New Trends in Psychoanalysis: Creative Therapies

Within the last twenty years, the field of psychoanalytic trauma studies has undergone its own analysis and has begun to question "the prevailing view in the field of trauma psychology [that] is weighted toward psychopathology rather than a more balanced understanding of the human capacity to cope with tragedy."[101] Psychoanalyst and psychologist Sophia Richman provides a check-up of the field by underscoring the disturbing trend to view subjects as forever damaged and to dismiss humans' capacity to cope with traumatic experiences. She asserts, "the problem with the widespread assumption (Laub & Auerhahn, 1989, and others) that catastrophic trauma destroys the ability to represent, symbolize, and integrate experience is that it does not hold up to scrutiny ..."[102] Simultaneous to a rejection of bleak views of trauma survivors, many psychoanalysts are now focusing on coping mechanisms and positive outcomes.

The themes of resistance, resilience, and growth once enjoyed much attention in psychoanalysis when associated with the topic of engaging in the arts. For some humanist psychoanalysts like Abraham Maslow and Donald Winnicott, creativity is the very essence of human existence. To Maslow's mind, art is not a question of having a purpose. It is rather intrinsic to the human experience. Art allows us to experience life more intensely and wholly.[103] Winnicott focuses on the experiences of children and puts forward that playing is a creative experience; it is a basic way of life. "Without play the child is unable to see the world creatively, and in consequence is thrown back on compliance and a sense of futility, or on the exploitation of direct instinctual satisfactions."[104] Creative play therefore becomes the very lifeblood of children. For other psychoanalysts, the creative process represents humanity's capacity for transformative change. The psychoanalyst Otto Rank sums up this idea most succinctly, "the artist not only creates his art, but also uses art in order to create."[105] And the creation of one's essence is a form of artwork. Nodding to Freud, Jung felt that art was a way to become acquainted with the unconscious realm. He writes about a patient who takes up painting and falls on "good terms with his unconscious."[106] This self-knowledge leads to (according to Jung) a heightened sense of self-confidence and social adeptness. Maslow, Winnicott, Rank, and Jung point to how human existence is at various stages and in various ways intimately tied to the arts.

Echoing Laub, Hartman, Felman, and Caruth to a certain degree, Richman proposed that engaging in the arts may help trauma survivors to form a testimony of their traumatic experiences.[107] She explains: "Art as a means of communication has the potential to reconnect the trauma survivor to others. It is immensely curative to feel known and recognized when one has felt alone and isolated."[108] Boris Cyrulnik expands on this idea by employing evocative vocabulary: "In all these cases, the feeling of selfhood, which is shaped by the gaze of others, can be reshaped and reworked by representations, actions, commitments, and narratives."[109] The self is "reshaped" and "reworked" through artistic acts? Cyrulnik prods us to envision the trauma survivor as a sculptor re-working the clay of her damaged identity and transforming it into a treasured ceramic to be displayed on a pedestal.

Richman and Cyrulnik have pulled back the curtain on the artist's workshop and revealed two explanations about how the artistic process might "work" for trauma victims. First since art is defined by symbols, it offers an indirect way to encounter emotions that may feel less threatening and hence more inviting. Symbols encapsulate feelings and physical sensations that the artist and viewer fail to confront head on. Richman sums up this process: "art can stimulate and assimilate potentially dangerous degrees of affect, thereby extending the limits of what is bearable, allowing processive integration within the safe holding presence of aesthetic structure."[110] Art thus bears the burden of trauma. The unknowns are made known in the stigmata of art, so to speak. It can liberate the body and mind from trauma-induced sensations and ill-defined emotions.

The artistic process for the trauma victim is also linked to dissociation, which may provide a conducive state to form a new story of trauma and a new identity.[111] "It is my contention here," writes Richman provocatively, "that dissociation is an integral part of the creative process, an essential aspect of making art, and is sometimes also experienced by the observer viewing artistic products and performances."[112] Dissociative states help facilitate artistic creations in two fundamental ways. They can serve as a source of inspiration. When reality is dismal and dark, daydreams can cast rays of hope that illuminate the way. Speaking about trauma survivors, Cyrulnik elaborates on this idea: "Their inner representations sometimes allow them to experience a great feeling of beauty, even though the real world around them is dreadful."[113] Furthermore, since the survivor is not perturbed by the distress of reality and inspired by her own therapeutic dreams, she might feel free to craft her trauma story anew. The victim of trauma becomes a survivor who changes her memories into a socially acceptable piece of artwork, rather than allowing it to fester in a pathological state of unconscious conflicts. It is important to point out that even though dissociation might offer "a means of mental escape at the moment when no other escape is possible, it may be that this respite from terror is purchased at far too high a price."[114] Simultaneous to a feeling that dissociation may be a dear price to pay for rest, Herman has held the position that it could turn out to be "a creative and adaptive psychological defense against overwhelming terror."[115] Thus, even if the trauma survivor might erase from her conscious mind the original traumatic event, the maladaptive strategy of dissociation ironically seems to render growth possible as the trauma survivor begins to take charge of constructing her own therapeutic story.

Though it may seem unrealistic to expect most trauma survivors to craft a socially "acceptable" piece of artwork, it is important to signal the established form of posttraumatic treatment called "art therapy." While Richman and Cyrulnik have looked under the hood of how the arts might help trauma survivors, research has been conducted to investigate how art therapy (drawing, painting, and pottery) fosters PTG. As reported by Michele Wood et al., it has been employed to manage stress symptoms and to ease psychological adjustment after traumatic experiences and was found effective mostly in younger populations.[116] Art therapy serves therefore as another tool in the clinician's toolbox. Combined with psychoanalysis, cognitive behavioral therapies, somatic-based therapies, and psychopharmacology, art therapy may very well offer trauma survivors alternative methods that suit their creative needs and artistic passions.

Recent Research Findings on Best Methods to Treat Posttraumatic Conditions

Many clinicians believe that Cognitive Behavioral Therapy is the most effective treatment for both PTSD and complex-PTSD; however, the evidence is inconclusive. On the one hand, Roger Pitman et al. in their 2012 article conclude that CBT is a most effective treatment.[117] Scaer elaborates on these findings: "Numerous studies suggest that these techniques [CBT] have a substantial therapeutic effect on reducing intrusive and cue-related arousal symptoms in PTSD."[118] On the other, Jonathan Bisson et al. underscore in their 2013 Cochrane Collaboration meta-analysis the inconclusive evidence of several studies on CBT for PTSD.[119] Writing in 2014, van der Kolk expands on this finding, "A thorough analysis of all the scientific studies of CBT shows that it works about as well as being in a supportive therapy relationship."[120] Another issue to stress is that for some patients, trauma-focused cognitive behavioral therapy (TF-CBT) seems effective; whereas conversely, present-centered therapy (PCT), a non-trauma-focused therapy incorporating common psychotherapeutic elements, may prove therapeutic.[121] Regarding somatic therapies, there is evidence that eye movement desensitization and reprocessing therapy (EMDR) is an effective treatment.[122] Conversely, a 2018 meta-analysis concluded that only a weak endorsement for yoga as a supplementary intervention for PTSD can be made at this time.[123] Research studies suggest that methods of deliberate rumination, self-disclosure, and narrative strategies cultivate posttraumatic growth.[124] This final result helps to support a Literary Arts Praxis, a cognitive training to be introduced in the next chapter.

As far as pharmacotherapy is concerned, the Food and Drug Administration (FDA) has approved (as of 2017) the use of two selective serotonin reuptake inhibitors (SSRIs) (Zoloft and Paxil) for PTSD, despite the mixed results about their efficacy.[125] Findings from a 2006 Cochrane Collaboration systematic review supports "the status of SSRIs as first line agents in the pharmacotherapy of PTSD, as well as their value in long-term treatment."[126] In their systematic review of 35 short-term randomized controlled trials of pharmacotherapy for PTSD (4,597 participants), Dan Stein et al. found a "significantly larger proportion of patients responded to medication (59.1%) than to placebo (38.5%) (13 trials, 1,272 participants) ..."[127] The largest trials showed efficacy for selective serotonin reuptake inhibitors. In sum, many researchers find that "Medication treatments can be effective in PTSD, acting to reduce its core symptoms, and should be considered as part of the treatment of this disorder."[128] Be that as it may, Stein et al. point out the presence of significant "gaps" in the evidence and the need to find more effective agents to treat PTSD.[129] To add to these ambiguous results, a 2015 systematic review and meta-analysis calls into question the efficacy of SSRI's.[130] While these findings are important, the author of this book can mention them only in passing to emphasize that no silver bullet exists to treat posttraumatic conditions such as PTSD. These findings also highlight the complexity of treating trauma survivors. This synthesis aims in fact neither to oversimplify research on treatments nor to convey a sense that recovery is straightforward. Ample references included should dispel such impressions. The tentative vocabulary (such as "appears") used throughout this chapter reflects moreover the tone of scientific research, which mirrors the complexity of posttraumatic conditions not to mention the human mind.

What remains striking about this list of therapies is how much trauma theorists and clinicians themselves have creatively imagined new therapies promoting creative exercises for survivors. Just as Mother Nature guarantees a chain of life by creating a wide variety of life forms and mutations, the sciences have created a wide variety of medical treatments to guarantee health, including healing methods for psychological trauma. Obviously, the humanities (religion, philosophy, literature, music, and art) have also contributed to sustaining mental health. A Literary Arts Praxis might offer another method to reach minds that otherwise cannot be reached by the standard methods discussed in this chapter.

Conclusions: Therapies or Memes to Foster Resilience, Resistance, and Growth

Although he does not use the word "trauma" in his writings, Charles Darwin personally understood what the term meant after two of his young children died. "What a book a Devil's Chaplain might write," Darwin predicts, "on the clumsy, wasteful, blubbering low and horridly cruel work of nature."[131] The expression "blubbering low and horridly cruel work" conveys how the naturalist was traumatized by nature's work. And yet, the Devil's Chaplain would have to also mention a powerful counterforce to the intrinsic traumatic nature of nature. Communities of animals, and most notably humans, gather their resources to care and protect the infirm in their struggle for survival. There is a therapy to life. In addition to genes, people transmit memes (cultural traditions, including therapies, transmitted from one mind to another) that promote resilience, resistance, and growth, perhaps even recovery after trauma.

As explored in this chapter, clinical memes are varied. Establishing a sense of safety through therapeutic alliances and a nurtured self; remembering the traumatic event and mourning what has been damaged and lost; and authoring one's own story may be therapeutic for some. Engaging in cognitive exercises that promote self-knowledge and self-expression; gaining awareness of one's thoughts, emotions, and bodily sensations; and participating in group therapies might prove therapeutic for others. Priming the body by engaging in dancing, chanting, drumming, and theatrical exercises before telling one's story may be essential for others, while art therapy may be considered a source of solace for still others. Whereas the meta-analyses and systematic reviews cited in this chapter do not report unequivocal evidence of a cure-all for PTSD, this chapter's summary of different therapies to treat trauma survivors attests to the creative enterprises of clinicians and scientists to help lighten the burden of trauma. This summary should also lead us to ponder what other forms of treatments, especially from non-Western communities, could inspire our therapies. It may very well be that to develop new therapies, we first need to observe carefully and locate new forms of trauma, such as those associated with prejudice and environmental degradation. For survivors of trauma, the consulting room or office might very well extend into narratives and literature, and even within a Literary Arts Praxis, as we shall discover in the pages that follow.

Notes

1 Sacks, *Anthropologist*, xix.
2 Herman, *Trauma*, 240.
3 See Tallis, *Aping*, 60, 29.
4 Rose and Abi-Rached, *Neuro*, 20–21.
5 By proposing a synthesis of clinical treatment methods for trauma survivors before introducing my creative and critical concept of a Literary Arts Praxis, I am not suggesting that my concept is a treatment method with therapeutic qualities. Instead, the objective of this chapter is to trace the origins of my Praxis. It draws ideas from Janet to Herman, Cyrulnik, Beck, van der Kolk, and Richman, among other clinicians.
6 While pharmacotherapy is a widely employed form of therapy to treat PTSD, the US Department of Veterans' Administration "recommends trauma-focused psychotherapy as the first-line treatment for PTSD over pharmacotherapy. For patients who prefer pharmacotherapy or who do not have access to trauma-focused psychotherapy, medications remain a treatment option." See Jeffreys, "Clinicians."
7 See Calhoun and Tedeschi, *Posttraumatic*, 6.
8 Tedeschi et al., *Posttraumatic*, 3.
9 There may be a potential controversy about the fundamental nature of the concept of posttraumatic growth. Psychologist George Bonanno refers to trauma survivors involved in meaning making. He reports that "Although there is clear evidence linking meaning making to positive adjustment, there are also abundant studies showing the opposite (Park, 2010)." Bonanno, *Meaning*, 151. I have yet to come across research that questions whether these findings might apply as well to the meaning making intrinsic to the conceptualization of posttraumatic growth.
10 See Calhoun and Tedeschi, *Posttraumatic*, 28–29.
11 Tedeschi et al., *Posttraumatic*, 40.
12 See ibid., 33.
13 See ibid., 36–37.
14 Ibid., 68.
15 See Bonanno, "Resilience," 135–136.
16 In Dantzer et al., "Resilience," 29.

17   Tedeschi et al., *Posttraumatic*, 71.
18   Agaibi and Wilson, "Trauma," 211.
19   See ibid., 199.
20   See ibid., 211; see Bonanno and Diminich, "Annual," 379.
21   Ibid., 378.
22   Ibid., 380.
23   Bonanno and Diminich, "Annual," 394.
24   Wu et al., "Understanding," 1.
25   Bonanno, "Resilience," 136; Wu et al., "Understanding," 1; Tedeschi et al., *Posttraumatic*, 72.
26   I am relying on Barbara Shapiro's concepts of growth and resilience. She writes in her essay "Resilience, Sublimation, and Healing" that "We see many severely traumatized people who come to us plagued with problems, who with help are better able to work, love, and play, although scars persist. That person's resilience makes him or her able to use the therapeutic opportunity for reflection and growth, and the growth then makes the person more resilient." Shapiro, "Resilience," 122.
27   See this chapter's discussion of Sophia Richman's research on dissociation.
28   Bonanno, "Resilience," 136.
29   For further information on the term *"liquidation médicale"* consult: Janet, *Médications III*, chapters II and III.
30   See ibid., 466. The original reads: *"Dans ces conditions il serait peut-être sage de conclure simplement qu'il est trop tôt pour se server de la psychothérapie et qu'on en reparlera dans un siècle."*
31   See ibid, 468. I am not suggesting that Janet categorically refutes psychotherapy, but there is ample evidence in his writings that he entertained substantial doubts about the field. Referring to observed psychological evolution in patients, he writes: *"Ces affirmations sur l'évolution régulière et immuable des névro-psychoses, ces répartitions sur leur évolution régulière et fatale me semblent encore plus téméraires que tous les rêves des psychothérapeutes les plus enthousiastes."*
32   See ibid., 470. My translation; the original reads: *"il fera mieux, il apprendra à ses maladies à augmenter leurs ressources, à enricher leur esprit."*
33   See Janet, *L'automatisme*, loc. 2077. My translation; the original reads: *"Les malades de M. Charcot ont eu besoin pour effectuer un pareil changement d'une longue rééducation."*
34   Ibid., loc. 2083. My translation; the original reads: *"Je répondrai: son éducation comme type moteur est déjà faite depuis longtemps, parce qu'elle est hystérique, c'est-à-dire le type de l'instabilité psychologique."*
35   See Janet, *Névroses*, loc. 5746.
36   See ibid., loc. 5845.
37   Heim and Bühler, "Pierre Janet," 197.
38   See Janet's *L'évolution* for an in-depth discussion of the concept of an *"évolution psychologique."* Most notably, he stresses the patient's evolution of mental activity and the development of initiative.
39   Van der Hart et al., "Pierre Janet's," 166.
40   Janet, *L'automatisme*, loc. 9205. My translation; the original reads: *"Du moment que vous pouvez guérir le sujet par suggestion, c'est qu'il est encore malade."*
41   Foa, "Guidelines," 580.
42   Janet, *Principles*, 196.
43   Van der Hart et al., "Pierre Janet's," 160.
44   See ibid.
45   Ibid., 170.
46   See Janet, *Médications III*, 213.

47 See Janet, *Médications II*, 297.
48 See van der Hart et al., "Pierre Janet's," 173–174.
49 Freud, *Interpretation*, 367.
50 Freud, *Introductory*, 99.
51 Freud, *Civilization*, chap. III.
52 Freud, *Introductory*, 186.
53 Wu et al., "Understanding," 6.
54 Herman, *Trauma*, 175.
55 Ibid.
56 See ibid.
57 Ibid., 177.
58 See ibid., 176–181.
59 Ibid., 176.
60 Ibid.
61 See ibid., 187–195.
62 Ibid., 195.
63 Ibid., 194.
64 See ibid., 196–213.
65 Ibid., 202.
66 Herman does state explicitly that "The traumatic event challenges an ordinary person to become a theologian, a philosopher, and a jurist." Ibid., 178. She refers to trauma survivors becoming the "author" of their recovery. Herman, "Recovery," S145. Though she points out that survivors can assume the role of storytellers, she indicates that "detailed storytelling" might need to be avoided. Herman, *Trauma*, 219.
67 Ibid., 203.
68 Ibid., 212.
69 See A. Beck, *Cognitive*, 1–3.
70 Ibid., 9.
71 Ibid., 2–3.
72 Much of the following description of cognitive behavioral therapy has been gleaned from Aaron Beck's *Cognitive Therapy and the Emotional Disorders* and Judith Beck's *Cognitive Behavior Therapy*.
73 Foa et al., "Challenges," 74.
74 Cusak et al., "Psychological," 10.
75 Scaer, *Body*, 164; Karen Cusak et al. elaborate on Scaer's statement about the efficacy of exposure treatment. "All of the existing guidelines agree that trauma-focused psychological interventions including exposure therapy and cognitive therapy are effective, empirically supported first-line treatments for PTSD." See Cusak et al., "Psychological," 4.
76 See van der Kolk, *Body*, 221.
77 See Scaer, *Body*, 164.
78 Ibid.
79 Foa et al., "Psychological," 11.
80 Foa et al., "Challenges," 2.
81 Ibid., 18.
82 Ibid.
83 Cloitre et al., *Treating*, 364.
84 Ibid.
85 Ibid., 152.
86 Ibid., 390.
87 Levine and Frederick, *Waking*, 132.
88 Scaer, *Body*, 22.
89 Scott, *CBT*, 12.

90   Lancaster et al. have found that "overly integrated trauma memories may lead to greater distress and not poorly integrated ones as suggested by Ehlers and Clark (2000)." Lancaster et al., "Path-analytic," 194.
91   See van der Kolk, *Body*, 157–158.
92   Levine and Frederick, *Waking*, 176.
93   Levine's treatment method is much more detailed than this summary provides. For more information about his Somatic Experiencing, consult Levine, *Unspoken*, 74–75.
94   Ibid, 77.
95   Van der Kolk, "Introduction," xvii.
96   Van der Kolk., *Body*, 335.
97   Ibid., 337.
98   Scaer, *Body*, 167.
99   See ibid., 167–170.
100 Ibid., 167.
101 Richman, *Mended*, 106.
102 Ibid., 93.
103 See Maslow, *Toward*, 55.
104 Winnicott, *Psycho-Analytic*, 60.
105 Rank, *Art*, 7.
106 Jung, *Modern*, 72.
107 Recall that Herman also stresses that in the first stage of recovery, trauma survivors are often encouraged to draw before they attempt to tell their story.
108 Richman, *Mended*, 7.
109 Cyrulnik, *Resilience*, 275.
110 Richman, *Mended*, 50.
111 Recall from this book's introduction that according to van der Kolk, dissociation consists of memories of the original traumatic event that are "split off and fragmented, so that the emotions, sounds, images, thoughts and physical sensations related to the trauma take on a life of their own." Van der Kolk, *Body*, 66.
112 Richman, *Mended*, 66.
113 Cyrulnik, *Resilience*, 49.
114 Herman, *Trauma*, 239.
115 Ibid.
116 See Wood et al., "What Research," 135–145.
117 See Pitman et al., "Biological Studies," 19.
118 Scaer, *Body*, 164.
119 Bisson et al. signal that there is inconclusive evidence on different treatment methods, including CBT for PTSD. Consult their meta-analysis article (and the entire authors' conclusions), Bisson et al., "Psychological."
120 Van der Kolk, *Body*, 221.
121 Belsher et al., "Present-centered," 2.
122 See van der Kolk, *Body*, 248–262; see Haour and Beaurepaire, "Summary," 284.
123 See Cramer et al., "Yoga," 8.
124 For research analyses on the efficacy of PTG treatments (deliberate ruminations, self-disclosure, and narrative developments), consult Tedeschi et al., *Posttraumatic*, 48, 49, 50, and 55.
125 American Psychological Association, "Medications."
126 Stein et al., "Pharmacotherapy," 8.
127 Ibid., 15.
128 Ibid.
129 Ibid., 8.
130 Hoskins et al., "Pharmacotherapy," 98.

131   Darwin, "Letter," July 13, 1856.

6 Metamorphoses of the Mind and a Literary Arts Praxis

The power of the metaphor of a metamorphosis is its ability to morph. It brings to life at once images of larvae, chrysalises (pupae in protective wraps), and butterflies. It evokes vulnerability and constriction as well as new life and new-found freedom. The potency of the metaphor lies not only in this duplexity, but also in its paradoxical nature. Larvae, chrysalises, and butterflies exist side by side, either hanging from silken threads on our neuronal branches or flying through the gardens of our mind.

This book's central thesis is inspired by metamorphoses in nature. Just as a larva and butterfly are dependent upon a chrysalis for a transformation, posttraumatic conditions are connected to the literary arts. The larva represents the vulnerable state of the trauma survivor. The butterfly is the posttraumatic survivor having experienced posttraumatic growth (PTG). The chrysalis represents the body and mind in the protective wrap of the literary arts.[1] Through exposure to the literary arts (such as, listening to and interpreting stories, storytelling, reading and decoding literature, and creative writing), the trauma survivor might create her own safe space. I refer to this exposure as a Literary Arts Praxis.

A Literary Arts Praxis is built on an interdisciplinary foundation. It is buttressed by clinical trauma theories on the importance of engaging in cognitive exercises (Pierre Janet, Aaron Beck, Edna Foa, Richard Tedeschi, Lawrence Calhoun, and Marylene Cloitre) and creative activities (Donald Winnicott, Otto Rank, Judith Herman, Peter Levine, Boris Cyrulnik, Barbara Shapiro, George Bonanno, and Sophia Richman).[2] The Praxis is also constructed on branches of philosophy (existentialism, phenomenology, and aesthetics) that have enjoyed a symbiotic relationship with the literary arts. I posit that an engagement in a Literary Arts Praxis may very well prod survivors to create testimonies of suffering followed by narratives (stories) rich in philosophical and imaginative content that breathe new life into their essence. The complexity of posttraumatic conditions obviously requires a wide range of treatments. This book does not seek to add a Literary Arts Praxis to the list, especially within the first stages of recovery.[3] As a literary theorist who has studied assiduously clinical posttraumatic treatments, I am positioned however to

DOI: 10.4324/9781003284642-10

imagine how creative engagements with the literary arts might reach trauma and foster metamorphoses of the mind, such as posttraumatic growth.

While pundits might argue that the image of a metamorphosis translates into a shallow interpretation of posttraumatic conditions from PTSD to PTG, I stress that the metaphor does not mean less distress or greater well-being necessarily, but rather that "persons who experience it are living life in ways that, at least from their point of view, are fuller, richer, and perhaps more meaningful,"[4] as Calhoun and Tedeschi claim. And responding to hopeless psychic posttraumatic states and trauma theories that focus on trauma and melancholy, the image of a metamorphosis may very well provide hope to trauma survivors.

Several research shortcomings in trauma studies have prodded me to envision a Literary Arts Praxis. First, prominent psychiatrists, psychologists, and psychoanalysts insist on a connection between trauma and the literary arts, as we shall unravel shortly. They suggest that trauma narratives help promote growth and/or even recovery. They have not investigated thoroughly how this might occur. I thus explore how the literary arts "can somehow get at trauma," a term from Dominick LaCapra.[5] He shares my reading of a need to explore more profoundly the relationship between the literary arts, history, and trauma. Speaking about this issue, he writes: "The apparent implication is that literature in its very excess can somehow get at trauma in a manner unavailable to theory—that it writes (speaks or even cries) trauma in excess of theory. It is not clear, however, precisely how it does so."[6] LaCapra's position that it remains unclear how literature "can somehow get at trauma" is an invitation to address this research gap. Second, and as we shall unfold, psychiatrists to psychoanalysts have called for trauma survivors to become philosophers, storytellers, and/or creative writers. And yet, these roles benefit from educational trainings that cultivate, like cognitive behavioral therapy, an independence of mind and thoughtful discernment. A Literary Arts Praxis is designed to resemble a "re-education" that responds to "psychic constriction," to rely on terms from Janet, already discussed in this book. Third, and as argued in Chapter 4, First Wave cultural trauma theorists tend to fixate on trauma, as opposed to forms of resistance, resilience, and growth, whereas clinicians have begun to move in the latter direction. A Literary Arts Praxis aims to address these three research gaps, while attempting to connect the fields of science, medicine, and the humanities. Finally, my motive to develop a Praxis and to investigate how the literary arts and specifically how the Praxis might "get at trauma" responds to the idea that, "PTG [post-traumatic growth] is better understood when the traditional biomedical model is combined with other models such as existential models, social-personality models, spiritual-philosophical models …"[7]

Definitions of Key Terms

Before exploring how a Literary Arts Praxis might get at trauma, let us define the term "Literary Arts Praxis." Again, the expression "literary arts" refers to listening to and interpreting stories, storytelling, reading and decoding literature, and creative writing. As for the term "praxis," Aristotle employs it in his *Nicomachean Ethics* to refer to an action or the achievement of an action.[8] Most importantly for the Greek philosopher, a praxis refers to activities whose goals are internal to themselves, whereas a practice describes activities with external goals. Engaging in the arts has a point during that engagement, but not necessarily one external to it. Similarly, self-realization constitutes a praxis for Aristotle.[9] Metaphorically speaking, the artist is not only the artist, but also the work of art she crafts. Drawing on Aristotle's conceptualization of a praxis as self-realization and Tedeschi's and Calhoun's concept of PTG, a Literary Arts Praxis consists of an educational training, a re-education, that may very well foster resistance, resilience, and psychological and philosophical growth through creative reading, story telling, and writing exercises that stimulate the imagination.

Let us now focus on LaCapra's expression that literature (and a Literary Arts Praxis) "can somehow get at trauma." Since "trauma" comes from the Greek word "wound," it seems instructive to approach the expression from a metaphorical medical perspective.[10] Doesn't the expression evoke an image of a surgeon using her scalpel to pull back layers of tissue to access an internal wound? Or might it imply that the literary arts can provide a metaphorical X-ray of a traumatized mind? Could the literary arts somehow help to void the mind of toxic memories, like drugs to induce vomiting? Might they provide a transfusion of novel images to bring new life to a weakened body and mind? Do they come closer to prophylactic treatments, such as vaccines, nourishment, and exercises to strengthen the mind and body? Or could they behave in all these ways? These questions point to ways to look at the main issues to be developed in this chapter, while philosophers and authors of literature might very well point us in still other directions.

The Devil's Advocate: How Trauma Undermines the Literary Arts

One might harbor doubts that a Literary Arts Praxis could serve as a multifunctional Swiss army knife for trauma survivors. Human biology appears to stack the deck against trauma survivors engaging in such a Praxis. After all, biology seems to refute links between trauma, posttraumatic conditions, and the literary arts, and most notably telling stories. As discussed in Chapter 3, language and storytelling are impaired by traumatic experiences. Scans reveal that the Broca's area of the brain, which is responsible for processing and producing language, goes "offline" during flashbacks of traumatic events. Research also indicates that trauma activates the right hemisphere of the brain and deactivates the left, which organizes experiences logically and translates emotions and perceptions into words. Therefore, "it is enormously difficult to organize one's traumatic experiences into a coherent account—a narrative with a beginning, a middle, and an end."[11] Moreover, in the state of dissociation, the thalamus's activity is compromised. This explains "why trauma is primarily remembered not as a story, a narrative with a beginning, middle, and end, but as isolated sensory imprints: images, sounds, and physical sensations that are accompanied by intense emotions ..."[12] If traumatic experiences weaken abilities to employ language creatively; think logically; translate feelings; and construct a story with a beginning, middle and end, then it is hard to imagine links between trauma, posttraumatic growth, and the literary arts. How could the literary arts access trauma, if some of the cerebral mechanisms that rely on language, logic, feelings, and storytelling are compromised? How could a trauma survivor engage in language-centered activities if her body's physiological reactions are the only form of communication she knows?

Clinicians: A Case for Employing the Literary Arts to Get at Trauma

While the above puts pressure on a connection between the literary arts and trauma, neurologists to psychoanalysts have insisted on links between them. It is perhaps Calhoun and Tedeschi who describe this intimate relationship the most poignantly: "A good way to judge whether an event is truly traumatic may be to consider the way it disrupts the personal narrative."[13] The more traumatic an event is, the more apt it is to undermine one's ability to tell a story about it, thus confirming the intimate relationship between trauma and stories. Referencing Janet's theories, van der Kolk unravels this tightly woven knot: "the memory traces of the trauma linger as what he called unconscious fixed ideas that cannot be liquidated as long as they have not been translated into a personal narrative."[14] In other words, it is not just the traumatic event itself and the conscious and physical recollection of the event that might undermine personal narratives; unconscious fixed ideas also appear to serve as roadblocks to new personal narratives. Although these statements project a dim light on the idea that the literary arts could get at trauma, they highlight all the same that the links between stories and trauma remain knotty. This is because stories originate in the very places (the conscious and unconscious realms) where the mind has been comprised by the traumatic event. If the well of one's mind has been filled with the collateral damage of trauma, then how could fresh stories be sourced from it?

But are there ways a damaged psyche might be restored? Herman argues that telling one's trauma story, while assuming the role of philosopher (or theologian), is an important step in recovery.[15] Calhoun and Tedeschi also highlight stories rich in philosophical content: "The [trauma] narrative must include all aspects of the client's experience, because growth does not come from denial, but from confronting the existential questions raised, and from sharing these experiences with appropriate others."[16] Wearing the philosopher's hat, the survivor attempts to make sense of a senseless horrid experience.

Beyond emphasizing the importance of trauma narratives from philosophical perspectives, Herman contends that recovery is dependent upon "a survivor's capacities for imagination and play."[17] Levine insists on literary aspects: "It is universally true that the renegotiation of trauma is an inherently mythic-poetic-heroic journey."[18] Cyrulnik echoes Levine's position implicitly. Writing poetically as if to prove a point about the link between his own trauma of being a Holocaust survivor and the literary arts, he contends, "The surest way to sew up a tear is to suture the wound with words."[19] How do words suture up wounds? His writing adorned with similes, analogies, metaphors, and symbols intimates that a literary style is the crux of the matter. The mind embarks on a creative exercise, interpreting literary features, not to mention philosophical content. Cyrulnik also relies on the nineteenth-century poet Charles Baudelaire to describe this creative process as "turning mud into gold."[20] This metaphorical perspective renders the topic even more nebulous as wizards engage in alchemical experiments before us. Perhaps this is Cyrulnik's point. He seeks to encourage survivors to embark on creative adventures. By creating a personal narrative rich not only in similes, symbols, metaphors, and analogies but also in philosophical musings, a victim might feel like she is gaining something from the creative process itself, to return to Aristotle's definition of a praxis

Similarly, Richman highlights the importance of artistic endeavors for trauma survivors. As explored in the previous chapter, she prefaces her argument by pouring scorn on the widespread belief that catastrophic trauma ruins subjects' ability to represent and integrate traumatic experiences.[21] She finds fault besides in the myopic view of survivors as irrevocably damaged. Such a limited reading fails to acknowledge the different ways humans react to traumatic circumstances. In her eyes, creative actions are a mechanism for survivors to express their experiences and to make meaning of them. The artistic product serves several roles: "It stands as a witness to the traumatic experience; it can be known by others; it can be admired by them; and it restores self-esteem damaged by the humiliation and shame attending victimization."[22] Richman, a Holocaust survivor and artist herself, puts squarely what is at stake, "It is immensely curative to feel known and recognized when one has felt alone and isolated."[23]

Akin to the psychoanalysts, psychologists, and psychiatrists mentioned above, Dori Laub puts forward that narratives are key to treating psychological trauma, even if he does cast doubt on this position, too. "Survivors did not only need to survive so that they could tell their story, they also needed to tell their story in order to survive."[24] Such a remark still begs the question about how narratives promote survival. He takes a stab at an explanation:

> "Trauma" is actually the word for "wound" in ancient Greek, so testimony is the healing of the wound by shaping and giving shape to an experience that's fragmented ... But to get it out in the interpersonal space there has to be a companion.[25]

Laub's comment provokes us to imagine that the traumatic narrative resembles a cubist painting in trauma survivors' eyes. It is "fragmented" or made up of incongruent forms and misplaced shapes like Picasso's cubist portraits. The companion helps survivors turn the portrait into a congruent image as symbols are decoded. The companion is not just outside the psyche; she is also an "internal companion, because the process of symbolization and the formation of narrative only happens within an internal dialogue."[26] Still, Laub is convinced of the "impossibility of telling."[27] The cubist painting is blown up and splatters on the museum walls.[28] Whether one states that there is an "impossibility of telling" or envisions a portrait blown to bits, the message is unequivocal.

Unlike Laub and closer to Herman, Barbara Shapiro states explicitly that "telling and retelling stories is central to healing and recovery from trauma."[29] She tempers this remark by adding that not all stories are created equal. Some prolong trauma. "They become rigid, fixed, or hateful and/or consist of fantastical elaborations that take on a life of their own and are not anchored in everyday reality."[30] Vocabulary such as "fantastical elaborations" and "not anchored in everyday reality" indicates that stories prolonging trauma seem to be related to fiction. And yet, other stories are "open, developing, growing, establishing links and meanings, with increasing freedom of thought, feeling, reflection, and understanding."[31] Shapiro delineates both a reshaping and retelling of stories over time. She describes how the process unfolds in the clinical setting: "One starts with raw experience, which especially with trauma is often chaotic, incoherent, and nonverbal. Over time, the feelings and content are put into words, and then into a story, which gets told, reshaped, and retold."[32] Though she sketches out a process, she does not explain how the chaotic, incoherent, and nonverbal are rendered a shade less chaotic, more coherent, or verbal. Nor does she examine if a story is not a story if it is chaotic, incoherent, and nonverbal. Although she leaves these important issues dangling, she tentatively offers one explanation. She shares Laub's opinion about the importance of a witness in the construction of stories. But she parts company with his insistence on an "impossibility of witnessing." She puts forward instead that through psychoanalytic therapy, the traumatic experience and story "are transformed, both by the co-constructed narrative itself and by the process of co-constructing the narrative."[33] It would make sense that Shapiro would highlight this narrative co-construction between therapist and victim of trauma. She is a psychoanalyst. Stories are the bread and butter of psychoanalysis. The field is predicated on the idea that personal narratives shared with an analyst both reflect and transform the client's experiences.

More recent research from Marylene Cloitre and her colleagues emphasizes the importance of narratives for trauma survivors. As introduced in the previous chapter, their research is based on a two-part treatment program called STAIR/NT. The premise of their Narrative Therapy (NT) module is that by narrating one's traumatic experiences, a survivor confronts, understands, and masters them.[34] While exploring her trauma through narratives, the survivor also develops a critical eye and hence is better positioned to locate the causes and deleterious consequences of the events. Since this module of therapy centers on narratives that have a past, present, and future, the survivor can establish a sense of "pastness" of the traumatic event, while imagining a future. "Through Narrative Therapy," Cloitre puts forward, "clients express themselves and become the owner of their life stories."[35] The relationship between the literary arts and trauma could not be any clearer, as survivors' narratives play a pivotal role in their treatment method. Her program however does not seem to include reading and decoding literary texts or creative writing exercises.

This synthesis leads us to conclude that although these traumatologists are convinced of links between the literary arts and trauma, they have failed to investigate in depth how this relationship might function. This is not surprising. These trauma specialists are scientists, clinicians, and social scientists, not literary theorists or authors of literature who might feel equipped to hazard explanations on the relationship between the literary arts and trauma. Some might insist furthermore that this relationship should remain veiled. The literary arts, unlike the mechanisms of monoclonal antibodies, are by nature ambiguous. To explore this relationship is therefore at best futile, at worst naïve. Nonetheless, this exploration is not simply an intellectual exercise. It is an ethical question. A more profound discussion of this topic may help clinicians and scientists to envision new creative therapies to treat trauma survivors.

Cultural Theorists: Masking and Unmasking How Literature Might Get at Trauma

Do cultural trauma theorists share clinicians' position about links between trauma and the literary arts? Do they believe that literature can access trauma? It seems self-evident that cultural theorists would point to connections. Cultural analysis with its hermeneutical approach serves as an academic counterpart to psychoanalysis. While cultural theorists explore these relationships, their explanations are also plagued by a distrust to investigate them deeply. Or seen from another perspective, their analyses are tentative responses that invite us to explore these issues more deeply and creatively.

As addressed in Chapter 4, Geoffrey Hartman, Shoshana Felman, and Cathy Caruth signal connections between trauma and the literary arts. They emphasize both the common interpretative mechanisms of investigation between psychoanalysis and literary theory and the production of testimonies that are shared material with other witnesses and originating from the unconscious realm. (This argument is cut from the same fabric as research from Sigmund Freud and Carl Jung, who claimed that art was a way to access the unconscious.) And yet, First Wave theorists have cast a long shadow on one's ability to gain conscious awareness of traumatic memories. Conversely, other cultural theorists have made less equivocal claims about the link between trauma and the literary arts. Psychoanalyst and literary theorist Françoise Davoine claims: "Understanding one's own story through a relation to, or in an interference from another's story, is healing."[36] Davoine's position is remarkable obviously because she states explicitly that an exchange of stories constitutes healing.

Though sociologist Jeffrey Alexander points to the therapeutic nature of the literary arts, his vocabulary is less explicit than Davoine's. As far as telling a story about the Holocaust is concerned, he claims that there is no way to transcend it. There is only catharsis.[37] According to Aristotle, catharsis clarifies emotions. This occurs when the audience identifies with characters on stage, sharing their suffering and learning from them. Viewers experience in their minds and with bodily sensations a perilous journey along with the protagonist. Though the hero might not survive, the theater goer returns home. She has survived and can purge herself of the feelings she has shared with the characters on stage. (This sounds very similar to how a gazelle shakes off the residual stress after escaping from a lion, a topic discussed in Chapter 5 regarding somatic-centered therapies.) Alexander also points out that literature plays a role in establishing "symbolic residues" of the Holocaust experience.[38] When individuals free-associate during psychoanalytic treatment, they recount as memories the symbols animating cultural artifacts (literature and film) about the Holocaust.[39] Literature therefore not only potentially provides a cathartic experience but also cultivates a bountiful harvest of images and metaphors otherwise absent from a barren mental terrain, one might say.

LaCapra offers some of the most enlightening explanations about how trauma and literature might be linked. He ponders first the differences between writing about trauma and writing trauma. Writing about trauma is part of historiography; writing trauma applies to the arts. Historians strive to reconstruct the traumatic event with as much objectivity as possible. LaCapra maintains nonetheless that truth claims are necessary but not sufficient conditions for historiography.[40] As far as how literature writes trauma, he proposes several tentative answers. He stresses that literature is characterized by ambivalence and undecidability and hence might provide a "safe haven"[41] where one can explore issues and emotions indirectly. Moreover, the arts can provide surrealistic situations that translate into imaginative openings to reinterpret reality from an uncanny angle. They can also offer raw commentary on social reality, thus provoking heightened awareness about problematic norms and possible new courses of action. Writing trauma is associated furthermore with enacting it, which includes artistic performances. This urge to act the trauma out occurs, because literature relishes in "pathos-charged writing that moves the reader."[42] These four explanations lead LaCapra to conclude that literature provides the "feel" of the traumatic experience, which "may be difficult to arrive at through restricted documentary methods."[43] Though he does not state explicitly that these elaborations are responses to the question about how literature gets at trauma, he does offer a thoughtful discernment about how literature writes trauma. By focusing on this issue, he is indirectly suggesting that the artistic approach (a truly radical constructivist model) to writing trauma has something important to teach historians who often employ a documentary research model.[44] His musings serve as an excellent segue to explore these issues from within the fields of both literature and philosophy, which we shall do in the next section.

How a Literary Arts Praxis Might Get at Trauma

Again, a Literary Arts Praxis is constructed on clinical theories and on three modes of philosophical inquiry that have benefited from mutually enriching relationships with the literary arts: existentialism, phenomenology, and aesthetics. A Praxis aims to be an active intellectual experience through a hermeneutical engagement with the literary arts. It may also serve as a wellspring of insight into the topic of emotions as well as phenomenological experiences that spur emotions. Between an active intellectual, phenomenological, and emotional engagement in literary texts rich in these three philosophical branches, a Praxis may very well help survivors to get at trauma and in nuanced ways that have not been put forward previously. Finally, it should be stressed that the exploration of a Literary Arts Praxis in the pages that follow aims to be descriptive, not prescriptive.

Existentialism and The Myth of Sisyphus

If metamorphoses define the very nature of Mother Nature (including flexible brains and creative minds), then it follows that her offspring, stories, would mutate and morph. The philosopher and Nobel prize-winning author Albert Camus sums up metamorphoses of narratives as: "Myths are made for the imagination to breathe life into them."[45] Such is the case of the myth of Sisyphus. The hero's story has never been etched in stone. Homer first breathed life into it. According to the Greek poet, Sisyphus is a clever and prudent mortal. In a later legend, he is both clever and cunning. Outsmarting the gods, he captures the god of the underworld, Hades. Whether one believes Homer or the later version matters less than the meaning of the punishment for Sisyphus's rebellious attempt to put to death, death itself. The gods condemned him to push a rock up a mountain, whence it would fall to the bottom for him to push back up again.

The clever mortal is morphed into a truly absurd hero.[46] His identity is defined by a nonsensical act. He has been mutated into the very object of his punishment: "A face that toils so close to stones is already stone itself!"[47] Sisyphus functions like a robot, shouldering a material burden and a psychic one too. That is, until Camus breathes new life into the myth and transforms the hero once again. The philosopher hits the pause button. Every time the rock descends the mountain, Sisyphus transcends his fate. Free from his burden on his descent, he is conscious of his being.[48] He chooses to think and to feel freely. "He is stronger than his rock."[49] To spite the gods and in defense of the absurd hero, Camus adds: "I leave Sisyphus at the foot of the mountain! One always finds one's burden again. But Sisyphus teaches the higher fidelity that negates the gods and raises rocks."[50] The clever mortal teaches us about revolting against cruel fates and carving out new ones. This lesson is not wishful thinking on the part of the author-philosopher. It aligns well with Sisyphus's personality before he was subjected to the burden of the boulder. By rebelling against the gods, he is cultivating a new identity both simultaneously and subsequently. After all, "There is no fate that cannot be surmounted by scorn."[51] His rebellion is triggered and fueled by remaining true to the aversion, revulsion, contempt, and other shades of scorn that make his blood boil. Thus, rather than remaining numb to the burden of his yoke, he allows himself to feel, which provokes a rebellion, a metaphysical protest against spiteful suffering.

Existentialism and Trauma Survivors

Sisyphus would be pleased to discover that his story appears as one of the cornerstones of a Literary Arts Praxis. What is behind such an uncanny claim? The Praxis moves beyond the walls of a clinic. By reading, absorbing, interpreting, questioning, and connecting profoundly with *The Myth of Sisyphus*, trauma survivors can find another setting where deeply wounded selves can be explored and perhaps even altered. This statement should not be construed as grotesquely removed from reality. Indeed, the rapport between existentialism and psychotherapy has been pronounced. Calhoun and Tedeschi write, "For other persons, however, the confrontation with a traumatic event can provide the context for significant change in the existential sphere, change that the individual regards as positive and perhaps highly significant."[52] The psychiatrist Irvin Yalom built the foundation of his psychotherapeutic model on existentialism, whereas neuro-psychiatrist and philosopher Viktor Frankl constructed his Logotherapy on a search to respond to philosophical questions, such as free will, self-awareness, and self-determination, themes resounding in Sisyphus's story.[53]

Alliances with Sisyphus

How might Camus's *The Myth of Sisyphus* speak intimately to trauma survivors and help them to get at trauma? Survivors might first engage in a highly imaginative escapade by developing an alliance with Sisyphus, which might help them to develop conscious awareness of their experiences. After all, his identity is built on three shared traits: a heavy emotional burden, a loss of personal control, and physical suffering. Survivors often feel that they too carry a yoke. This burden might take the form of traumatic memories defying control. Or it may center on a realization that society causes their chronic traumatic suffering, a victimization phenomenon Pierre Briquet put on the map. Or they may feel overwhelmed when they struggle to control their emotions and destiny. Further, the physical condition of the Greek hero might speak intimately to trauma survivors. Sisyphus seems to embody the feeling of what happens posttraumatic experience. The post-traumatized body carries so often a burden in the form of physical tension, triggered by a continuous secretion of stress hormones. In sum, survivors might cultivate a bond with Sisyphus as they grow cognizant of a shared condition. Through this connection, fortified by similar emotional experiences and physical sensations, they may begin to observe and feel themselves more clearly. Metaphorically, they might view their own condition as if they were observing an Xray and grow in conscious awareness.

This alliance is fortified furthermore as trauma survivors become aware of Sisyphus's personality dichotomy. This dichotomy plays out as the Greek hero rolls the boulder up and down the mountain. On his ascent, he has no choice but to shoulder the boulder. On his descent, he transcends the yoke and becomes a hero of resistance. By reading the myth over and again, following Sisyphus up and down the mountain, survivors might experience a prophylactic treatment, such as daily emotional nourishment and motivational exercises. This process may make them aware of their vulnerability (on their ascent) and their strengths (on their descent) as well as a sense of resilience to revolt against the cruel fate befallen them and against death itself.

Revolts

Sisyphus's determined will to engage in a revolt might also serve as a source of inspiration for trauma survivors. A revolt in Camus's eyes is not necessarily violent.[54] It can consist of a historical, metaphysical, or artistic rebellion.[55] The rebuilding of the self is, for example, an artistic rebellion. Sisyphus's revolt is also metaphysical in that the rebel's act reflects the conundrums of existence. It consists of first a "yes" to engage in life, then a "no" to nihilism. By exposing themselves to Sisyphus's story and to the philosophical positions he evokes, survivors might be inspired to resist nihilism and embrace life. By acknowledging their traumatic suffering in testimonies and then refusing trauma to have the last word in their stories, they might resist it and perhaps even abate its debilitating effects.[56] I acknowledge that Herman has stressed that narratives should first be factual in nature and then followed by more creative ones. A Literary Arts Praxis may very well provide the necessary tools to facilitate this transition from composing versions of a factual testimony to a creative story.

It is important to stress that the absurd hero's acts of resistance are directed against not only the gods (and death itself) but also a self-imposed norm of remaining numb to his own suffering. One might say that it is a psychological revolt. He remains true to his core personality. Though Sisyphus may need to remain affectless on his ascent to shoulder his boulder, he comes alive on his descent as he watches it fall. Thus, Sisyphus might inspire trauma survivors to resist artistically, by rebuilding themselves; metaphysically, by defying death and nihilism; and psychologically, by remaining true to their feelings and core personality traits and values.

Testimonies as Acts of Rebellion

After a thoughtful engagement with Sisyphus's story, survivors might even move beyond trauma while crafting a testimony of their experiences. How might this work? As argued above, Sisyphus's example of rebellion might inspire survivors to rebel against their suffering and this includes formulating a testimony. Furthermore, a rebellion is a collective experience, according to Camus. Before Sisyphus was transformed into a hero who negated the gods and raised rocks, he suffered in solitude.[57] When Camus breathed life into the Greek hero's myth, he assumed part of Sisyphus's burden. "The malady experienced by a single man becomes a mass plague,"[58] the philosopher claims. This idea finds resonance in trauma survivor support groups, a topic explored in the previous chapter. Sisyphus may very well provide an imaginary support group that encourages survivors to speak out by way of a testimony against individual and collective suffering. Why testimonies and not stories? Testimonies tend to be rooted in accepted facts and evidence.[59] A trauma survivor who gives a testimony can become more of an objective witness, attesting to events or to conditions. Hence, there might be a degree of emotional distance between the survivor and the testimony.[60] Stories and poems, conversely, thrive on imaginative interventions, including pathos charged language and lively metaphors that animate a page or discourse. It may be that for some survivors writing first a testimony of individual and collective suffering could be a first act of rebellion. They can then move on to write a more imaginative story, another act of revolt and a topic to unravel shortly.

Not every trauma survivor is fortunate enough to have an award-winning editor to modify her narrative the way Sisyphus did. Nor is every survivor endowed with the mental or physical strength to raise stones against the gods. These objections may be moot points, as Sisyphus's punishment is not necessarily eternal. On his ascent, he wears away the mountain, not to mention the rock. His burden appears lighter as he confronts less friction and less weight. Besides, what happens if we stepped in where Homer and Camus left off? Aren't readers invited to breathe new life into the ancient Greek myth? We might hand our hero a pully and watch him use his wits to outwit the gods. Our task as bystanders is to give the absurd hero the tools to transform his story and alter his destiny. Sisyphus's metamorphosis occurs therefore thanks to the intervention of a community of writers, no matter how renowned or obscure, combined with the hero's own creative powers. This suggests that it is not just a question of telling or writing testimonies, but also creatively reading, including survivors' own testimonies and stories of trauma.

Phenomenology and Nausea

Sisyphus left a legacy of existentialist heroes and heroines. The philosopher and Nobel-prize winning author Jean-Paul Sartre's character Roquentin from *Nausea* (first published in French in 1938) follows Sisyphus by attempting to carve out his own path. The novel assumes the form of a diary, thus reinforcing the existentialist theme of self-construction. By writing a diary, one not only captures the self but also constructs it. However, Roquentin transforms the diary into an act of deconstruction and construction. He deconstructs himself while experiencing an existential crisis through the body (phenomenologically) and builds himself back up through an aesthetic awakening.

Acts of deconstruction and construction of the self are tightly woven together, if not contingent upon each other. While Roquentin is writing a book about a certain Marquis de Rollebon, he becomes a secondary character in his own life. If the marquis needs Roquentin to exist, the latter needs the former in order not to feel his existence.[61] From this external position, the existential hero gains keener self-awareness and deconstructs himself with a more critical eye, which triggers in turn an existential crisis.

This crack-up occurs as a phenomenological experience. Phenomenology explores consciousness spurred by subjective interactions with objects. These interactions are phenomena. In the French phenomenological tradition (inherited in large part from Martin Heidegger), one's living body is the center of experience and thus the site where conscious awareness develops. Roquentin experiences an existential crisis in the body and through feelings transmitted by the body. His corporal relationship with objects changes first. "I recall better what I felt the other day at the seashore when I held the pebble. It was a sort of sweetish sickness … It came from the stone, I'm sure of it, it passed from the stone to my hand. Yes, that's it, that's just it—a sort of nausea in the hands."[62] The pebble has infected the existential hero. Is he infected with a case of stone-cold emotions? He complains of having plunged into frozen waters. In addition to psychic numbing, his malady consists of an aggravated sense of existence. This new condition contrasts with his pre-infection state when he wrote about the Marquis de Rollebon to evade his own existence. His whole physical being assumes an intensely strange character. His hands are like two beasts wrangling at the end of his arms. After a while, their weight feels intolerable and no matter what he does, they continue to exist. He can suppress neither them nor the sensations coming and going in and out of his body. He suffers not only from nausea, but also vertigo.

Burdened by the weight of his existence, he focuses on his face. Gazing at himself in the mirror, his eyes, mouth, and nose all disappear, leaving behind an object resembling the moon with slopes, crevices, and mole holes. He discovers that "a silky white down covers the great slopes of the cheeks, two hairs protrude from the nostrils: it is a geological embossed map."[63] His self-portrait is, to put it lightly, unrecognizable. While contemplating his physical being, he feels nauseous and dizzy. He decides that what is left for him to do is to outlive himself. That is, "Eat, sleep, sleep, eat. Exist slowly, softly, like these trees, like a puddle of water, like the red bench in the streetcar."[64] Roquentin contrasts the basic and organic existence of the trees, puddle of water, and the streetcar bench with the values of the Enlightenment. The world of existence is not the world of reason. Feelings make the world go round at dizzying speeds.

Existence is therefore not so much a heady affair in the existentialist world. It is a phenomenological one involving flesh and bones. The body is "our living link" (*notre lien vivant*)[65] with nature, according to the philosopher Maurice Merleau-Ponty. The feminist philosopher Simone de Beauvoir expands on this idea: "The body is not a thing, it is a situation, it is the instrument of our grasp upon the world, a limiting factor for our projects."[66] To understand the world in real and imaginative form, therefore, one must acknowledge the body and its signals about the world.

The bridge between the human body and nature is reinforced by the alloy of emotions.[67] Put more squarely, if the body is our link with nature, so too are emotions. This is because emotions dwell and sometimes thrive in the body. They also speak through the body. Smiles, grimaces, sweat, and tears communicate feelings through bodily sensations. Even if Roquentin confesses to inhabiting frigid waters, he eventually develops intense bodily feelings and emotions about his own existence, as witnessed in his becoming beastly. One might say that Sartre's hero replaces Descartes's dictum *cogito ergo sum* with "I feel the horror of my existence, therefore I am." Existence is defined by emotions over reason. Sartre nuances this idea in his war diary from 1939–1940. He admits that it is very easy to remain a stoic. He can guess, explain, put in black on white what people might feel. But he cannot feel what they feel. He is nothing more than a "desert."[68] Sartre translates Hamlet's "to be or not to be" into another opposition: "to feel or not to feel."[69] We are free, in theory, to choose the intensity of our emotions.[70] We can become a stoic or respond more authentically to our bodily feelings and emotions. This is an invitation to freedom that Sisyphus would gladly accept.

Phenomenology and Trauma Survivors

How might *Nausea* speak intimately to trauma survivors and help them to get at trauma? Alliances based on a shared existential crisis might form between survivors and Roquentin. Survivors might undergo phenomenological experiences while reading *Nausea* and develop keener awareness of their bodies. Furthermore, the novel might provoke in readers a host of emotions in a setting that is safer or less threatening.

Alliances with Roquentin

There are several ways in which trauma survivors might develop bonds with Roquentin, even though *Nausea* may not be a story of trauma. Firstly, they might feel a kindred state of being and notion of time. "Being traumatized is not just an issue of being stuck in the past; it is just as much a problem of not being fully alive in the present."[71] Van der Kolk's description of traumatized states finds resonance in Roquentin's condition; that is, before he experiences an existential crisis and awakening. Sartre's hero not only remains stuck in the past (researching and writing about the Marquis de Rollebon) but also experiences cognitive constriction in the present. In addition, when Roquentin undergoes an existential crisis followed by an awakening, his identity is thrown out of kilter. Similarly, traumatic life events often consist of extreme challenges to one's core life beliefs, an argument advanced by Calhoun and Tedeschi.[72] While the first part of *Nausea* focuses on Roquentin being stuck in the past and disconnected from the present, the second centers on an existential crisis disrupting his core identity that manifests itself through the feeling of an alienated body. Third, it is not only a shared existential crisis, but also a phenomenological experience involving alienation that may also trigger survivors to develop a bond with Roquentin. Trauma survivors might not feel as if their hands are hairy paws with darkened claws, but enduring stress often makes bodies feel foreign. Recall furthermore that Levine, van der Kolk, and Scaer advocate somatic-centered therapies, precisely because traumatic stress dwells in the body, wreaking havoc on viscera and triggering hormonal imbalances. By contemplating profoundly Roquentin's portrait, not least his existential and phenomenological crises, survivors might view a metaphorical scan of their own existence and experience conscious awareness and cognitive growth.

Phenomenological Experiences while Reading Nausea

Even more noteworthy is that *Nausea* might trigger bodily feelings in readers and help survivors to get at trauma. As the title alludes, the novel is about phenomenological experiences. This includes readers' phenomenological experiences. Readers might feel horror as they sense Roquentin's horror. Disgust, when they picture disgusting images. The themes are grasped both cognitively and through and in the body. Further, by contrasting his stone-cold existence with his "I feel the horror of my existence, therefore I am," Roquentin creates a spectrum of emotional reactions upon which readers can place their own emotional profile. Whether it is an exposure to the topic of physical sensations and emotions or a direct participation in the stimulation of those sensations and emotions, *Nausea* might provide survivors with both a scan of their own condition and a type of inoculation. That is, the stimulation of emotions and bodily sensations while reading might help them to develop the emotional "antibodies" needed to confront their own experiences.

Detractors might object that it is foolhardy, if not insensitive, to expect trauma survivors to read and interpret a story about a privileged white man experiencing an existential crisis while writing a biography and his own diary. Nonetheless, the novel is not so much about Roquentin's existential crisis, but about readers' phenomenological experiences. The act of reading *Nausea* provokes a stimulation of emotions and bodily sensations that might mirror survivors' own emotions and sensations but only obliquely. This notion of obliqueness finds resonance in Levine's research. He advises against frontal confrontation of trauma memories and advocates for body-centered therapies. "In directing our attention to these internal body sensations, rather than attacking the trauma head-on, we can unbind and free the energies that have been held in check."[73] If posttraumatic responses (viz. hyper-arousal or hypo-arousal states) can lead to feelings of fear and helplessness and a resistance to confront the traumatic event head on, then survivors might gravitate toward a story that makes known that which one does not wish to know. Exposure to Roquentin's story may serve therefore as a prophylactic treatment. Survivors might learn about themselves in a less emotionally and physically intense fashion (compared to memory "flooding" experiences), and this may help them to access gradually their trauma.

Perhaps it seems to make little sense to engage trauma survivors in a Literary Arts Praxis featuring *Nausea*. They might need to address their own bodies before reading about and pondering Roquentin's. To be sure, the suppression of physical forms of traumatic procedural memory is key to recovery and may very well need to occur before survivors engage in reading literature replete with existential and phenomenological themes.[74] I do not deny the centrality of the body in posttraumatic conditions, a topic explored in Chapter 5. I fully recognize that the body stores traumatic stress in it and that reading about a traumatic experience might provoke memories laced with physiological and other physical responses. It is short of amazing however that traumatologists have not contemplated how trauma can be reached through a body that is stimulated while reading. The topic merits our attention as another mechanism to access trauma, and hence the reason for including a piece of literature rich in phenomenological themes and experiences in a Literary Arts Praxis.

As reviewed in Chapter 2, Hartman gave a stab at the body, reading, and trauma issue in his article "Traumatic Knowledge and Literary Studies" (1995). Again, he contends that "Perhaps the only way to overcome a traumatic severance of body and mind is to come back to the mind through the body."[75] While reading Samuel Coleridge's poem "The Rime of the Ancient Mariner," the reader's imagination provokes somatic feelings. Hartman's ideas about this stimulation of somatic feelings obviously do not apply exclusively to Romantic poetry. *Nausea* might provide another field of investigation about how reading literature might help trauma survivors "to come back to the mind through the body," as Hartman would say. The novel can easily translate into an intense phenomenological experience for readers. Readers can feel literally nauseous while reading about Roquentin's nausea. They can live his nausea vicariously. Consequently, reading *Nausea* may serve like a drug to induce a release of toxic feelings and memories and help survivors to access trauma in a physical way. Compared to Romantic poetry, literature rich in phenomenological and reader-induced phenomenological experiences may very well speak more intimately to trauma survivors.

Emotional Experiences

Related to the issue of how reading is a phenomenological experience, and thus a possible source of enlightenment about stored trauma in the body, is the topic of emotional stimulations. In his *How to Read Literature* (2013), literary theorist Terry Eagleton elaborates on a misunderstanding regarding emotional experiences. To his mind, some literary theorists claim that one cannot "really pity, admire, fear or abhor a fictional character, but can only 'fictionally' experience such emotions."[76] In more mundane terms, if we scream while watching *The Exorcist*, we are not truly afraid but only fictionally so. A Literary Arts Praxis—centering on an engagement with *Nausea*—is built on the idea that the distinction between "fictional" and "real" emotions is negligent. All felt emotions are "fictional." They are creative acts occurring on the stage of the mind. It takes imagination to comprehend one's own emotions and those of others. (Lest some harbor skepticism about the imaginative acuity needed to interpret one's own emotions, one ought to consider the emotional numbness (alexithymia) prevalent in trauma survivors.) This discussion of how emotions are stimulated during reading has relevance to trauma-survivor treatments. Recall from Chapter 5 that according to traumatologists, an emotional engagement with traumatic memories is necessary for the processing of the original event and eventual recovery. Foa and her colleagues point out consequently that clinicians can prepare trauma survivors for exposure therapies (ET) by training them to label and manage emotions.

Reading and interpreting literature, such as *Nausea*, may very well serve as a preparation to label and manage emotions that are stimulated when reading, so that survivors can label and manage them better in real-life situations.

Aesthetics *and* Nausea

One final important issue is missing from this discussion of how *Nausea* might speak intimately to trauma survivors and help them to reach trauma. We neglected to review the novel's ending. Even though Roquentin feels nauseated by his existence, he discovers meaning in life. By developing a sense of his bodily sensations and emotions, he at least feels alive. It is better to feel disgust and despair than to feel nothing at all. Eventually, he feels even more alive upon experiencing an epiphany about art.

This awakening is not so much about art but about the relationship between existence and art and occurs in two steps. It takes place when he hears the voice of a black woman singing the jazz tune "Some of these Days" on a phonograph. The song first provokes a piercing thought: "To think that there are idiots who get consolation from the fine arts."[77] Though this statement rings with cynical tones about humanists' faith in the arts to serve as a balm, it must be taken in a larger context. Sure, Roquentin reproaches his aunt for turning to Chopin for consolation at the time of his poor uncle's death. He also disdains concert goers who "imagine that the sounds flow into them, sweet, nourishing, and that their sufferings become music, like Werther; they think that beauty is compassionate to them."[78] To Roquentin's mind, art consumed in this way does not soothe suffering; it masks it with a shiny coat of shellac. He confesses that he too used to hide his existence behind Tintoretto's paintings and Stendhal's character Julien Sorel.[79] If art can nourish, Roquentin would rather go hungry. If it can turn his suffering into sweet sounds, he would rather hear groans.

It only takes four notes from the jazz tune for him to awaken and to edit his opinion about the arts. The sounds appear to say: "You must be like us, suffer in rhythm. All right! Naturally, I'd like to suffer that way, in rhythm, without complacence, without self-pity, with an arid purity."[80] Once his voice joins the chorus of suffering, he imagines a Jewish composer in New York penning the music and verse. He thinks to himself: "But when I hear the sound and I think that the composer made it, I find this suffering and sweat … moving."[81] Roquentin marvels that the composer made it through the sticky messy stuff of existence. If Camus helped to rewrite Sisyphus's story, if the musician penned his tune, if the jazz singer performed her piece, then Roquentin will embark on a creative enterprise. He will write a book about his existence, thus carving out his essence, rather than writing about the Marquis de Rollebon who helped him escape it. Creative writing is as real as a pebble in a hand, the very justification of his existence.[82] "The only goal of an absurd existence," writes Sartre in his war diary from 1939, "is to produce indefinitely works of art that escape that absurdity."[83] What the writer fails to become in life, he can become vicariously in his novel. And this applies to both Sartre and his character Roquentin as well as to readers.

Aesthetics and Trauma Survivors

Many traumatologists stress the importance for trauma survivors to create a testimony. However, what about reading literature, such as *Nausea*, and engaging in creative writing exercises? What is at stake when one reads literature (besides phenomenological experiences) and writes creatively? Against the background material on testimonies and creativity presented previously in this book, we shall offer new explanations.

Interpretative Reading

Just as Roquentin has an awakening as he listens to the jazz tune, is it not possible for trauma survivors to experience their own awakening while reading *Nausea*? Roquentin would scoff at such an idea, as made clear above from his snide remark about his aunt finding comfort in Chopin's music at the time of her husband's death. However, works of art do not have transformative effects, according to the existential hero. The production of art does. But how does one define a production of art? Isn't reading literature a creative act? Isn't the reader an artist or writer? Doesn't she dabble in paint on the palette of her mind or write verse on leaves of gray matter? As she reads nestled on the couch near an open window covered by gauze curtains dancing in the breeze, she creates images in her mind. The breeze touching her skin comes from the south and is laced with a salty mist from the sea. Roquentin is also at the seaside about to skip a stone along the water. He pauses and throws it back on the seashore. The reader picks it up and throws it into the sea, watching circular waves form as it falls to the sandy bottom. Of course, reading is a creative exercise; the act of reading literature is kindred to a workshop (comprised of novices and master artists) creating a masterpiece together. Furthermore, just as Sisyphus's rebellion against the gods could be inspirational, it may very well be that Roquentin's epiphany about the production of artwork and his determination to write a novel could inspire trauma survivors as well to create first stories in their heads while reading.

Creative Writing

How might creative writing get at trauma? First, it "works" in many of the same ways as interpreting creative works of art. It jumpstarts the mind. By engaging in both interpretative reading and creative writing exercises, the mind is infused with new words and new images that seed new ideas into a mind that has remained dormant. Second, words and images appear to cut like a knife through memories lodged in stone. The word "lapidary" in fact comes from the Latin term "*lapidarius*," which means stonecutter. A tomb of memories is assigned a name as the stonecutter cuts through granite. The past has not been buried after all like a corpse in the underground. It can be brought to life through words. Memories can be excised, and cerebral tissues can rejuvenate in the absence of energy consumed by the past. Third, recall from our discussion of Cyrulnik's research that the neuropsychiatrist seems to intimate that literary writing constitutes an important creative exercise for trauma survivors. By creating a personal narrative replete not only with similes, symbols, metaphors, and analogies but also philosophical musings, survivors are invited to luxuriate in masked meaning. The survivor becomes the sphinx and the riddle solver. She may be prepared to solve the riddle of her own traumatic memories and experiences. Fourth, while inventing a new life story from new images and words, the survivor crafts her being like a work of art. This may infuse her with a heightened sense of dignity, as Richman put forward. She has become an alchemist turning mud into gold, rather than feeling like dust on the ground upon which (potentially) the perpetrators of her trauma have trampled.

It is important to stress nonetheless that not all forms of creative endeavors are created equal, as Shapiro points out earlier in this chapter. Writing stories, composing poems, and even assuming a role in a play may very well serve different purposes, than composing a testimony for trauma survivors. Stories and poems demand imaginative interventions. Whether it is linguistic, literary, or plot features, poetry and stories consist of inventive forms that may very well help trauma survivors to rewrite their trauma story. By assuming authorship of their life story, survivors may gain a sense of jurisdiction over their own identity. They can rewrite the memory of their past (a testimony) and renegotiate that testimony by creating a new story of their present and future. And kindred to Sisyphus's revolt and Roquentin's plan to write an imaginative book, survivors rebel against their traumatic past through creative writing and join a community of artists and writers.

Creative Stories Replace Testimonies

The replacement of a testimony with creative stories is another possible way in which survivors might get a trauma. (Again, to my mind a "testimony" comes closer to a factual attestation of events, whereas a story is an interpretation replete with emotional content and creative adjustments.) Moving beyond a testimony allows a survivor to move beyond a wounded spirit. As she creatively constructs a story, concentrating on acts of resistance and resilience, she builds herself and thus helps to repair her damaged identity.

Referring to patients who have suffered the trauma of disease, Arthur Frank describes a process that moves beyond catharsis:

First they resist the call: the disease, or trauma, or chronic pain that is being forced upon their bodies. As their stories develop and as they develop in their stories, they resist the silence that suffering forces upon their bodyselves. Finally their resistance finds a voice; they make suffering useful. In the wounds of their resistances, they gain a power: to tell, and even to heal.[84]

Frank's statement is pertinent for several reasons. His expressions "they resist the call"; "they resist the silence"; "their resistance finds a voice"; and the "wounds of their resistances" put into plain language existential engagement (creative revolts). In addition, trauma theorists have referred to healing the wound of trauma by testimonies. But the idea of rebellion is missing from their argument. And yet Frank intimates that acts of resistance fuel the development of one's story, leading to empowerment and perhaps even to healing.

By reshaping testimonies into creative stories in an act of conscious resistance, survivors re-experience the traumatic event, but on their own terms, including the time, amount, and personal reactions to it. In practical terms, they make suffering "useful," as Frank claims above. This creative process consists of establishing new openings, new ways of viewing the past, present, and future. The literary theorist Roland Barthes refers to this phenomenon when writing about his mother's death: "Not to suppress mourning (suffering) (the stupid notion that time will do away with such a thing) but to change it, transform it, to shift it from a static stage (stasis, obstruction, recurrence of the same thing) to a fluid state."[85] Barthes's reference to shifting away from obstruction and stasis brings to mind psychoanalysis and cognitive behavioral therapy. These treatment methods are based on the premise that they take place not only in the therapist's office, but also in the subject's mind, thus altering neuronal networks.[86] From a physiological perspective, telling creative stories might restore the brain, because neurons fire in novel ways, which triggers the brain to secrete dopamine, the pleasure hormone.[87] Constructing stories might not only translate into an act of empowerment, but also a cognitive act that promotes growth that helps survivors redefine themselves in new ways.

Conclusions

Following clinicians' invitation for trauma survivors to wear a philosopher's hat, following their recommendations for survivors to engage in creative activities, and following their insistence on employing cognitive exercises to combat psychic constriction, I have developed the concept of a Literary Arts Praxis and considered how it might "get at trauma." The Praxis is built on literature seeped in existential, phenomenological, and aesthetic themes as well as clinical research. I have argued that engagements with literature rich in these branches of philosophy may help trauma survivors to get at trauma, which might in turn foster resistance, resilience, and posttraumatic growth. These mental metamorphoses may very well occur as trauma survivors engage in imaginative escapades, including forming alliances with characters; interpretative exercises while reading *The Myth of Sisyphus* and *Nausea*; and creative writing endeavors, such as turning testimonies into imaginative stories.

While Sisyphus may inspire readers to engage in acts of artistic, philosophical, and psychological rebellion, *Nausea*'s final message about creating works of art may very well serve as a source of inspiration for trauma survivors to chip away at the marble of their mind to find a new sculpture of identity. Aesthetic experiences, as seen in Roquentin's intent to write creatively, may help survivors to get at trauma as they: infuse their minds with novel words and images that foster novel ideas; cut through encrusted memories; become accustomed to masked meaning to solve the riddle of their own traumatic memories and experiences; and restore a sense of dignity by crafting their essence like a work of art.

What creative contributions do I bring to the field of trauma studies through a Literary Arts Praxis? How do I build and expand on other musings on the relationship between trauma and the literary arts and how a Praxis might get at trauma? While I have relied on LaCapra's positions, I have adjusted and added to them. First, though I share his opinion that literature might provide a haven, I emphasize that this is possible because of alliances formed between existential characters and trauma survivors. Second, I echo his position that the arts can provide imaginative openings to reinterpret reality from an uncanny angle; however, I do not point so much to surrealistic situations, but rather to psycho-philosophical content presented in ways that are easier to decipher than an essay by Martin Heidegger. Sisyphus and Roquentin might inspire trauma survivors to resist artistically, by rebuilding themselves; metaphysically, by defying death and nihilism; and psychologically, by remaining true to their feelings and core personality traits and values. Third, whereas I agree with LaCapra that literature can provide raw commentary on specific social realities, I argue that existential literature offers universal portraits of the human condition that strike above all a profound chord in readers. Fourth, my explanations on phenomenological and phenomenologically induced emotional experiences find resonance with his position that writing trauma prods readers' actions and emotions; still, I stress that a stimulation of emotions and bodily sensations while reading might help survivors to develop emotional and physical "antibodies" needed to confront the memories of their own traumatic experiences.

Beyond amplifying LaCapra's arguments, I have also developed creative arguments in response to other traumatologists' research. Most notably, though I agree with Hartman's position that reading induced bodily experiences may be a way to access trauma, I shine a spotlight on literature rich in phenomenological themes and experiences as it may speak more intimately to trauma survivors. A Literary Arts Praxis distinguishes itself moreover from clinical treatments in that the place of action takes place in a highly imaginative realm; I have yet to hear of the possibility of forming therapeutic alliances with literary characters. Further, while I do refer to testimonies (borrowed from First Wave theorists and Davoine), I have put forward that they might serve as precursors to creative stories. The Praxis also makes an adjustment to the idea that trauma is a wound that is sutured up (Cyrulnik) or given shape (Laub) by words. More than a wound, posttraumatic experiences can behave like a malignant cancer. They can grow to be just as harrowing and painful as the original traumatic event. Hence, I have proposed instead the idea of excising the cancer of posttraumatic states through an engagement with creative words and images. Finally, and perhaps most importantly, the Praxis is founded on the idea of a revolt, a concept I have yet to encounter among other theorists, save for Frank. These revolts do not take place in the streets, but in the imaginative space between our ears and through testimonies that metamorphize into creative stories.

If metamorphoses are to happen, if trauma survivors are expected to alter their trauma narratives and memories, think like philosophers, and compose creative works, they ought to be trained to assume these roles. While this may seem like a given to any humanities professor, a training in philosophy and literature seems to be absent in treatments reviewed in this book. A Literary Arts Praxis may very well help survivors to engage more profoundly in these activities. This position flies in the face of psychiatrist Peter D. Kramer's staggering comment (reviewed in this book's introduction) that a near-obsessive devotion to reading literature, including pieces from Camus, were alarm bells for psychopathologies in his patients.[88]

With this comment in the rearview mirror, it becomes apparent that a Literary Arts Praxis may confront several roadblocks. Clinicians may have neither the time nor the knowledge to engage their patients in such an educational training. Cultural trauma theorists may dismiss it as governed by a tyranny of lucidity, as opposed to a tyranny of opaqueness and even pseudo-profundity.[89] This may be an easy criticism to level when one is not confronted with the rude reality of trauma, especially suffered by youngsters who do not have the resources to treat their mental suffering. An even greater barrier is a current reality in which literature and art are not exactly prized commodities in contemporary culture. Consequently, it is almost as if scientists and clinicians are left solely responsible for treating psychic suffering through psychotherapeutic or pharmacotherapy, while the arts are relegated to a back closet covered in dust or to an ivory tower for the privileged few at universities and museums. The Praxis attempts precisely to encourage survivors to build their own museum of the mind. And readers are invited to take a tour in the pages that follow to discover pieces of world literature in which characters seem to get at trauma through a Literary Arts Praxis.

Notes

1 Psychologist Peter Levine makes a similar distinction: "When dealing with a physical trauma, the physician's job is to support healing (wash the wound, protect it with a bandage or cast, etc.). The cast doesn't heal the broken bone; it provides the physical mechanism of support that allows the bone to initiate and complete its own intelligent healing processes. Similarly, in integrating the psychic polarities of expansion and contraction, the felt sense supports us in orchestrating the marvel of transformation." Levine and Frederick, *Waking*, 196–198.

2 I lean heavily on the idea that resilience is linked to regenerative experiences, such as "engaging in new creative activities"; see Bonanno, "Resilience," 136.

3 I am suggesting that safety must be cultivated first in trauma survivors, as Janet and Herman have insisted. A Literary Arts Praxis might prove of interest to clinicians at a later recovery stage. For further information about recovery stages, consult Chapter 5.

4 Calhoun and Tedeschi, *Handbook*, 7.

5 LaCapra, *Writing*, 183.

6 Ibid.

7 Tedeschi et al., *Posttraumatic*, 9.

8 Aristotle, *Nicomachean*, loc. 5949–5959.

9 See Aristotle, *Éthique*, Livre VI, 157–162. The notion that the Greek word "praxis" refers to self-realization or an "accomplishement of existence," consult the following translator's note: "*Hè praxis sera donc traduit par l'accomplissement (de l'existence), la manière d'accomplir …*" Aristotle, *Éthique*, 162. The French translator's note translated is: "'*Hè praxis*' is thus translated as accomplishement (of existence), the manner of accomplishment …"

10 Recall that Geoffrey Hartman refers to a criticism that decodes the wound of trauma; see Hartman, "Traumatic," 549; Boris Cyrulnik also relies on the image of wounds that are stitched up by words; a discussion of his work appears later in this chapter.

11 Van der Kolk, *Body*, 70.

12 Ibid.

13 Calhoun and Tedeschi, *Handbook*, 9.

14 Van der Kolk, "Trauma and Memory," 7.

15 See Herman, *Trauma*, 178; though Herman mentions the role of "theologian," I feel less qualified to comment on it and do not include it in my discussions.

16 Calhoun and Tedeschi, *Posttraumatic*, 103.

17 Herman, *Trauma*, 202.

18 Levine and Frederick, *Waking*, 119.

19 Cyrulnik, *La nuit*, 10. My translation; the original reads: "*Le plus sûr moyen de récoudre la déchirure, c'est de suturer la plaie avec des mots.*"

20 Baudelaire, "Épilogue," 219–220. My translation; the original reads, "*Tu m'as donné ta boue, j'en ai fait de l'or.*"

21 Richman, *Mended*, 93.

22 Ibid., 96.

23 Ibid.

24 Felman and Laub, *Testimony*, 78.

25 Laub, "Record," 48.

26 Ibid.

27 Felman and Laub, *Testimony*, 79; Laub's view of testimony and the "impossibility of telling" finds resonance in the ideas of Felman and Caruth, explored in Chapter 4.

28 The idea of blowing up art was the modus operandi of the Dadaists. Their destructive spirit was triggered by a deep sense of disappointment in all sacred cows, from science and technology to art itself post World War I.

29 Shapiro "Resilience," 121.
30 Ibid.
31 Ibid.
32 Ibid., 120.
33 Ibid.
34 Cloitre et al., *Treating*, 345.
35 Ibid.
36 Davoine and Gaudillière, "Mad Witness," 102.
37 Alexander, *Trauma*, 61.
38 Ibid., 11.
39 Alexander, *Meanings*, 89.
40 LaCapra, *Writing*, loc. 357.
41 Ibid., 185.
42 Ibid., 186–187.
43 Ibid., 13.
44 LaCapra offers an insightful discussion on how historiography was grounded in a "documentary or self-sufficient research model" at the end of the nineteenth and early twentieth centuries and that historians "dissociated" from literature. He contends that this model has "persisted" in historiography, even though its value has been questioned. LaCapra, *Writing*, 2.
45 Camus, *Myth*, 120.
46 I write "truly" since Camus claims that Sisyphus was an absurd hero before he was subjected to the punishments of the gods in his passionate devotion to attempting to defy them.
47 Camus, *Myth*, 121.
48 Camus writes, "That hour like a breathing-space which returns as surely as his suffering, that is the hour of consciousness." Ibid.
49 Ibid.
50 Ibid., 123.
51 Ibid., 121.
52 Calhoun and Tedeschi, *Posttraumatic*, 11.
53 See Yalom, *Existential*; see Frankl, *Man's Search*.
54 I am not suggesting that Camus was averse to violence in all circumstances. He had fought in the French Resistance and understood the necessity of violence when fighting the Nazis. However, he did object to comfortable violence. This is carried out from one's armchair in the name of ideology, not in the name of starving children or persecuted peoples.
55 Camus outlines these different types of rebellion in separate chapters with the same names in his essay *The Rebel*.
56 See Herman, *Trauma*, 176.
57 See Camus, *Myth*, 123.
58 Camus, *Rebel*, loc. 418.
59 While testimonies can include obviously creative writing, the term "testimony" carries more of a sense of public profession of facts. I lean more on the latter sense, because I would like to propose a distinction between testimonies and stories in trauma survivor treatments.
60 The notion that a testimony might provide a more factual narrative, and hence a first step towards creative stories does not correspond to Herman's position: "The recitation of facts without the accompanying emotions is a sterile exercise, without therapeutic effect." Herman, *Trauma*, 177. However, this is an idea that I am putting forward for clinicians to contemplate.
61 Sartre, *Nausea*, loc. 2185.
62 Ibid., loc. 444.
63 Ibid., loc. 569.

64 Sartre, *Nausea*, loc. 3406.

65 See Merleau-Ponty, *Visible*, loc. 573.

66 Beauvoir, *Second*, 46.

67 Merleau-Ponty does not employ this metaphor. I devised it to encapsulate his ideas from the following passage: *"Comme la chose, comme autrui, le vrai luit à travers une expérience émotionnelle et presque charnelle, où les 'idées',—celles d'autrui et les nôtres—, sont plutôt des traits de sa physionomie et de la nôtre, et sont moins comprises qu'accueillies ou repoussées dans l'amour ou la haine."* Merleau-Ponty, *Visible*, loc. 304.

68 My translation. The original reads: *"Tout ce que les hommes sentent, je peux le deviner, l'expliquer, le mettre noir sur blanc. Mais non pas le sentir. Je fais illusion, j'ai l'air d'un sensible et je suis un désert."* Sartre, *Carnets*, loc. 4305.

69 Jacques-Henri Bernardin de St. Pierre coined the formula, "I feel, therefore I am" (*Je sens donc je suis*) in response to Descartes's axiomatic expression. See Bernardin de St. Pierre, *Œuvres*, 105.

70 This idea originates from Sartre's war diaries: *"L'authenticité exige qu'on accepte de souffrir, par fidélité à soi, par fidélité au monde. Car nous sommes libres-pour-souffrir et libres-pour-ne-pas-souffrir. Nous sommes responsables de la forme et de l'intensité de nos souffrances. Il est très facile d'être—très facile aussi d'être stoïque."* Sartre, *Carnets*, loc. 4083.

71 Van der Kolk, *Body*, 221.

72 Calhoun and Tedeschi, *Posttraumatic*, 16.

73 Levine and Frederick, *Waking*, 66–67.

74 I make this assertion based on the following remark from van der Kolk: "The act of telling the story doesn't necessarily alter the automatic physical and hormonal responses of bodies that remain hypervigilant." Van der Kolk, *Body*, 21.

75 Ibid.

76 Eagleton, *How*, 24.

77 Sartre, *Nausea*, loc. 3731.

78 Ibid., loc. 3734.

79 See ibid., loc. 3760. He refers more specifically to Julien Sorel, the main character from Stendhal's novel.

80 Ibid., loc. 3742.

81 Ibid., loc. 3788.

82 Roquentin confesses that his book would help him perhaps to "remember his life without repugnance." See ibid., loc. 3817.

83 Sartre, *Carnets*, 102.

84 Frank, *Wounded*, 182.

85 Barthes, *Mourning*, 142.

86 See Doidge, *Brain*, 221.

87 See ibid., 216.

88 See our discussion in this book's introduction on Kramer's insinuation.

89 The wording of this sentence has been inspired by Alan Sokal and Jean Bricmont's *Fashionable Nonsense*, 1–16.

Part IV

Engaging in a Literary Arts Praxis and World Literature

Introduction

The Foreign and Familiar of World Literature

World literature seems well-positioned to morph our understanding of traumatic and posttraumatic experiences. However, before provoking such a mental metamorphosis, let us explore the concept of world literature. Wolfgang von Goethe seems to have coined the term *Weltliteratur* (world literature) in the early nineteenth century.[1] Goethe's definitions of world literature are useful starting points. His vision does not apply simply to geography or culture. It also encompasses a universality of form, as "poetry is the universal possession of mankind."[2] In his *What is World Literature?* (2003), David Damrosch stretches this notion of world literature beyond cultures of origin and literary forms (poetry) to include time:

> Over the centuries, an unusually shifty work can come in and out of the sphere of world literature several different times; and at any given point, a work may function as world literature for some readers but not others, and for some kinds of reading, but not for others.[3]

A literature defined by a temporal, cultural, linguistic, and spatial elasticity? This makes it seem as if world literature stretches to include too much or remains too flaccid to encircle any culture, geography, genre, or time. Damrosch acknowledges in fact a "ghostly or vampirish concept of world literature."[4] This ghostly or vampirish concept seems to apply to most literature and the arts, whose intrinsic nature is hard to pin down.

In his recent *Comparing the Literatures: Literary Studies in a Global Age* (2020), Damrosch proposes that if the definition of world literature remains shrouded, the author of world literature may very well lift the shroud. Turning to Gabriel García Márquez, Damrosch relays how a gigantic insect piqued the Colombian writer's interest in writing:

DOI: 10.4324/9781003284642-11

One night a friend lent me a book of short stories by Franz Kafka. I went back to the pension where I was staying and began to read *The Metamorphosis*. The first line almost knocked me off the bed. I was so surprised. The first line reads, "As Gregor Samsa awoke that morning from uneasy dreams, he found himself transformed in his bed into a gigantic insect ..." When I read the line I thought to myself that I didn't know anyone was allowed to write things like that. If I had known, I would have started writing a long time ago. So I immediately started writing short stories.[5]

All it took was the first line of Kafka's *Metamorphosis* for García Márquez to envision his own metamorphosis into a novelist. Even a limited encounter with "a world author can have a transformative effect," Damrosch argues, "if it comes at a critical moment for a young writer looking for an alternative to the reigning norms at home."[6] The key to this interpretation is the dichotomy between the "alternative" and "reigning norms at home." World-literature authors have the power to transform a reader through their writing that is strange enough to intrigue and yet familiar enough to reach the reader to begin with. The insect introduces an alternative reality, while Gregor Samsa's family reflects a recognizable one. These images were foreign and yet familiar enough to stick to García Márquez's wall of imagination. But doesn't this apply to literature in general? Isn't literature precisely a tango dance of foreign and familiar tones and rhythms of fiction and reality?

Before addressing these questions, it is important to signal that Damrosch nuances the definition of world literature further in his discussion of the author Kenzaburō Ōe. Speaking about the Japanese author, he writes: "For him, world literature has been a refuge, a resource, and a weapon."[7] In other words, world literature provides just as much the harbor, as the treasure chest and the cannons aboard Ōe's vessel. It also provides shipmates who steer and guard his ship through rough waters and against attacks. Ōe relies upon authors from across the globe who have employed their pens like swords to fight political injustices. They have given the creative writer a sense of "brotherhood."[8] World literature has the power therefore to unite readers behind a common cause while edifying and fortifying. The familiar may be the urge to combat injustices; the foreign is found in the details of the combat.

Damrosch's implied definition of world literature as a combination of the familiar and the foreign needs to be explored from the other end of the scope. Can the foreign not be familiar and the familiar foreign? The first line from *The Metamorphosis* is not any old line: "As Gregor Samsa awoke one morning from uneasy dreams he found himself transformed in his bed into a gigantic insect."[9] The potency of Kafka's writing obviously lies in the metaphor. There is a universality about metaphors or "commonplaces," as they are called in rhetoric. They readily transport images and emotions to readers' minds, reaching conscious and even far-to-reach unconscious realms. The universality of the metaphor of an insect or spider is staggering as seen in its use in idiomatic expressions in other languages such as French and Japanese.[10] García Márquez's reaction to Kafka's insect suggests that world literature is animated by metaphors that can travel to readers' psyche, despite cultural and linguistic barriers. The foreignness of the image of an insect is familiar enough to seize the imagination of readers. An "insect-hood" replaces Ōe's sense of "brotherhood."

While the metaphor of an insect carries universal images and feelings, it also transmits psycho-philosophical messages. Consider that Gregor simply awakes as an insect, whereas in Apuleius's *The Metamorphoses*, the jealous goddess Minerva changes Arachne into a spider. It is one thing to have a jealous goddess change a mortal into a spider condemned to spin webs. It is still another to awake one morning covered in a crustacean carapace. The etiology of Gregor's grotesque disfigurement may be found in his obsessional worries about arriving late to his job. Obviously, his greater concern should be his invertebrate form not his job. He is stuck in the state of abjection. If his job is not to blame for making him feel so abject, it may be that existence by definition is alienating.

This sense of self-estrangement is made apparent not only by his grotesque form but also by his family's silence. Nobody asks why or how he changed into an insect. The mother faints upon seeing him. The father pelts him with apples. The sister delivers him trays of food that remain untouched. The cleaning lady taps his eventual corpse with a broom. This absence of meaningful interaction adds to the alienation that his anthropoid form conveys. Gregor has become the living embodiment of an existential crisis. He symbolizes "every man, without any support or help whatever... condemned at every instant to invent man," as Sartre contends.[11] Be that as it may, the symbol of the insect binds the abstract psycho-philosophical message to bodily concreteness, thus bringing to life phenomenological themes in bug form as opposed to Sartre's stone held in the palm of a hand.

García Márquez's encounter with Gregor's metamorphosis suggests that world literature is defined by its ability to reach people universally, as it treats psycho-philosophical topics found at the heart of the human condition. To quell any doubt of the universality of Kafka's message, one could consult various dictionaries to witness how a kindred term to "kafkaesque" appears in German, French, Spanish, Japanese, and Chinese. Kafka's work is so universal that it defies the Tower of Babel. Thus, the foreign is neither the insect nor the metaphor of the insect. The foreignness appears instead when the content is made known and yet remains unknown given the complexities of character, voice, style, form, and theme.

Like existential, phenomenological, and aesthetic issues, traumatic and posttraumatic experiences are universal themes that world literature portrays with both foreign and familiar colors and strokes of paint. Trauma may seem foreign not only in its depth and breadth of suffering but also in its textures and tones of ambiguity. Besides, the sense of alienation common in traumatic experiences may feel so real and yet so unreal that it can only be conveyed in stories about insects and intense phenomenological experiences. That is, the body becomes another body, a concept Frantz Fanon explored regarding the traumatic experience of colonialism for the colonized.[12]

In the next three chapters, we shall examine world literature that explores different forms of traumatic experiences. Miguel de Cervantes offers a vivid portrayal of the trauma of aging; Albert Camus paints a portrait of traumatic suffering during an epidemic; and Jean-Marie Gustave Le Clézio transmits a visceral sense of childhood trauma. The main characters from these masterpieces, Don Quixote, Rieux, and Lalla, also provide examples of creative mechanisms to transcend trauma. These novels are not so much "trauma fiction" but rather "resistance, resilience, and posttraumatic growth fiction."[13] Characters seem to engage in a Literary Arts Praxis to get at trauma, forge resilience, engage in acts of resistance, experience growth, and perhaps even recover. While we have contemplated how a Literary Arts Praxis can somehow get at trauma through imaginative escapades, interpretative reading adventures, and creative writing exercises in the previous chapter, we will examine how fictional characters seem to transcend their trauma through other creative mechanisms. And by contemplating portraits of trauma from world literature, familiar stories may very well seem foreign, while the foreign may seem familiar. (Beyond Camus and Sartre, other world literature authors to consult include: Beauvoir, Castellanos, Dostoyevsky, García Márquez, Gogol, Kafka, Kierkegaard, Kundera, Murakami, Ōe, Unamuno, and Zweig.) This might in turn stir the pot of our received ideas on trauma, posttraumatic conditions, trauma narratives, and even trauma studies.

Notes

1 I write that Goethe seems to have coined the term "*Weltliteratur*" (world literature) to acknowledge that perhaps other cultures had developed such a term to refer to literary writing that was universal in nature, and that we remain blind to this history.
2 Goethe and Eckermann, *Conversations*, 264.
3 Damrosch, *What*, 6.
4 Damrosch, *Comparing*, 68.
5 García Márquez, "Interview."
6 Damrosch, *Comparing*, 270.
7 Ibid., 272.
8 Ōe in Ibid.
9 Kafka, *Metamorphosis*, 67.
10 In French, "*J'ai le cafard*" means "I am depressed," but literally translated means "I have a cockroach."
11 Sartre, *Existentialism*, 29.
12 See my discussion of Fanon's work in Chapter 2.
13 By employing the term "trauma fiction," I am referencing Anne Whitehead's book on the topic.

7 The Trauma of Aging and Reading Adventures with Miguel de Cervantes

Keeping in mind that world literature often makes the familiar foreign and the foreign familiar, we explore the Spanish writer Miguel de Cervantes's canonical *Don Quixote* (published first in Spanish in 1605/1615). This chapter on Cervantes's work and the trauma of aging responds to a current resistance to ponder the issues of aging and dying. In his *Being Mortal* (2014), surgeon Atul Gawande highlights that while he learned a lot about anatomy and physiology during medical school, the topics of mortality, aging, frailty, and dying were neglected: "How the process unfolds, how people experience the end of their lives, and how it affects those around them seemed beside the point."[1] Related to Gawande's concern about medicine's failure to address the topics of aging and death, oncologist Siddhartha Mukherjee points out in his *Laws of Medicine* (2015) that his medical education taught him "plenty of facts, but little about spaces between facts."[2] By spaces, Mukherjee is referring to life's ever-present ambiguities, contradictions, and conundrums, which were absent in his medical education. Cervantes's masterpiece addresses both Mukherjee's and Gawande's concerns. The novel explores the themes of diminishment and dying through masked and hidden content demanding slow and thoughtful readings. While humans may not be living longer, some are certainly dying longer. How people experience the end of their lives remains thus a topic of ethical importance demanding creative and interdisciplinary attention.

But can physical and cognitive diminishment and dying be considered traumatic? The *DSM-5* does not seem to indicate this, as it states explicitly that "A life-threatening illness or debilitating medical condition is not necessarily considered a traumatic event. Medical incidents that qualify as traumatic events involve sudden, catastrophic events …"[3] However, the use of the words "not necessarily" leave some room for us to consider physical and mental diminishment a traumatic event; besides, experience and intuition may confirm this reality. Relying on notions from both clinical trauma theories and cultural trauma studies, I put forward that the pre-Don Quixote character, Alonso Quijano, has experienced a trauma of aging. The second main critical position centers on Quijano's Literary Arts Praxis, a

DOI: 10.4324/9781003284642-12

term I developed previously to refer to a training to address traumatic suffering. Quixote's Praxis involves: (a) reading about traumatized characters (to build a lexicon of emotions); (b) engaging in a phenomenological practice; that is, he stimulates emotions through performances with the body; (c) listening to others' stories of trauma; (d) sharing his expressions of grief with others; and (e) building bonds of empathy that stimulate collective empathy toward his own traumatized self. This study takes three original turns in trauma studies. First, it emphasizes a unique form of posttraumatic growth as Cervantes's hero engages with characters in the books he reads; those he encounters on his adventures; and most significantly with his own former traumatized self. Second, it adds to LaCapra's notion of "empathic unsettlement,"[4] a sense of compassion for others' traumatic experiences. I argue that "empathic unsettlement" is effective, because it addresses the "central dialectic of psychological trauma"[5] or the urge to keep the traumatic experience a secret and yet to reveal it. Namely, the character Alonso Quijano assumes the identity of Don Quixote thanks to reading about knights. He then embarks on an imaginative adventure, transforming himself gradually into another who is liberated from the traumatic experience. He knows without knowing and speaks without speaking. Third, from outside the reality of trauma or inside the "unreality" of creative expression, Don Quixote seems to develop resilience and to experience growth and somehow seems to get at trauma.[6] While some of these topics were unpacked in Chapter 6, our discussion of *Don Quixote* will offer nuanced and expanded views.

Measuring Alonso Quijano's "Madness" and the Trauma of Aging

A standard reading of Cervantes's masterpiece does not refer to the theme of trauma, nor, for that matter, Quixote's trauma. A typical interpretation is that Alonso Quijano has gone mad and transforms himself into the besotted knight errant Don Quixote. Apparently, an obsessive-compulsive tendency to read books of chivalry is to blame for Quijano's madness or in clinical terms, his "monomania," "paranoid," or "delusional disorder."[7] The narrator sums up the circumstances surrounding his condition: "he became so absorbed in his books that he spent his nights from sunset to sunrise, and his days from dawn to dark, poring over them; and what with little sleep and much reading his brains got so dry that he lost his wits."[8] Other characters, such as Quijano's niece, the housekeeper, the curate, and the barber, among others, blame books for his madness and consequently, burn almost all the contents of his library. Their motivation to burn especially his poetry books is spurred by the fear that his condition will only worsen: "what would be still worse, to turn poet, which they say is an incurable and infectious malady."[9] And yet, our hero confesses that he reads books to get up in the morning. This intimates that books have not caused his madness, but rather have provided a "remedy."[10]

This confession leads us to question the standard interpretation of Quijano's madness and to argue that he is traumatized by his diminished state associated with aging; absorbs himself in books; and then assumes the identity of Don Quixote. His madness (interpreted as avid reading and assuming a foreign identity) is a form of therapy. This idea finds resonance in the research of psychiatrist Jodi Halpern who argues that "healing involves grieving, a process that includes phases of emotional irrationality."[11] To categorize Quijano's psychic disturbance as simply madness denies the possibility for irrationality to play a positive role in trauma recovery.

Is there other evidence to indicate that Alonso Quijano has been traumatized by the experience of aging? Françoise Davoine appears to be one of the few critics to read trauma in *Don Quixote*. She argues that Cervantes's two volumes "are the best antidepressants to heal trauma ..."[12] The text makes us laugh, thus stimulating the unconscious, including the "cut-out" unconscious, while Sancho Panza shows us how to talk and work through hardships. She also claims that the text itself serves a cathartic role for Cervantes who experienced trauma.[13] Referring to the complete title (*Don Quijote de la Mancha*) and to the fact that *la mancha* means "stain," she argues that the author felt the stain of "war trauma" and transfers and transforms that burden into an epic. This is how Don Quixote allegedly heals his author: "the hero's work and science is devoted to the building of free speech and of thought, this despite the disasters of a century plagued by epidemics, religious wars, genocides, hijackings, and abuse ..."[14] Much of Davoine's thinking about trauma revolves around the traumatic war experience of the author and how the "son" (Don Quixote) was put in charge to heal his "father" (Cervantes). Such a focus undercuts the traumatic experience of Alonso Quijano (the pre-Don Quixote character). This research centers directly on the dyad character Alonso Quijano/Don Quixote to grasp the history of his trauma, "folly," and posttraumatic states.

Even if it seems tempting for psychoanalysts to approach Don Quixote from a Freudian perspective—by analyzing the relationship between the "father" (Cervantes) and "son" (Don Quixote)—it should be stressed that Don Quixote is not so much the son, but rather Cervantes's "stepson." In the author's note, he confesses: "for though I pass for the father, I am but the stepfather to 'Don Quixote'."[15] By denying total responsibility for his hero, the author forcefully creates a distance between Don Quixote and himself.[16] One of Cervantes's most remarkable literary coups confirms the prevalence of this distance: The narrator informs us that the story of Don Quixote does not actually belong to him. He learned about it through a "mysterious Arabic manuscript" penned by Cide Hamete Benengeli. Moreover, Don Quixote belongs to Alonso Quijano. He is the brainchild of Cervantes's Quijano, and this fact creates a sense of distance between the author, narrator, and hero. Since the authorial hand has lost some of its force, Don Quixote appears freer to roam the world quixotically and to heal his previously traumatized self. The distance is established to give the traumatized room to write his own script, not so much as a story, but as an embodied experience of transformation, as "trauma is much more than a story about something that happened long ago. The emotions and physical sensations that were imprinted during the trauma are experienced not as memories but as disruptive physical reactions in the present."[17] Don Quixote gets to work dislodging those physical disturbances as he embarks on adventures.

Cervantes scholar Carroll Johnson hints in fact at the possibility of a complex past that caused Quijano's madness: "psychosis is not a cause, but an effect, the last and most drastic weapon in the arsenal of defenses we humans can mobilize to cope with intolerable reality."[18] Johnson argues that Quijano's life had been boring, devoid of meaning, and defined by unbridled erotic desires. To deny this unsettling reality, Quijano "mobilizes as a first line of defense an all-consuming passion for books of chivalry, which offers the possibility of a vicarious experience of a more fulfilling life."[19] While Johnson rightly emphasizes an "intolerable reality" of the past, he ignores the symbolic importance of the knight, which is not defined by "egoism" but rather by "self-sacrifice," as the historian Johan Huizinga points out in reference to the Late Middle Ages.[20] Huizinga's research propels us to argue that Quijano reads books about errant knights living on the cusp of death in order to prepare himself for his own demise. The thought of death torments Quijano: "When in my mind I muse, O Love, upon thy cruelty, To death I flee, In hope therein the end of all to find ... Thus life doth slay, And death again to life restoreth me; Strange destiny, That deals with life and death as with a play!"[21] It is precisely this combination of contemplating an impending diminished future—along with a keen sense of loss of what was and will never be—that proves traumatic for Quijano.

Kindred to Davoine's argument on Cervantes's traumatic experiences, Josep Beá and Victor Hernández claim that Cervantes (who was in his fifties and sixties when he penned his masterpiece) created Don Quixote in order to work through his "anxieties of approaching old age and death."[22] They judge Alonso Quijano nevertheless more critically, arguing that Don Quixote is the "psychopathological answer to his inability to overcome the same conflict ..."[23] It is curious that Don Quixote is a "healthy" and "fertile" response to the author's anxieties about aging, whereas the quixotic character is a "psychopathological" answer to Quijano's same anxiety.

From time to time, Don Quixote hints at a previous existence defined by trauma. He confesses to his squire Sancho that he "was born to live dying."[24] This could mean that he has suffered his whole life long from alexithymia or felt physically and/or cognitively depleted. Either way, his condition resembles an ill-defined pathology. His life story remains sealed in a protective envelope, and hence the nebulous definition of the pre-Don Quixote character: "They will have it his surname was Quixada or Quesada (for here there is some difference of opinion among the authors who write on the subject), although from reasonable conjectures it seems plain that he was called Quexana."[25] The narrator's uncertainty about the original character's name speaks volumes about the latter's insignificance (at least ostensibly). His identity "is of but little importance to our tale."[26] Readers finally meet Quijano at the end of the epic. Don Quixote has shed his armor literally and figuratively when his real self is prepared to die. Otherwise, Quijano is always presented as the other, the one who dwells in the shadow of his alter ego Don Quixote.

The very existence of a proxy character that dwells in the imagination of the character Quijano is the first piece of circumstantial evidence that he had experienced trauma. Don Quixote, the so-called brave knight, and Dulcinea, his imagined noble mistress, are remnants of his trauma. Such a reading is rooted in theory. Psychiatrist and trauma specialist Mark Epstein writes: "The traumatized individual lives outside time, in his or her own separate reality, unable to relate to the consensual reality of others."[27] To drive home the message of separate realities, we should recall that Don Quixote makes up stories that defy the so-called reality in which he dwells. Instead of telling the truth that she along with the housekeeper, curate, and barber burned Don Quixote's books, his niece dreams up a story of a magician, a certain Sage Munaton, who arriving on a cloud, dismounted a serpent and committed an act of mischief in the library. Don Quixote snatches the bait of his niece's overactive imagination, responding that it must have been Friston, not Munaton, and that he is a sage magician, his great enemy. This illustrates how Don Quixote's reality is not only unreal, but surreal, while fiction becomes even more fictional. Both extreme conditions point to separate realities and signs of lingering trauma, as Epstein reminds us.

Related to this first piece of evidence, the missing character Quijano is also the epitome of depersonalization, one of the symptoms of the massive dissociation created by trauma.[28] Dissociation is characterized by sensing that some other force (other than one's own) is in control of one's thoughts, feelings or even actions. In metaphorical terms, it is kindred to being a passenger on one's own ship instead of being the captain. Rather than labeling his condition madness, it seems more fitting to argue that he has lost executive functioning. As reviewed earlier in this book, psychiatrist Bessel van der Kolk explains that trauma deactivates the left hemisphere, which is responsible for analytical reasoning and organizing experiences into logical sequence. This describes Don Quixote's behavior as he undertakes adventures such as dueling over the exquisite beauty of his fictitious Dulcinea; fighting the supposed giants (the windmills); or battling the apparent armies (the flocks of sheep covered in dust clouds) (chapters 4, 8, and 18 of part 1). The absurdity of these acts reflects the intensity of his trauma, but their intensity could very well promote a steeling effect. If might have fostered resilience to accept the impending reality of physical diminishment in aging.

In her *The New Wounded* (2012), philosopher Catherine Malabou claims that cerebral pathologies such as dementia can be among the most perplexing and intense forms of suffering.[29] This leads us to question whether Quijano might have experienced a form of cognitive decline and felt consequently traumatized. In their article "Neurology and Don Quixote," neurologists Jose-Alberto Palmab and Fermin Palmab point out that,

> Cervantes portrays some of the characteristics of cognitive impairment, including … time disorientation: "three days passed in one hour" (part II, ch. 23); misidentification of people, such as the episode where he identified the modest priest of his town, an old acquaintance, as the "Archbishop Turpin" (part I, ch. 7), and agitation: "When they reached Don Quixote he was already out of bed, and was still shouting and raving, and slashing and cutting all round, as wide awake as if he had never slept" (part I, ch. 7).[30]

One could easily advance the argument that Quijano's madness is the result of cognitive impairment, induced by physiological changes in the brain. Following Malabou's position of the "new wounded," this research puts forward nevertheless that while Quijano might have experienced cognitive impairment, he also might have experienced psychic disturbances (trauma) associated with that cognitive decline. And to return to Halpern's research, to categorize Quijano's psychic disturbance as simply madness denies that "unrealistic moments within grief make it possible for a person to arrive at a more realistic emotional state."[31] Counter to our Cartesian thinking, irrationality might pave the way for sharpened emotional reasoning. If skepticism still abounds about the possibility of Quijano's encounter with trauma, this imagery may offer a final segue into such an interpretation: "As in the Greek myth of Medusa, the human confusion that may ensue when we stare death in the face can turn us to stone. We may literally freeze in fear, which will result in the creation of traumatic symptoms."[32]

Readjusting Alonso Quijano's Emotional Compass Through Reading Adventures

Having laid the groundwork for understanding Quijano's traumatic experience associated with aging, we focus now on his reading practices while drawing on literary theorists' and affective scientists' research. At first glance and as pointed out earlier, Quijano seems to be propelled by a passion for reading. The narrator warns us that our hero reads books of chivalry with such "ardor and avidity that he almost entirely neglected the pursuit of his field-sports, and even the management of his property; and to such a pitch did his eagerness and infatuation go that he sold many an acre of tillage land to buy books of chivalry to read."[33] The terms "ardor," "avidity," "entirely neglected," "to such a pitch," "eagerness," and "infatuation" convey in no uncertain terms an obsessive-compulsive tendency. Doesn't it make sense to contend that reading harms him, as the niece, housekeeper, barber, curate and most critics maintain? His niece offers a more precise and critical reading of her uncle: "It was often my uncle's way to stay two days and nights together poring over these unholy books of misadventures, after which he would fling the book away and snatch up his sword and fall to slashing the walls ..."[34] The fact that he is "poring over" intimates again compulsive behavior, whereas his snatching up his sword and slashing the walls transmits an image of madness.

The author sounds a word of caution about judging Quijano's reading eagerness. In the "author's preface," Cervantes relays to readers advice received from a friend: "Strive, too, that in reading your story the melancholy may be moved to laughter, and the merry made merrier still; that the simple shall not be wearied, that the judicious shall admire the invention, that the grave shall not despise it, nor the wise fail to praise it."[35] Even if it remains unclear whether reading is therapeutic for Quijano, *Don Quixote* itself appears designed to be therapeutic for readers. It is easy to consider the text as a *mise en abîme*: Quijano appears to be moved from melancholy to laughter by reading books, just as readers of the masterpiece may very well be moved from melancholy to laughter.

Although the narrator might have described Quijano's reading as obsessive, he is also careful to draw a tempered conclusion about our hero's mental condition. Don Quixote navigates between apparent madness and lucidity: "their master was now and then beginning to show signs of being in his right mind" and "he is a madman full of streaks, full of lucid intervals."[36] The narrator also offers a cautious and subtle interpretation of our hero: "His fancy grew full of what he used to read about in his books, enchantments, quarrels, battles, challenges, wounds, wooings, loves, agonies, and all sorts of impossible nonsense; and it so possessed his mind that the whole fabric of invention and fancy he read of was true ..."[37] On the one hand, Quijano has been "possessed" by material that just is not true. On the other, he is an extremely careful reader who relishes ("his fancy grew") the complexities of reading. He engages in a close reading, distinguishing between "quarrels" and "battles"; "loves" and "wooings"; "wounds" and "agonies," while comparing "enchantments" with "all sorts of impossible nonsense." This description of his reading practice finds resonance in van der Kolk's findings about hallucinations. The psychiatrist asks: "But if the stories I'd heard in the wee hours were true, could it be that these 'hallucinations' were in fact the fragmented memories of real experiences?"[38] This rhetorical question intimates that hallucinations—kindred to Quijano's belief in "all sorts of impossible nonsense"—may not simply be concoctions of a deranged mind, but rather creative endeavors designed to soothe. Such a statement leads us to ponder whether there is a "clear line between creativity and pathological imagination."[39] Quijano does not seem to engage in this creative enterprise simply for art's sake. His mind creates an atmosphere of creativity and health while reading. As we shall discover, he entertains new thoughts; builds new images; finds a new voice; inoculates himself with new emotions; and eventually forms "therapeutic alliances" with characters. These steps are precursors to Quijano's transformation into Don Quixote.

Before Quijano becomes Don Quixote, he transforms his identity by reading. How do new thoughts, images, voices, emotions, and eventual therapeutic alliances with characters provoke a metamorphosis of the mind? Although we discussed the act of reading in Chapter 6, let us expand on these concepts by turning to literary theorists. The act of reading is an experience of personal amplification. More precisely and as literary theorist Wolfgang Iser contends, reading literature stimulates new thoughts in the reader's mind, thus provoking a greater sense of self-awareness.[40] Quijano entertains the thoughts of the knights of the fictional tales and yet reformulates them on his own terms. Literary theorist Georges Poulet describes this process as: "Because of the strange invasion of my person by the thoughts of another, I am a self who is granted the experience of thinking thoughts foreign … I am the subject of thoughts other than my own."[41] Quijano obviously does not disappear, since without him the imagined characters could not come alive. Still, Quijano's identity begins to fade away. It becomes imbibed with the knights' thoughts and experiences. Iser also argues that reading literature stimulates new images in the mind that are then juxtaposed with past images. This juxtaposition of new and old images results in an expansion in thinking. This mental process may very well help trauma survivors to get at their trauma, as they often do not display "the mental flexibility that is the hallmark of imagination."[42]

Thus, when I read, I utter an "I" that does not completely belong to me. Referring to this experience, Iser contends that the reader (composed of an alien "I" with "alien thoughts") "places his mind at the disposal of the author's thoughts."[43] The literary theorist should have written "narrator's thoughts" (as opposed to author's thoughts), since the author is not necessarily the "I" of the narrative. It is obviously important to distinguish between the author and narrator, even if Iser fails to do so. The "I" as narrator dwells in an imaginary realm; it exists within the limits of the reader's imagination, as opposed to some unknown reality of a real author. If the reader is truly engaged in the act of imaging and re-telling the story in his mind, then she becomes the author of the story as well as the narrator transmitting the story. By reading the imaginary narrative, the reader engages in a creative exercise of establishing firmly her voice in the story, which should serve as a training for the traumatized to give a voice to the unspeakable. Thanks to a new voice, new images and new ideas, the trauma survivor might approach the hidden story of her own trauma. Perhaps, it is more fitting to claim that she might discover almost unwittingly her own story of trauma by reading pieces of literature. And yet, she discovers it on her own terms, as she formulates thoughts and images in her mind and listens to different registers of her own voice. In this respect, she knows without knowing and speaks without directly speaking, while stimulating in turn new emotions.

The topic of emotional stimulation and reactions while reading literature has caused much ink to flow in both the humanities and the sciences, as witnessed in the birth of affect theory and affective science, which cannot be reviewed within the confines of this chapter. (Besides, we elaborated on the role literature plays in the production of emotions in Chapter 6 when reviewing Alexander's notions on catharsis and LaCapra's concept of a haven.) Instead, I should like to put forward that the act of reading has the power to introduce a new lexicon of emotions and especially a mental encyclopedia of human experiences. By forming "therapeutic alliances" with characters, readers can encounter their own private trauma, while learning about others' trauma. More precisely, just as trauma survivors are urged to form "therapeutic alliances" with their mental health-care provider (as reviewed in Chapters 5 and 6 and particularly in relation to Sisyphus and Roquentin), Quijano finds resonance in the characters' experiences, especially in those of the knights confronting death. These alliances become apparent as Quixote assumes the identity of the knights Amadis or Roland (chap. 26, part I) and are characterized by both projection (he projects his emotions onto others) and contagiousness (he assumes the emotional experiences of others).

Perhaps more accurately, reading is kindred to a vaccine. By inhabiting the mental space of characters, Quijano exposes himself to characters' emotional reactions and thus develops emotional antibodies (in the absence of a real emotional immunity). Unconsciously, Quijano uses his own physiology—the part of his brain altered by reading—to prepare his body for the attack of trauma of aging and dying. It is by engaging in reading that he is able to grasp better and mourn his own impending death, for "effective mourning requires total emotional responses ..."[44] Just as children are exposed therapeutically to fairy tales, designed to luxuriate in topics such as death, aging, faithfulness, and erotic desire, Quijano exposes himself to chivalry tales in order to confront that which his conscious mind is afraid to explore, diminishment and death. Relying on Bruno Bettelheim's theories regarding the therapeutic effects of fairy tales, I propose that Quijano's unconscious mind is revealed to him through the images of the chivalry tales.[45] As his conscious and unconscious minds unite with the books of chivalry, meaning is no longer simply an object to be defined, it develops as an experience. This leads Quijano to assume another identity—Don Quixote—and to engage in another literary arts mechanism that is phenomenological in nature (from the Heideggerian and French branch of the philosophical movement). That is, the mechanism is performative centering on the intersection between the body and emotions.

Before expanding on these ideas, we should stress that reading seems to be a first step toward posttraumatic growth for Quijano. He develops creative new images, new voices, and new emotions through therapeutic alliances with characters. This is a collective experience of treating trauma. He reads and interprets his own trauma through characters. He approaches his own hidden pathos and suffering associated with the trauma in a masked form, in the form of other characters' emotional experiences. He remains both inside and outside the traumatic event and "to occupy a territory while loitering skeptically on the boundary is often where the most intensely creative ideas stem from."[46]

Don Quixote's Phenomenological Experience to Stimulate Emotions

Could Quijano's transformation into Don Quixote really be both a consequence of traumatization as well as a form of therapy?[47] The narrator informs us that Don Quixote had contemplated on several occasions whether it would be: "better and more to his purpose to imitate the outrageous madness of Roland, or the melancholy madness of Amadis."[48] In fact, Don Quixote exclaims: "Long live the memory of Amadis and let him be imitated so far as is possible by Don Quixote of La Mancha."[49] Quijano assumes the identity of a knight who ventures into the world, experiencing it in intense physical ways. He does not simply mistake windmills for giants, flocks of ewes for enemy armies. He attacks the windmills with a joust and hits himself against the blades. He charges at the so-called enemy armies of dust-covered ewes and spears them, while the shepherds peg him with stones and almonds that knock out his grinders and crush two fingers. He even performs somersaults or capers naked from the waist down on a mountaintop. Since the residue of trauma is stored in bodily tissues, therapies that involve the body serve an important role. Don Quixote engages in a phenomenological experience, fueled by the imagination to respond to that stored trauma. While his body is absorbed in these adventures, he also tells tall tales. His imagination is so rife that he is able to devise glorious names and attributes of imaginary armies that he wages war against: "Ho, knights, ye who follow and fight under the banners of the valiant emperor Pentapolin of the Bare Arm, follow me all; ye shall see how easily I shall give him his revenge over his enemy Alifanfaron of the Trapobana."[50] His stories nonetheless should not be interpreted as simply products of an overactive imagination. He constructs himself by telling stories about himself, since stories not only depict parts of the self but also construct it. This means however that his moral repair takes place within a lie, which seems contrary to accepted practices of trauma recovery, if not unethical.[51] Peter D. Kramer reminds us all the same that "Lying is just a necessity of human discourse, and the therapeutic relationship is not exempt from having to depend on it now and again."[52]

There are other ways to read this unorthodox form of behavior. It may be that Don Quixote navigates his body through harmful circumstances to master fear and break the anxiety of helplessness. "When anxiety is associated with helplessness, it may be experienced as distressful, but in association with other feelings—for example, optimistic expectation—it is usually downright pleasure."[53] By putting his body into a vulnerable and dangerous position, he quells his anxiety about aging and a related sense of helplessness to redefine the past and future. These intense physical experiences prepare him for the impending pain of dying. Instead of feeling nothing, he also welcomes physical pain to feel still alive, a phenomenon we witnessed in Sartre's Roquentin.

Whether it is provoking the body to come alive through pain or an excited state; or whether it is creating new images and a new voice in his mind; or learning a new lexicon or encyclopedia of emotions through a collective reading experience, Don Quixote has prepared himself for his next steps of a Literary Arts Praxis. He reaches out to other traumatized victims, who populate his community rather than the pages of books.

Don Quixote's Collective Literary Arts Praxis and Empathic Unsettlement

There are two features that stand out about this next stage of Don Quixote's Literary Arts Praxis: a new forged relationship with a community (outside his books) and a heightened sense of empathy for others and eventually for his traumatized self. Unlike his previous engagements—that take place mostly within his own mind and body—this next one occurs within a community, but a community that will need to be nuanced. As reviewed in Chapter 5, Herman maintains that both reconnection and commonality remain key to posttraumatic growth: "The solidarity of a group provides the strongest protection against terror and despair, and the strongest antidote to traumatic experience. Trauma isolates; the group re-creates a sense of belonging … Trauma dehumanizes the victim; the group restores her humanity."[54] How shall we understand the term "community"? Could it not include an imaginary one in books? Could it include different dimensions of the psyche of trauma? Before connecting with a community, Don Quixote finds first a visceral sense of safety by embarking on his journey with his trusted squire Sancho, who listens time and again to his master's imaginative stories and follows him along in every pursuit. Sancho is so faithful that he appears to serve a therapeutic role. Indeed, he likens himself to Don Quixote's doctor: "Surely, senor, I'm the most unlucky doctor in the world … but with me though to cure somebody else costs me drops of blood, smacks, pinches, pinproddings, and whippings, nobody gives me a farthing …"[55] Though Sancho and his unwavering dedication to his "master" may appear at times unhealthy, it does serve as an example of a therapeutic alliance. Sancho combines both dedication and leeriness; intimacy and objectivity; empathy and distance to provoke Don Quixote to reveal and eventually tell his story.

Don Quixote's Praxis is not limited to a talking cure, however. He becomes a faithful if not voracious consumer of oral stories, transforming himself into a knight who both listens empathically to the downtrodden and rescues them from physical distress. To understand how Don Quixote reacts empathically to others, it is necessary to outline how these connections develop. Empathic connections can be forged by stories.[56] In a literary coup, the narrator unveils the rich, complex, and multilayered nature of stories, almost as if to emphasize the need to chip away slowly and methodically at the hidden content of narratives cemented by numbed emotions or masked by visceral ones. For example, the goatherd Pedro tells Don Quixote about the tragic love story of Chrysostom and the shepherdess Marcela. The next day, our hero encounters travelers on the road and insists that they share their version of the same tragedy. The following day, Don Quixote attends the burial of the broken-hearted Chrysostom. There he is captivated by Ambrosia's rendition of the tragedy and by Vivaldo's reading of Chrysostom's poem "Lay of Despair" that echoes through the mountains and provokes Marcela to appear. She shares her side of the story, summing up her position: "If Chrysostom's impatience and violent passion killed him, why should my modest behavior and circumspection be blamed?"[57] No sooner does Marcela vanish into the thick of the woods than Don Quixote exclaims that the fair lady should not be held in contempt, but rather esteemed for her virtuous resolution, which intimates that he has responded empathically.

Don Quixote's longing to hear others' stories and his resolution to listen with an empathic ear are present throughout the epic. He is captivated by the story of the ragged knight of the Sierra. Again, the theme of the importance of stories as a transformative force is underscored when Don Quixote unearths an old valise containing a book full of letters and poems. The written artifacts are a treasure finer than the booty of fine linen and nuggets of gold accompanying the book. The literary treasure trove contains, "complaints, laments, misgivings, desires and aversions, favors and rejections, some rapturous, some doleful."[58] A sonnet is one of the diadems crowning the book, and Don Quixote makes haste to admire it. Pages of moving pathos propel him to seek out the author who hides in the mountains. Eventually, our hero meets the ragged knight, a nobleman named Cardenio, and assures him of his most noble intents:

> Mine is to be of service to you, so much so that I had resolved not to quit these mountains until I had found you and learned of you whether there is any kind of relief to be found for that sorrow under which from the strangeness of your life you seem to labor; and to search for you with all possible diligence, if search had been necessary. And if your misfortune should prove to be one of those that refuse admission to any sort of consolation, it was my purpose to join you in lamenting and mourning over it, so far as I could; for it is still some comfort in misfortune to find one who can feel for it.[59]

These words serve as a powerful sign of Don Quixote's motivation to build a bridge of understanding with others. He longs to be of "service" at all costs by providing "consolation." He seems to understand so well the stranger's yoke of "sorrow." Even more remarkable, he vows to share the stranger's "mourning," adding compassionately that suffering is more easily endured when others share it.

The narrator employs a literary trick to suggest how difficult it is to share and decipher the meaning of both stories and trauma. Namely, Cardenio grows so vexed by Don Quixote's interruptions that he abruptly departs leaving his troubles trailing in the wind. Left with Cardenio's book of sorrows, Don Quixote pens in the book a love letter to the object of his desire, Dulcinea, and incorporates Cardenio's penname signature "Knight of the Rueful Countenance" into his letter. In other words, Don Quixote assumes another identity in addition to his already assumed one. He takes on a new identity of author. He thus gains a new level of independence as he writes a separate script of identity. This act alone suggests how the vocabulary of sorrow is contagious. As soon as he finishes the love letter and sends Sancho off, supposedly to deliver it to his imaginary lady love, he pens new verses, "writing and carving on the bark of the trees and on the fine sand a multitude of verses all in harmony with his sadness, and some in praise of Dulcinea."[60] Cardenio, Marcela, and Chrysostom mirror Don Quixote. By listening to and reading their stories of regret, Don Quixote understands from a collective perspective his own misfortunes or better yet, those that plagued his life as Alonso Quijano. But is this any different from his collective fictional reading exercise? Doesn't reading stimulate self-awareness, too? The principal difference: Don Quixote feels a sense of empathy when he encounters real life stories, when traumatic suffering is embodied.

The role of empathy in posttraumatic growth is at the very heart of this novel reading of the canonical work. What is the relationship between trauma survivors and empathy? By feeling empathy for others, Don Quixote/Don Alonso can begin to apply it to his own traumatized self who might remain sequestered in a no-man's land of self-identity. LaCapra believes that empathy is a "counterforce to numbing" recapturing the "possibly split-off, affective dimension of the experience of others."[61] To describe an affective connection with others, he has coined the term "empathic unsettlement."[62] This leads us to question how Don Quixote becomes "unsettled" to respond to others' emotional states. To respond to this question, we must first return to Quijano's reading Praxis. Recall that he first formed therapeutic alliances with characters by locating a resonance of experiences and emotions and by inheriting (or catching by contagion) new emotions from those characters.

Thanks to his "obsessive compulsive" passion for reading, Quijano had accrued emotional information to understand others' misfortunes and eventually his own. However, does this reservoir of emotions guarantee an empathic response? Could one not benefit from a lexicon of emotions—having observed and mused on them in books and in reality—but respond to others in a detached and purely cognitive manner? It is not so much that a sense of empathy is fostered when people share the same experiential histories. Rather, it is cultivated when one person can creatively imagine common human "possibilities" with another. It is not so much that Don Quixote relates to the exact experiences of Cardenio, Marcela, and Chrysostom. Rather, he appears first and foremost curious to learn about those experiences (he is in the right mood) and relates to the underlying pathos of regret and sorrow, having grown "aware" of those through reading.

Finally, and most importantly for the critical suggestion of this research on posttraumatic growth and how the literary arts might get at trauma, Don Quixote can feel empathy toward himself once he feels empathy for others. How does this work? Empathy is feeling as someone, whereas sympathy is feeling for them. In metaphorical terms, the distinction between empathy and sympathy is kindred to the difference between an actor on stage engaging fully in a role and an actor in a photograph dressed in a costume. As an actor performing on stage, one is aware that one is not truly the character. That is, "the emotional response comes with respect for the other and the realization that the experience of the other is not one's own."[63] When Don Quixote feels as others, not only does he learn new vocabulary and experience new emotions, but he also becomes acquainted with an ethos of care, as evidenced in his reaction to Cardenio. This is a vital step toward his growth, since traumatized individuals often remain sealed off and become unreliable about caring for themselves.[64] By assuming the role of the empathic listener, Don Quixote interprets gradually his own traumatic story with empathy. In the simplest terms, growth occurs when the self that has begun to heal cares for the traumatized self that lingers.

In summary, Don Quixote engages in a cognitive and emotional training. He learns to: read himself from outside himself; care for his traumatized self by caring for others; feel empathy for himself by feeling empathy for others encountered in his books and "reality"; and imagine new ways of understanding his traumatic experiences and moving beyond them by learning about others' experiences. Even if his traumatic experiences might be individual in nature, his Literary Arts Praxis is distinctly collective. And the fact that Don Quixote finally accepts himself as Alonso Quijano before his dying days suggests that the dyad-character experienced growth and could somehow get at trauma through a Literary Arts Praxis.

Conclusions: "Quixotic" Psychic Resilience and Growth

Focusing first on the pre-Don Quixote character Alonso Quijano, this chapter has explored the traumatic experience of aging that might have triggered Quijano's "madness." It was argued that his "obsessive" reading and transformation into an imaginary errant knight should not be interpreted as simply a sign of psychopathology. On the contrary, it is an attempt to move beyond psychic suffering. By assuming the role of Don

Quixote, Quijano was able to entertain creative thoughts; build new images; and establish new emotional responses, all reinforced by therapeutic alliances with fictional characters. This first part of his Literary Arts Praxis centered on reading literature and collective experiences with imagined characters. It was a first step toward growth or a "changed sense of sense,"[65] to employ the words of Tedeschi and Calhoun. The second step entailed a phenomenological experience. Since trauma is stored in bodily tissues, Don Quixote confronts his trauma of aging through the body, as he chases down ewes or charges at windmills. This intense bodily experience might have dislodged the stress of trauma and hence served as solace rather than as a sign of "madness." The third stage of his Praxis consists of encountering other trauma survivors (from his "real" as opposed to "fictional" community) and building empathic bonds with them. This in turn led us to one of the main critical suggestions of this research: Once Don Quixote felt empathy for others and experienced "empathic unsettlement," he felt empathy for his previously traumatized self, Quijano. Since Quixote is a role played by Quijano, the former works through the traumatic experience for the latter. The team addresses the "central dialectic of psychological trauma"[66] or the desire to keep the traumatic experience veiled and yet to unveil it.

The fact that Don Quixote acknowledges himself as Alonso Quijano on his deathbed suggests that the dyad-character accessed his trauma and experienced growth through a Literary Arts Praxis. To be sure, Quijano/Quixote's Praxis should not be seen as a prescription for all trauma survivors. On the contrary, the kingdom of suffering remains mysterious, and Cervantes's hero reminds us just how incomprehensible it can be. Yet he also reminds us not to underestimate the power of the human imagination. By assuming a new identity and living in freedom exempt from the trauma of aging, Don Quixote knows without knowing and speaks without speaking and begins to experience growth. Obviously, such a conclusion leads us away from a current emphasis on melancholy in trauma studies toward an understanding of "quixotic" psychic resilience and growth.

Notes

1 Gawande, *Being*, 1.
2 Mukherjee, *Laws*, 6.
3 American Psychiatric Association, *DSM-5*, 274.
4 See LaCapra, *Writing*, loc. 131 and 267.
5 Herman, *Trauma*, 1.
6 Recall from Chapter 5 that posttraumatic growth consists of positive transformations resulting from mental struggles with a traumatic life event and challenges to one's core beliefs. The growth experience can involve cognitive, emotional, behavioral, and physical changes and more specifically, might include alterations to one's philosophy of life, relationships with others, and self-identity. This transformation boils down to ego development and self-actualization, as survivors struggle psychologically; cope with emotional distress and intrusive

ruminations; gravitate toward deliberate and concerted ruminations; and disclose themselves through narratives or other creative processes. See Calhoun and Tedeschi, *Handbook*, 16–18. Recall as well that we discussed extensively Dominick LaCapra's expression "can somehow get at trauma" in Chapter 6.

7 Gracia Guillén, "Discreet," 106.
8 Cervantes, *Quixote*, 70.
9 Ibid., 109.
10 Ibid., 97.
11 Halpern, *Detached*, 6.
12 Davoine, "Quixotic," loc. 2779.
13 Ibid., loc. 2854.
14 Ibid., loc. 2865.
15 Cervantes, *Quixote*, 22; the original passage in which Cervantes admits to being only Don Quixote's stepfather reads: "*Pero yo, que, aunque parezco padre, soy padrastro de Don Quijote …*" Cervantes, *Ingenioso*, 3.
16 To defend against the temptation to focus on the author-hero relationship, it is useful to turn to Eagleton: "*Don Quixote* is not 'about' the character of that name: the character is just a device for holding together different kinds of narrative technique." Eagleton, *Literary*, 3.
17 Van der Kolk, *Body*, 206.
18 Johnson, *Madness*, 64.
19 Ibid., 65.
20 Huizinga, *Autumn*, 81–82.
21 Cervantes, *Quixote*, 1238.
22 Beá and Hernández, "Don Quixote," 143.
23 Ibid.
24 Cervantes, *Quixote*, 1155.
25 Ibid., 68.
26 Ibid., 69.
27 Epstein, *Trauma*, 149.
28 See van der Kolk, *Body*, 72.
29 Malabou, *Wounded*, xii. I am not confusing suffering with trauma. Instead, I am stressing the distinct possibility that diminishment and dying can be considered by some as traumatic experiences.
30 Palmab and Palmab, "Neurology," 250.
31 Halpern, *Detached*, 6.
32 Levine and Frederick, *Waking*, 19.
33 Cervantes, *Quixote*, 69.
34 Ibid., 100.
35 Ibid., 65.
36 Ibid., 646 and 796.
37 Ibid., 70.
38 Van der Kolk, *Body*, 25.
39 Ibid.
40 Iser, *Act*, 157–158.
41 Poulet, "Phenomenon," 56.
42 Van der Kolk, *Body*, 17.
43 Iser, *Act*, 154.
44 Krystal, "Trauma," 88.
45 See Bettelheim, *Uses*, 31.
46 Eagleton, *After*, 40.
47 By suggesting that Quijano's transformation into Don Quixote could be both a consequence of traumatization as well as a form of therapy, this brings to mind

the concept of Plato's *pharmakon*, which advances the idea that something can be both a poison and a cure.

48 Cervantes, *Quixote*, 310.
49 Ibid., 311.
50 Ibid., 210.
51 Herman maintains that "Remembering and telling the truth about terrible events are prerequisites both for the restoration of the social order and for the healing of individual victims." Herman, *Trauma*, 1.
52 Kramer, *Moments*, 25. Related to the issue of telling lies, Ruth Leys contends that "it must be acknowledged that the relative merits of forgetting and remembering in any given case are a matter of therapeutic possibilities and tact, as well as of political circumstances." Leys, *Trauma*, loc. 4088.
53 Krystal and Krystal, *Integration*, 94.
54 Herman, *Trauma*, 214.
55 Cervantes, *Quixote*, 1256.
56 Obviously, stories can provoke other emotions, such as "connections" of contempt.
57 Cervantes, *Quixote*, 173.
58 Ibid., 273.
59 Ibid., 281.
60 Ibid., 312.
61 LaCapra, *Writing*, 40.
62 Ibid., 41.
63 Ibid., 40.
64 Herman, *Trauma*, 165.
65 Calhoun and Tedeschi, *Posttraumatic*, 7.
66 Herman, *Trauma*, 1.

8   The Trauma of a Plague and Creative Writing Exercises with Albert Camus

The COVID-19 pandemic has brought to the forefront of our minds the pressing issue of the well-being of healthcare providers. One pertinent mental-health topic is how clinicians react emotionally to patients and to themselves as persons at risk. At the heart of the issue lies a paradox. Providers are schooled in the "art" of medicine and to practice an ethos of care built on emotional connections. However, during a pandemic when clinicians experience extreme physical exhaustion and the trauma of witnessing suffering on a massive scale, they might remain affectless as a form of self-protection. Objectivity, logic, and statistics can also trump affects since an emotional connection with patients could translate into an inability to perform well. Yet, emotionally connected providers may have a placebo effect, as they assuage patients during recovering and encourage resilience and healing. In addition to these complex topics, it is not clear what happens to healthcare providers themselves if they are disconnected from their patients and from themselves. How do they process traumatic experiences—such as witnessing suffering, dying, and the associated moral questions—if they remain disconnected emotionally? How can they engage empathically with a patient if they struggle to understand emotionally (feel empathy for) their own traumatic experiences? In metaphorical terms, how can they help a patient prepare for death, if they themselves have experienced a type of psychic death?[1] Do these questions simply point to philosophical conundrums, or do they assume an ethical dimension as well?

In search of answers to these questions, we turn once again to Albert Camus and to his novel *The Plague* (originally published in French in 1947).[2] Camus was born in French Algeria to impoverished *Pieds-Noirs* parents, people of European descent living in colonial Algeria. His *Algerian Chronicles* (2013) contain his "pleas on behalf of Arab misery."[3] *The Plague* is another plea on behalf of human misery. It takes place in Oran, Algeria, amid a pandemic, as the title suggests. Many interpret the plague as a symbol of Nazism. This interpretation carries historical weight since both France and French Algeria were occupied by the Nazis during World War II. I propose to plunge into the meaning of the plague, not so much as a metaphor of a political crisis, but rather as health crisis that triggers traumatic experiences. I wish to understand

DOI: 10.4324/9781003284642-13

the traumatic experiences of the main character Doctor Rieux and how he navigates through his own emotional death by engaging in a Literary Arts Praxis that involves creative writing. Although Rieux does not explicitly state that he undergoes a traumatic experience during the plague, readers can draw this conclusion from circumstantial evidence. He loses his wife and his friends, while his community is decimated. He witnesses the suffering of his patients while being overwhelmed with a sense of despair about his futile attempts to treat them. He seems to suffer from alexithymia, a common manifestation of enduring trauma.[4] This results in an inability to feel emotions and to express them.

We explore first the essence of Doctor Rieux's traumatic and posttraumatic experiences by scoping out the genre of the novel. It takes the form of intimate literature: Rieux's chronicle coupled with another character's (Tarrou's) notebook.[5] Even though the doctor seems to write an "objective" chronicle, as Shoshana Felman asserts, he first creates a "metaphysical" chronicle to capture the essence of a shared existential crisis and personal emotional experiences.[6] This more subjective chronicle provokes empathy, since the narrator-doctor feels *as* his patients (empathy), not just *for* his patients (sympathy).[7] The second main argument is that Rieux creates a "narrative" chronicle. That is, a chronicle laced with stories of characters who are dispersed dimensions of the masked doctor himself. Related to this critical suggestion, I argue that these alter-ego characters serve as metaphors, laying bare emotions that otherwise would remain hidden and cut off from conscious awareness. Finally, these noncanonical interpretations of *The Plague* suggest that a Literary Arts Praxis founded on intimate literature (namely a metaphysical and narrative chronicle) might somehow help trauma survivors to get at trauma and experience growth. Kindred to Don Quixote's Literary Arts Praxis, Doctor Rieux fosters emotional awareness and a sense of empathy toward others and himself. However, there is a slight difference in their empathy producing strategy. Instead of relying on fictional characters and "real" people as Don Quixote did, the doctor creates a literary haven where he crafts alter-ego characters who adjust his emotional compass. Kindred to Sartre's Roquentin, Rieux engages in an existential act of building his essence posttraumatic existence by engaging in a creative act.

A Metaphysical Chronicle

According to the *Merriam-Webster Dictionary*, a chronicle is "a historical account of events arranged in order of time usually without analysis or interpretation." In her chapter "Camus' *The Plague*, or a Monument to Witnessing," Felman contends that, "[e]merging out of the very urgency of history, *The Plague* presents itself as a pure 'chronicle,' an objective reproduction of historical events."[8] At first glance, Doctor Rieux's narrative seems to be indeed an objective account without analysis or interpretation.

This chapter seeks to question however Felman's reading and offer a nuanced definition of the doctor's chronicle as a composite metaphysical and narrative one.

On the one hand, the narrator certainly employs the writing devices of a chronicler. To convey a sense of an objective transmission of events, the narrator does not even reveal his identity as Doctor Rieux until six pages before the end of the book. This distance between himself as narrator and himself as actor is often referred to as an "autobiographical gap,"[9] as described by physician Rita Charon. Two characters dwell within one and create a gap: the narrator of the plague and the doctor trying to heal those stricken by the plague. The narrator manages this deception by referring to himself as "Doctor Rieux" (as opposed to an explicit "I") and by employing the third-person pronoun ("he"), a narrative coup designed to give a sense of distance. This gap may also be evidence of trauma. It suggests, as mentioned earlier, that the doctor is suffering from alexithymia. Furthermore, the chronicle follows a chronological order, which gives it an appearance of objectivity. The narrator does not privilege certain events over others. He allows time to dictate the unfolding of events in narrative form. It appears objective also by virtue of the narrator's claims: "His business is only to say: this is what happened, when he knows that it actually did happen, that it affected the life of a whole populace, and that there are thousands of eye-witnesses who can appraise in their hearts the truth of what he writes."[10] This statement and the fact that chroniclers are supposed to write in a historical and chronological order without analysis or interpretation provide weight to Felman's reading of the chronicle as "objective." By simply reporting events, the narrator creates a sense of order in an otherwise chaotic world where innocent people suffer and die randomly from microbes that doctors fail to understand and control. Rieux conveys not only a message of control but also a degree of emotional disengagement from his patients, which might be vital for his own survival. After all, if he grows emotionally engaged with others, he risks putting himself in a vulnerable position, he could falter emotionally and compromise his rational and objective practice of medicine.[11]

On the other hand, the narrator is trying to trick readers (and/or himself) into believing that his chronicle is objective. Contrary to what the narrator states explicitly and what Felman contends, the chronicle is far from objective. It contains traces of objectivity and subjectivity. Rieux can remain both distant and affectless and/or connected and emotionally engaged. The following comment alone gives us reason to harbor suspicion about the chronicler's objectivity: "To be an honest witness, it was for him to confine himself mainly to what people did or said and what could be gleaned from documents. Regarding his personal troubles and his long suspense, his duty was to hold his peace."[12] Again, he certainly sounds like an objective chronicler. He claims to be an "honest witness." He "confines" himself to what others say. He employs "documents." About his personal life (his "suspense" and his "troubles"), not a word is uttered. His vocabulary nonetheless is so ambiguous that one struggles to understand "personal troubles and his long suspense." It is true that he speaks very little about his sick wife, who is being cared for away from plague-stricken Oran. "His long suspense" (*son attente*) might in fact refer to her. Still, the chronicler employs the word *épreuves,* translated as "troubles," which is an expansive term in both French and English. Some of the transmitted conversations between Tarrou and Rieux elucidate the nature of the chronicler's "troubles." When Tarrou asks Rieux whether he believes in God, he admits to "fumbling in the dark, struggling to make something out."[13] Rieux is "fighting against creation as he found it."[14] He vows not to "give up the struggle."[15] Yet, he admits to "a never ending defeat."[16] Fumbling in the dark? Struggling to make something out? Fighting against creation? Vowing never to give up? These expressions most certainly convey "troubles" of a very intimate, if not existential nature. This leads us to conclude that he does indeed expose his "troubles," even though he claims otherwise.[17] This in turn indicates that the chronicler is not the most reliable narrator (hardly objective, as Felman contends) and more importantly for my purposes, he is out of touch with his emotions or does not disclose them readily. He seems to keep them masked. In the next section of this chapter, we shall discover that he does unmask his "troubles" and "his long suspense" but not explicitly. He finds another mechanism to expose them to himself and to readers—through characters that serve as metaphors of his complex state of being.

Rieux's hypercritical readings of Oran and its residents serve as another indicator of nonobjectivity in his narrative of the plague. He writes, "How to conjure up a picture, for instance, of a town without pigeons, without any trees or gardens, where you never hear the beat of wings or the rustle of leaves—a thoroughly negative place, in short?"[18] By using the negative terms "without" and "never" repeatedly and by explicitly stating that Oran is simply a "negative place," the chronicler establishes right from the start a nonobjective tone. That a city could have no pigeons, trees, or gardens seems hardly possible. This is an exaggeration pregnant with subjective meaning and also apparent as he describes the residents of Oran:

> The truth is that everyone is bored and devotes himself to cultivating habits. Our citizens work hard, but solely with the object of getting rich. Their chief interest is in commerce, and their chief aim in life is, as they call it, "doing business." Naturally, they don't eschew such simpler pleasures as love-making, sea-bathing, going to the pictures. But, very sensibly, they reserve these pastimes for Saturday afternoons and Sundays ...[19]

Considering that the narrator uses superlatives such as "everyone," "solely," and "chief," it is hard to interpret his point of view as objective. He also speaks in a condescending tone laced with sarcasm. Evidently, the people of

Oran "naturally" partake in "simpler pleasures," but "very sensibly" reserve those pastimes for the weekend. Why does the chronicler say "naturally"? Beneath the adverb, lies a snide rhetorical question: "What else would you expect?" Moreover, he refers to "simpler pleasures" as if he were somehow above those activities. The ironic expression "very sensibly" is a jab at the people of Oran for constraining themselves to pleasures only on the weekend. These two examples indicate that the chronicler can be ironic and, thus, nonobjective. This less-than-flattering subjective reading may establish an emotional distance between the residents of Oran and the doctor. It might feed his state of alexithymia. If people are not very noble to begin with—the chronicler might reason—then it makes no difference if he remains emotionally disengaged from them.

In staggering contrast to this position, he does seem to strive to identify with others. He employs the plural first-person pronoun ("we"), thus creating a semantic union. One might object that the use of the plural first-person pronoun does not necessarily mean that he feels a sense of existential solidarity with the people of Oran. But this sense of solidarity is highlighted in other ways. When the plague strikes, he confesses that everyone, including the narrator himself, "was in the same boat."[20] A connection between the chronicler and other people is further strengthened by the act of writing imaginatively. The dry ink on the pages of his chronicle is evidence that he spent time imagining the condition of others, which means connecting with them, at least first mentally. He bonds with them as he writes about their shared traumatic experiences, as the following passage demonstrates:

> What is more exceptional in our town is the difficulty one may experience there in dying. "Difficulty," perhaps, is not the right word; "discomfort" would come nearer. Being ill is never agreeable, but there are towns that stand by you, so to speak, when you are sick; in which you can, after a fashion, let yourself go. An invalid needs small attentions, he likes to have something to rely on, and that's enough.[21]

In this passage, Rieux sounds more like a psychologist or better a philosopher than a medical doctor. He centers on the emotional "discomfort" of dying in utter solitude. He refers to "small attentions," such as the support of a hand. By using the pronoun "our," he exposes his own struggle to comprehend dying. He can stand by his dying friend Tarrou and experience those final moments or let his mother guard over him instead. He can embrace the emotionally wrenching moment or retreat. He can feel empathy or feel apathy. He can stay and "watch the natural history of an illness unfold in real time" or practice a "therapeutic nihilism."[22] That is, he can feel and act or feel nothing and do nothing.

These issues are made even more acute as Rieux appears cognizant of humanity's absurd fate. The plague renders our shared absurd existence more immediate and pertinent. We live and die like all living creatures. Our life is just as meaningful or absurd as any other. A stream of ants busily labors on our path of life, and we trample it underfoot, while microbes stream into our blood and wipe us out from one day to the next. The problem is not that life is rendered absurd because we are all going to die, but rather because "we are free to stoke the crematory fires or to devote ourselves to the care of lepers. Evil and virtue are mere chance or caprice."[23] What difference does it make if we stand by to witness the dying agony of another, if virtue is capricious and a matter of chance as opposed to moral principle?

By exploring these metaphysical issues in the chronicle, Rieux takes a first step to rebel like Sisyphus. He rebels against emotional dilettantism and disengagement toward another's suffering and death. His revolt is not in the form of violence, as in the case of the Roman emperor in Camus's play "Caligula." It consists rather of documenting and witnessing the dying agony of others, such as Tarrou's and the magistrate's son's death. This points to a shared emotional experience, proof that this reading of *The Plague* is defined by the notion of solidarity, as seen in Camus's "I revolt, therefore we are."[24]

By venturing into a subjective reading of a shared existential crisis, Rieux is stepping outside his normal identity (as a doctor) and objective position (as a chronicler). He centers on the psychological subtleties of illnesses rather than on the physical symptoms of disease, for the field of medicine must eventually resign itself to the power of diseases. While he can practice sanitation measures by quarantining the city and eventually administering a serum that might work, he can neither alleviate the suffering of a child on his death bed nor prevent the child's death. If his vocation is subverted continuously by death, Rieux must feel defeated, growing conscious of the fundamental nature of medicine's impotence. Faced with the devastating power of the plague, he abdicates his role as healer of physical pathologies and becomes a perceptive observer of the art of dying and the existential questions dying raises.

As narrator of the chronicle, Rieux is no longer Doctor Rieux. He must deny his role as a doctor. This is another reason why the narrator does not admit to being himself. He doubts his own identity and must assume a new one within his community. His metaphysical chronicle allows him to imagine the psycho-philosophical state of others. His new identity resembles a philosopher or poet, which corresponds with the positions of traumatologists, such as Herman, Tedeschi, Calhoun, Cyrulnik, Levine, and Richman discussed in Chapter 6. In this new role, he strengthens emotional ties with others and heals himself from the isolation and alienation of his vocation as a doctor. This need to build bonds with others is made especially acute at the end of the plague with the deaths of his friends Tarrou and Paneloux and his wife.

Rieux's metaphysical chronicle describes both an illness predating another illness, and a war festering within individuals, followed by another one erupting in the greater community. These wars of the mind cannot be understood by MRI scans or even by so-called objective chronicles. They demand an imaginative reading that stems from creative mental resources, which obviously will be subjective in nature. His metaphysical chronicle becomes an exercise in empathy, for it encourages the doctor to imagine generously the inner lives of the people in Oran, rather than to quarantine them off emotionally.

This leads us to contemplate Rieux's empathic responses toward others, whereas we shall address the topic of his empathic responses toward himself in the next section of this chapter. The issue of empathy dominates the pages of *The Plague*. Though we discussed the topic of "empathic unsettlement" in the chapter on *Don Quixote*, we should expand on the topic since Rieux and Don Quixote foster it in different ways. Dox Quixote cultivates it by reading literature and listening to stories, whereas Rieux triggers the emotion through creative writing. Empathy is vital to healing from trauma, since it serves as a "counterforce to numbing," recapturing the "possibly split-off, affective dimension of the experience of others."[25] Psychiatrist Helen Riess offers a detailed definition of empathy: it is a "process with both cognitive and affective components, which enables individuals to understand and respond to others' emotional states and contributes to compassionate behavior and moral agency."[26] Her definition organizes empathy into three distinct phenomena: it is based on both cognitive and affective experiences, fostering in turn understanding and responses as well as compassionate conduct. How is Rieux "enabled" (to use Riess's vocabulary) to understand, respond, and react empathically to others? What happens cognitively and emotionally to him? Psychiatrist Jodi Halpern puts forward that "the empathizer must be in a mood that is interested in the human predicament that another faces."[27] Rieux assumes a new mood of understanding the predicament of others when he seizes upon the plague's moral complexity. He comprehends cognitively that the issue is not so much treating medically the incurable. The key issue is witnessing and paying tribute to the dignity of the dying individual. While Riess highlights that empathy is not only a cognitive, but also an emotional experience, Halpern narrows the term down further as an "emotion-guided activity of imagination."[28] A sense of empathy is cultivated not so much when people share the very same experiences, but rather when they imagine common (and not-so-common) human experiences. In sum, Rieux's critical remarks about the people of Oran underscore his sense of distance toward others. While composing a metaphysical chronicle, as opposed to an "objective" one, he finds himself in the right mood to envision creatively the underlying shared trauma of a plague and the prevalence of a sense of an existential crisis. Furthermore, by writing a metaphysical and narrative chronicle, Rieux participates in an emotional, as well as intellectual, exercise of imagination.

A Narrative Chronicle

Rieux also builds emotional and empathic connections with himself and with others by crafting characters in a "narrative chronicle," a term I have coined to refer to a hybrid form of intimate literature and fiction. As explored in our discussion of *Don Quixote*, LaCapra's expression "empathic unsettlement,"[29] which refers to emotional responses triggered by the impact of trauma, can shed light on characters' strategies to move beyond numbing. While LaCapra applies the term to "secondary witnesses (including historians) to traumatic events,"[30] I argue that Rieux, the trauma survivor, benefits from empathic settlement toward himself, just as Cervantes's hero did, but through a different mechanism.

The individuals populating the chronicle are condensed forms of Rieux's compartmentalized personality and yet are constructed from previous encounters with other individuals. The characters Tarrou, Rambert, Grand, and Paneloux are all facets of Rieux. They make up his masked and multifaceted identity, which resembles the psychological state of dissociation.[31] These characters are neither the doctor nor the narrator. They are rather those who live in Rieux when the doctor is not serving the needs of his patients and the narrator is not writing his chronicle. While the narrator masks himself in his "objective" chronicle, he investigates his identity through the construction and development of these characters. Moreover, when he states that his "identity will be made known in due course," he is referring not only to his identity by name.[32] He is hinting at a self-portrait that requires time and effort to paint. This position can be advanced with confidence, since the narrator employs the French verb "*connaître*," which means above all to "know," as in to understand, rather than just to meet.

It takes time for readers to become acquainted with the narrator. And it takes time for the narrator to become acquainted with himself. Like any other character who constructs himself psychologically (as in a *bildungsroman*), Rieux constructs himself by narrating stories about himself. The characters have the power to tell the doctor and readers just as much as a confessional memoir, mostly because they assume the dirty work. That is, they reveal to him and to readers that which the doctor does not or cannot reveal explicitly. As we shall explore in more detail, secondary characters also stimulate in Rieux self-awareness and awareness of others and, hence, an eventual feeling of empathy. The character Grand, a frustrated writer, symbolizes the doctor-chronicler's inability to express that which escapes expression. To add weight to the argument of how Grand encapsulates a part of the doctor's hidden personality, one should recall that when Rieux must write a letter, he "found it a laborious business, as if he were manipulating a language that he had forgotten."[33] The imaginary Grand helps Rieux lighten his load, just as Camus breathed new life into Sisyphus's myth and rendered his yoke less burdensome.

Father Paneloux symbolizes and uncovers another hidden dimension of Rieux's personality. While the priest lives through a crisis of faith, Rieux experiences a crisis of vocation. There are hints of Paneloux's doubts when the preacher dallies with "heresy."[34] As we shall examine shortly, the doctor experiences a crisis of vocation, as there is always a moment when medicine confronts the power of death. The doctor feels "helpless" as medical care is "impotent."[35] Most noteworthy, both Paneloux and Rieux turn to chronicles about the Black Plague when confronted with this crisis, another proof that the priest represents a segment of the doctor's ego.

Rambert exposes Rieux's masked feelings about love and "the long suspense."[36] This link stems from Rambert's situation. He is a journalist from Paris who becomes trapped in Oran during the quarantine and desperately seeks to rejoin his wife in the French capital. The doctor confesses to Rambert that he understands what separation feels like for people who are so fond of each another. The fact that Rieux is so silent about his mental anguish and his deep physical longing for his sick and absent wife underscores that Rambert fulfills a very important role. The journalist expresses a pain and frustration that defy expression. The dislocation and agony provoked by the absence of the doctor's wife could be so raw that it could only be absorbed second-hand, as it were. Rambert becomes a spokesperson of pain, so that the doctor does not have to confront it directly. Conversely, the narrator claims, "At Oran, as elsewhere, for lack of time and thinking, people have to love one another without knowing much about it."[37] Since Rieux is from Oran, and since he speaks about the townspeople as "we," it appears that he may also be ignorant or unsure of his emotions about his wife. He therefore relies on Rambert to unveil and communicate them.

Finally, Tarrou, an outsider who was on vacation in Oran when the plague struck, uncovers the most about the inner workings of Rieux. He serves as the doctor's alter ego and therefore merits special attention. Excerpts from Tarrou's notebooks (*carnets*) in the doctor's chronicle clearly indicate that their relationship is knotty. Rieux uncovers his double identity while describing the outsider's notebooks:

> His notebooks comprise a sort of chronicle of those strange early days we all lived through. But an unusual type of chronicle, since the writer seems to make a habit out of understatement, and at first sight we might almost imagine that Tarrou had a habit of observing events and people through the wrong end of a telescope. In those chaotic times he set himself to recording the history of what the normal historian passes over. Obviously we may deplore this curious kink in his character and suspect in him a lack of proper feeling.[38]

There is evidence to indicate that the doctor is speaking about himself in this passage. Tarrou is writing a "type of chronicle"; this is kindred to the ambiguous status of the doctor's chronicle.[39] The outsider's writing is characterized by understatement; Rieux's writing also distinguishes itself by a reserved style, as seen in his tendency for "objective," restrained descriptions. Tarrou tends to look at people as through "the wrong end"[40] of a telescope. Faced with the devastating power of the plague, Rieux also looks at the world from the so-called "wrong end." The doctor must relinquish his stethoscope. The importance of his role as a doctor grows obsolete as the plague decimates populations. He concentrates instead on the psychopathologies of the people, and, for this reason, he must use the wrong end of the telescope, looking at the devasting situation from a different angle.

Referring to Tarrou's descriptions of Oran in his diary, the doctor claims they contain "appropriate comments on the lack of trees, the hideousness of the houses and the absurd lay-out of the town."[41] As highlighted earlier, the doctor writes, "How to conjure up a picture, for instance, of a town without pigeons, without any trees or gardens, where you never hear the beat of wings or the rustle of leaves—a thoroughly negative place, in short?"[42] It is hard to distinguish Tarrou's opinion from Rieux's precisely because they both originate in the latter's mind.

The doctor highlights an apparent idiosyncratic feature of the outsider's personality: one suspects in him "a lack of proper feeling."[43] This is another example of Rieux serving as an unreliable narrator. The outsider appears more in touch with his emotions than the doctor as they witness the death of the magistrate's son. When the doctor and outsider stay to witness the death of the child, the former looks at the latter, searching for guidance.

> They had already seen children die ... but they had never yet watched a child's agony minute by minute ... The pain inflicted on these innocent victims had always seemed to be what in fact it was: an abominable thing. But, hitherto they had felt its abomination in, so to speak, an abstract way.[44]

How is it possible that Rieux had never stayed to witness a child's agonizing death? How could he have only understood the abomination of an innocent child's suffering in an abstract way? This doctor claims that "the thing was to do your job as it should be done."[45] Does he believe that to be a good doctor, one should only view and understand suffering in an abstract way? Is he suggesting that a good doctor does not become involved emotionally in the suffering of patients?

These questions suggest that Rieux has stifled his emotional experiences as a doctor. Consequently, he needs his friend to serve as a coach to guide him through emotionally wrenching experiences. In the simplest of terms, Tarrou is the very heart of Rieux. Indeed, as they look upon the dying child, this "parody of crucifixion," the outsider strokes "with his big paw the small face stained with tears and sweat."[46] Like a dog, Tarrou has paws. Like any other animal (save for humans, perhaps), he can neither suppress nor rationalize away his emotions. The doctor seems to make a step toward understanding the suffering child in more than just an abstract way:

> Now and then Rieux took his pulse—less because this served any purpose than as an escape from his utter helplessness—and when he closed his eyes, he seemed to feel its tumult mingling with the fever of his own blood. And then, at one with the tortured child, he struggled to sustain him with all the remaining strength of his own body. But, linked for a few moments, the rhythms of their heartbeats soon fell apart, the child escaped him, and again he knew his impotence.[47]

This passage intimates that an emotional union between Rieux and the suffering child remains problematic if not impossible. The doctor takes the pulse of the child to dispel his own sense of impotence to abate the child's suffering. The doctor moreover was only linked to the child for a "few moments" as the "rhythms of their heartbeats" grew discordant and the "child escaped him."[48] Perhaps, however, links between the dying and the living are weak and few, as only the dying know what it feels like to die.

The impossibility of an emotional union between the living and the dying seems even more pronounced in the case of Tarrou's death. Tears blind the doctor's eyesight as he watches his friend die: "And thus, when the end came, the tears that blinded Rieux's eyes were tears of impotence; and he did not see Tarrou roll over, face to the wall and die with a short, hollow groan as if somewhere within him an essential chord had snapped."[49] This passage, like the excerpt about the dying child, emphasizes the doctor's sense of impotence. It also underscores a shared emotional experience between the two as the doctor sheds tears for his friend. And yet, it also reveals that his friend's actual final moments escape Rieux. Upon his friend's death, the doctor expresses emotions, but does so referring to himself in the third person: "Thus, too, he had lived at Tarrou's side, and Tarrou had died this evening without their friendship's having had time to enter fully into the life of either."[50]

Curiously, Rieux uses the pronoun "we" when speaking also about his friend: "We gather that Tarrou was agreeably impressed by a little scene that took place daily on the balcony ..."[51] Who is this "we"? Rieux and who? It refers to the doctor and his other dimensions, including the narrator, the doctor, and Tarrou. It also refers to the other characters and the rest of the community, even to readers, as we involve ourselves in interpreting the chronicler's words. The doctor claims in fact: "No longer were there individual destinies; only a collective destiny, made of plague and the emotions shared by all."[52] He might have been playing with the double entendre of the term "*histoire*," which conveys a sense of both "history" and "story" in French.

How exactly does the process of constructing alter-ego characters and imagining their emotional experiences promote conscious awareness and a sense of empathy and help the doctor to get at trauma? The characters are pared down versions of the doctor. Each one encapsulates one specific issue that the doctor struggles to confront. They are dissociated versions of the self. Again, Rambert unveils Rieux's conflicted emotions about love; Grand unsheathes the topic of writing and the difficulty of self-expression; Father Paneloux speaks explicitly about doubting his vocation; and Tarrou serves as a rawer image of Rieux, unveiling emotions more readily.

These characters create what the philosopher Paul Ricœur calls a "narrative identity."[53] Rieux needs to foster a "narrative identity" because he has experienced a "self-divestiture" or "zero identity."[54] In trauma studies parlance, he has experienced a constriction of cognitive functions such as memory, judgment, and personal identity This phenomenon becomes evident in his masked identity as narrator of the chronicle. By constructing characters to carry the load of his emotions, he renders his own emotional experiences more readable (*lisible*) when they are interpreted in function of characters' stories. Rieux's characters help him to uncover the hidden content of his mind. They help him to cultivate heightened conscious awareness of himself, especially regarding his emotions.

Referring to Franz Kafka, the psychiatrist Thomas Ogden argues: "The experience of writing fiction was a principal medium through which he achieved moments of human consciousness ..."[55] But how exactly does writing fiction promote consciousness? As unfolded previously, metaphors and phenomenological experiences help to cultivate conscious awareness. Rieux's alter-ego characters are metaphors of realms of his being. According to psychiatrist Leonard Shengold, a metaphor is a map of both the world inside the mind and the world outside.[56] Metaphors link the mind with representations of the external world, which are pregnant with sensations and emotions. "They are the first steps toward our thoughts, language, memory and insight," Shengold argues.[57] Rieux's metaphorical characters both reflect and build the mind through new thoughts, words, emotions, memories, and insights, just as dreams reflect the mind and construct it anew. In short, the chronicle populated by his alter-ego characters represent a safe space where the chronicler-doctor can begin to access his hidden emotions. Over time, he develops conscious awareness at the intersection of the imaginary and the real in a haven of mental creativity.

While I share LaCapra's notion that literature, pregnant with ambivalence and undecidability, provides a "safe haven," I would stress that the metaphorical characters also play another important function in posttraumatic conditions. Rieux's creative exercise provokes empathy toward himself. To grasp this argument, it is instructive to return to Riess's and Halpern's definitions. Riess maintains that empathy is both a cognitive and affective experience, whereas Halpern claims that it is stimulated by an imaginative experience. Rieux engages in a cognitive and affective experience in his "metaphysical chronicle" and an imaginative and affective one in his "narrative chronicle." In simpler terms, he feels empathy for others, including himself, in "real" life, because he has first fostered both cognitive and highly emotional relationships with imagined characters that are metaphors of his own personality through creative writing activities.

Although one might object that this interpretation (that the characters are metaphors of Rieux's multidimensional personality) undermines the exploration of different responses to a shared crisis and experience of suffering, nothing could be further from the truth. The potency of this interpretation is based on links between emotions and empathy, which is at first an "emotion-guided activity of imagination."[58] Rieux becomes aware of his own traumatic experiences of witnessing suffering and death on a mass scale and simultaneously bonds with others and himself more profoundly and authentically by writing a highly creative chronicle as opposed to an objective one. After all, how can one emotionally connect with others if one fails to connect emotionally with oneself first?

Moreover, the doctor experiences phenomenologically these alter-ego characters. Since Rieux is the narrator of the chronicle, he cannot simply empirically examine the characters as objects "out there." They are "in there," in his head. They become a mental experience. The positions of philosopher Edmund Husserl may offer elucidation about this point. He underscores that the subject is the source and origin of all meaning.[59] Individual experiences (with others in reality) are always subjective phenomena permeated with an individual's emotions, thoughts, and images and are thus distinct from the "actual" experiences themselves. The process of constructing the characters in his narrative chronicle helps Rieux to capture meaning about his own experiences and to grow consciously aware of his emotions about himself and others.

This brings us back to the current issue raised at the beginning of this chapter. Namely, we asked whether being emotionally disconnected from others simply points to an interesting psycho-philosophical issue and whether it also assumes an ethical dimension. Rieux teaches us that dehumanizing moral experiences (consisting of being emotionally disconnected from others) do indeed contain an ethical imperative, as it involves empathic responses that might help humans to grow and even to recover from traumatic experiences.

This discussion leads us to question Raymond Stephanson's claim that in *The Plague* "pestilence finally defeats man's power to imagine."[60] His reading neglects the very structure of the novel. Rieux is not defeated; he engages in a creative writing project to describe his personal journey. His metaphysical and narrative chronicle serves as an artifact of his attempt to make sense of his traumatic experiences. The stories transmitted through his alter-ego characters enrich the tissues of Rieux's mind. After all, "[w]e nourish ourselves with the stories we hear and read; we metabolize them and incorporate them into our tissues, derive energy from them, become more of who we are by virtue of their fuel."[61] Though some might object that this comment refers to how others' narratives nourish us, Charon encourages doctors "to understand how urgent it is for them as healthcare professionals to reflect on and tell of their own lives."[62] This chapter on Rieux's chronicle and its characters also demonstrates the intersubjective nature of narration, which echoes Freud's notion that it takes two to witness the unconscious.

Conclusions: Encouraging Stories through Metaphysical and Narrative Chronicles

Interpreting *The Plague* as Rieux's creation of alter-ego characters to help him to understand his traumatic experiences is a powerful illustration of a Literary Arts Praxis centering on creative writing exercises. He creates a metaphysical chronicle to capture the essence of a shared existential crisis and emotional experiences. This metaphysical chronicle helps him to develop in turn a sense of empathy towards others and himself. He also crafts a narrative chronicle featuring characters who mirror the doctor's "real" acquaintances and friends as well as his splintered mind. Furthermore, the construction of these characters is a phenomenological experience. By chronicling shared experiences with others, the doctor devises a playbook, so to speak, on human reactions to suffering. The characters also reflect (and hence offer elucidation) about otherwise-masked dimensions of his own mind. These alter-ego characters serve as metaphors, laying bare emotions that otherwise would have remained hidden and cut off from conscious awareness. The doctor experiences these characters phenomenologically. Since Rieux is the chronicler of the fictional narrative, these characters cannot simply be objects "out there" to be objectively examined, but rather are "in there," in his mind and body. And the process of constructing such characters helps him to capture meaning about his own experiences. This writing endeavor translates into not only a phenomenological process but also an existential one. The doctor carves out his essence posttraumatic experience rather than allow his existence to be determined by the suffering he endured. In sum, these noncanonical interpretation of *The Plague* intimates that a Literary Arts Praxis founded on writing intimate literature might help trauma survivors to access their traumatic experiences by cultivating emotional awareness and a sense of empathy toward others and themselves.

Are such speculations about a fictional doctor warranted, though? Are healthcare providers interested in learning that they can stimulate emotional connections with others by chronicling universal existential issues (in a metaphysical chronicle) and by writing stories about their traumatized composite selves (in a narrative chronicle)? Do they care to discover that writing creatively can help them to decolonize their minds from an exclusively "medical" way of thinking? Are they motivated to discover in intimate literature other practices to stimulate a sense of empathy?[63] And ways to confront traumatic experiences, such as those experienced during a pandemic?

While we have explored the issue of doctors' emotional responses to suffering as portrayed in fictional intimate literature, the question of how healthcare professionals react emotionally to patients has been researched and documented in scientific fields. Zak Kelm and colleagues point out in their meta-research on emotions and empathy that even though they examined over 1,000 studies on methods to stimulate empathic reactions in doctors, scientific rigor and results were lacking. These studies were characterized by "relatively small sample sizes and vague reporting of intervention durations and outcome-assessment frames."[64] The work of Charon, Therese Jones, and others suggests nevertheless that narrative medicine is a highly effective method for clinicians. Describing how healthcare professionals wrote reflectively about their practice, Charon states, "As these authors wrote the biographies of their patients, they came to understand how urgent it is for them as healthcare professionals to reflect on and tell of their own lives."[65] Jones and colleagues report some of the most interesting data about how doctors experiment with narratives. They find that medical residents tend to tell "homeostatic" and "rebalancing" stories in which there is healing for the patients and some cognitive and moral enlightenment for the doctor.[66] Another challenge is that doctors are trained not only to understand pathologies from an objective or scientific position, but also to view "the word 'anecdote' [as] particularly poisonous since it refers to a subjective memory,"[67] as oncologist Siddhartha Mukherjee confesses. Literary critic Anatole Broyard confirms doctors' aversions to anecdotes while lamenting his own experience with cancer by pointing out: "doctors discourage our stories."[68]

This chapter on Doctor Rieux's experiment with a narrative and metaphysical chronicle provides a succinct example of how clinicians can undertake creative-writing exercises in intimate literature to gain conscious awareness, establish empathy with others and themselves, and locate psycho-philosophical narratives to address the issues of traumatic experiences. Rieux makes it clear that he has not constructed a restitution story. It is not neatly resolved. He reminds us that the plague will reappear. With this final insight in mind, *The Plague* may very well serve as a source of inspiration for clinicians as they endeavor to understand and navigate their emotional responses to traumatic experiences.

Notes

1 This statement is not meant to sound insensitive to the mental anguish and physical exhaustion physicians experience. It is drawn instead from a doctor's comment found in Arthur Kleinman's *Illness Narratives*: "I feel the need to protect myself, my involvement with patients. If I could only do, just do the cognitive side and leave the emotions, the family, the whole mess to someone else. If this keeps up, I'll either burn out in another year or two or become a danger to patients and myself." Kleinman, *Illness*, 214.

2 Recall that Camus's philosophical work was used to build the concept of a Literary Arts Praxis in Chapter 6.

3 Camus, *Algerian*, loc. 517.

4 Again, alexithymia refers to a psychic constriction characterized by an indifference to the original traumatic experiences.

5 The topic of intimate literature—chronicles, diaries, journals, essays, thoughts, eulogies, memoirs, confessions, souvenirs autobiographies, notebooks, and letters—was a near-obsession among existentialist French writers. Hence it seems fitting to probe this feature of *The Plague*. To prove this point, one should consider the following: André Gide experimented with diaries and letters in his novel *The Counterfeiters* (1925); Georges Bernanos's story of a dying priest and suicidal doctor in his *Diary of a Country Priest* (1936) is buttressed by diary form; Sartre, of course, explored the genre by crafting a parody of a diary in his novel *Nausea* (1938); and Simone de Beauvoir explores the disintegration of a woman's marriage and identity in diary form in her *The Woman Destroyed* (1967).

6 See Felman and Laub, *Testimony*, 99.

7 I am borrowing this distinction between empathy and sympathy from Terry Eagleton, who writes, "Sophocles is not inviting us to empathize with Oedipus. The play expects us to feel pity for its doomed protagonist, but there is a difference between feeling for someone (sympathy) and feeling as them (empathy)." Eagleton, *How*, 76.

8 Felman and Laub, *Testimony*, 99.

9 Charon, *Narrative*, 70; the French literary theorist Philippe Lejeune investigated in depth the issue of an autobiographical gap in his *Le Pacte autobiographique* (1975).

10 Camus, *Plague*, 6.

11 The neuroscientist Antonio Damasio describes the tendency for doctors to constrain emotional responses. In his *Descartes' Error: Emotion, Reason, and the Human Brain*, he writes: "Mind you, restraint of this sort is often most welcome, from the point of view of the physician-listener, since it does reduce one's emotional expense." Damasio, *Descartes'*, 44.

12 Camus, *Plague*, 301.

13 Ibid., 126.

14 Ibid., 127.

15 Ibid.

16 Ibid., 128.

17 Some may object that the term "troubles" is modified by "personal" and, hence, it seems as if Rieux is referring to something other than an existential issue. Still, the original reads: "*Mais ce que, personellement, il avait à dire, son attente, ses épreuves, il devait les taire.*" Camus, *Peste*, 242. The English translation of this phrase is problematic. First, the word *épreuves* in French has a different connotation than "troubles." The plural form comes closer to "trials and tribulations" than to "personal troubles." Second, the adverb *personnellement* is translated by the adjective "personal," and this transforms the meaning of the sentence completely. For instance, consider the difference between: "I personally have nothing to say about my troubles" versus "I have nothing to say about my personal troubles."

18 Camus, *Plague*, 3.

19 Ibid., 4.

20 Ibid., 67.

21 Ibid., 5.

22 Mukherjee, *Laws*, 13–14.

23 Camus, *Rebel*, 7.

24 See Chapter 6's discussion of Camus's the *Myth of Sisyphus*.

25 LaCapra, *Writing*, 40.
26 Riess et al., "Empathy," 1280.
27 Halpern, *Detached*, 76.
28 Ibid., 11.
29 LaCapra, *Writing*, loc. 355.
30 Ibid., 47.
31 Bessel van der Kolk claims that dissociation occurs when an individual suffers from a traumatic event and the ensuing traumatic experience of the mind is "split off and fragmented, so that the emotions, sounds, images, thoughts and physical sensations related to the trauma take on a life of their own." Van der Kolk, *Body*, 66.
32 Camus, *Plague*, 6.
33 Ibid., 260.
34 Ibid., 224.
35 Ibid., 215.
36 Ibid., 302.
37 Ibid., 4.
38 Ibid., 24.
39 Ibid.
40 Ibid.
41 Ibid.
42 Ibid., 3–4.
43 Ibid.
44 Ibid., 214.
45 Ibid., 41.
46 Ibid., 240.
47 Ibid., 216.
48 Ibid.
49 Ibid., 289.
50 Ibid., 291.
51 Ibid., 25.
52 Ibid., 167.
53 Ricoeur, "Narrative," 73.
54 Ibid., 80.
55 Ogden, "Kafka," 392.
56 See Shengold, "Insight," 291.
57 Ibid., 302.
58 Halpern, *Detached*, 11.
59 See Husserl, *Ideas*, 15.
60 Stephanson, "Plague," 234.
61 Charon, *Narrative*, 125.
62 Ibid., 75.
63 For a thoughtful (and alarming) analysis of how medical school students are not trained or encouraged to cultivate human qualities such as empathy, see Shimon Glick's essay "The Empathic Physician: Nature and Nurture."
64 Kelm et al., "Interventions," 7.
65 Charon, *Narrative*, 75.
66 Jones et al., "Minding," 120.
67 See Mukherjee, *Laws*, 46.
68 Broyard, *Intoxicated*, 52.

9 Childhood Trauma and Imaginative Escapades with J.M.G. Le Clézio

The genealogy of literature is characterized by a most striking feature. Don Quixote, Robinson Crusoe, Manon Lescaut, Pamela, Candide, Werther, Jean Valjean, and on and on the family tree has grown. Neither the tree's prolific blossoming nor the dominance of male characters on its branches is so remarkable.[1] Most alarming was the near absence of children characters on the pedigree until the nineteenth century. Along with Charles Dickens, Victor Hugo did more to raise awareness about the condition of children in modern European society than any other writer, philosopher, or early sociologist. Who has not felt a deep affinity and concern for Gavroche and Cosette from Hugo's *Les Misérables*? What reader has not welcomed these orphans into her living room? Following Oliver Twist, David Copperfield, and Hugo's characters, a proliferation of children characters has appeared in the twentieth century from the Little Prince to Lolita.

If children failed to appear on literature's ancestry chart until the nineteenth century, the same could be said about their absence from the mental-health field until the end of the same period. The history of children's mental health services in the United States provides evidence of this neglect. The country established the Society for the Prevention of Cruelty to Animals (1866) before the Society for the Prevention of Cruelty to Children (1875), the first child protection agency in the world. While Freudian psychoanalysis might have helped to design child mental health services in the form of individual talk therapy, it addressed the needs mostly of upper- and middle-class children.[2] Services for children did not improve much immediately after World War II when most clinicians were devoted to treating combat veterans, if at all. Gradually, government agencies called attention to this neglect, but neither laws nor funds could match children's mental health needs.[3] These facts have prompted psychologist Murray Levine to advocate for more community-based and holistic mechanisms (including recreational, educational, and vocational programs) to address child well-being. He adds that this would require "political activism, something that most mental health personnel do not see as falling within their job descriptions."[4] But does it take only political activism? What about activism from the

DOI: 10.4324/9781003284642-14

humanities in the form of novels that serve as megaphones and pens as swords to cut through hypocrisies?

Authors of literature have often considered political activism as part of their job description. Many have followed Dickens and Hugo to raise conscious awareness about the condition of children through lyrical prose. A chief concern today is the prevalence of childhood trauma and ACE (Adverse Childhood Experiences). As reviewed in Chapter 5, there are many different types of childhood trauma, including parental loss; emotional and physical abuse and neglect; sexual abuse; domestic violence; bullying; community violence; sex trafficking; and refugee trauma, among others.[5] If some traumatologists have insisted on the "unknowable" nature of trauma, imagine how children must feel?[6] Without the linguistic or emotional maturity to interpret events and feelings, without the wherewithal to approach a psychotherapist, how do they tell their trauma story? They beckon for their stories to be told, while they await the day to tell their own, not only of trauma, but of resistance, resilience, growth, and even recovery.

We turn to the Franco-Mauritian author Jean-Marie Gustave Le Clézio (b. 1940) to capture portrayals of childhood trauma and posttraumatic experiences in marginalized communities. His literature is an invaluable resource to address these issues. Le Clézio could be called a world citizen. He carries a passport from both France and Mauritius and has lived in Great Britain, Korea, Mexico, Nigeria, Thailand, and the United States. Between his binational, multilingual, and multicultural background, his oeuvre offers not only a striking example of world literature but also insights into the condition of those outside the boundaries of dominant Western and especially Anglo-American cultures. In fact, upon receiving the Nobel Prize in 2008, he was praised for being an "explorer of a humanity below the reigning civilization."[7]

Focusing on Le Clézio's *Desert* (published first in French in 1980), I explore the themes of childhood trauma in post-colonial communities. While these topics may appear vast and dispersed, they are tightly woven in the novel. The three orphaned-adolescent characters (Lalla, Nour, and Radicz) represent trauma triggered by a post-colonial geopolitical crisis. I pull apart the Literary Arts Praxis in which the main character Lalla engages to access her trauma. She embarks on imaginative escapades consisting of listening to stories and fairy tales; recalling comforting memories and creating memory-stories; listening to music; and soothing the body through physical contact with nature. To buttress these arguments, I rely on the research of literary theorist Joseph Campbell, psychoanalyst Melanie Klein, and sociologist Albert Memmi, among others. Building on existentialism and aesthetics (topics discussed in Chapter 6), I also propose the term "benevolent retaliation," which conveys a unique form of resistance against perpetrators of trauma through aesthetics.

A Triptych of Trauma in a Post-Colonial World and New Concepts of Trauma

Desert resembles a trauma triptych, a painting with three separate and yet attached panels often adorning the altars of medieval churches. Each panel traces the footsteps of three orphaned adolescents who are on the move, forced to flee their homes by factors beyond their control. In the center panel, appears the novel's main character Lalla. She lives in the projects in a town on the coast of Morocco. On the right, we meet Nour. He is a nomad and belongs to the tribe of Lalla's ancestors, the desert nomadic warriors of North Africa who were chased out of their native lands and massacred by the colonizing French. On the left, we encounter Radicz, an enslaved gypsy whom Lalla meets in Marseille. Like so many other immigrants living in Europe, Lalla and Radicz both struggle as they face intense feelings of deracination and alienation in an era of globalization. The three characters appear as icons of a traumatic reality in a post-colonial world. And yet, Lalla, Nour and Radicz attempt to survive in and thrive despite traumatic personal, cultural, and environmental events.

Does it make sense to interpret individual trauma as global in nature? Doesn't such an expansive view of trauma water down the individual experience? By highlighting the global nature of trauma, Le Clézio does not minimize or discount individual experiences. On the contrary, he seeks to underscore how individual, cultural, and community traumatic experiences are interconnected. Perhaps, the dominant definition of trauma leaves us with the impression that a wider perspective on traumatic experiences is problematic. Indeed, the current individual-centered concept of trauma could be modified if one considers how much individual traumatic experiences are associated with historical and cultural realities, such as colonialism, globalization, and the associated phenomena of community violence, cultural denigration, environmental destruction, and migration. Whereas the entry on trauma in the *DSM-5* consists of an "elimination of the subjective component to the definition of trauma" (from the *DSM-IV*), trauma theorists such as Laura Brown and Kai Erikson provide more comprehensive definitions of trauma that correspond with Le Clézio's global perspective. Brown questions that trauma occurs only when a "person has experienced an event that is outside the range of human experience."[8] Erikson describes a traumatic experience as something "alien [that] breaks in on you, smashing through whatever barriers your mind has set up as a line of defense."[9] In contrast with the *DSM-5* entry, these definitions expand the notion of trauma beyond a life-threatening event. The prepositional phrases "outside the range of"; "breaks in on you"; and "smashing through" insinuate that trauma occurs when something from the outside targets an interior facet of being. Moreover, these definitions underscore that the attack is highly ambiguous and hence complex. It is outside the range of "human experience"; it is "something alien"; and "it smashes through whatever barriers." How does one define these terms? What is an "experience"? What is "something"? What are examples of those "barriers"? This expansive (and subjective) vocabulary indicates that trauma could not only consist of an attack on an individual's body, brain, and mind, but also on a community, culture, or natural environment—those places we call intimately our own. By portraying the traumatic experiences of these three youngsters in a vast cultural landscape, as opposed to the space between their ears, Le Clézio makes it clear that individual trauma so often is a consequence of a geo-political and cultural reality.

Lalla's Traumatic Experiences and Mechanisms to Move beyond Trauma

Lalla appears to have been traumatized as a young child by the death of her mother. Surviving this loss is continuous. The trauma remains in the mind, persistent like the scorching sun of the desert. As Henry Krystal reminds us: "Since separation from the mother quickly becomes a matter of life and death, the whole affective apparatus of the child is mobilized, the child becomes frantic and noisy and assumes a search pattern."[10] Lalla's personality is governed by patterns triggered by trauma. As a young adolescent, she would ask her aunt to tell her stories about her mother, which intimates that she still searches to comprehend her loss. She also asks her aunt to sing repeatedly the songs her mother would sing, since her mind struggles to repeat what she fails to recall. It is a song of lamentation and hope for better days. When her aunt sings, Lalla is transported to another realm. The voice no longer belongs to her aunt, but rather to some "unknown young woman who is singing through the curtains of flames for Lalla, just for Lalla."[11] In the absence of her real mother, she finds a mechanism to comfort herself through music.

Lalla also finds a way to communicate with her deceased mother. She relies on memories, which develop into stories, as psychiatrist Robert Coles reminds us.[12] And relying further on Cole's theories, these memory-stories help her to survive.[13] Let us examine how Lalla's memory-stories function. She relives the experience of being lost as a young child before her mother's death. Imagining that she is in a field of stones and dust, she chances upon a snake slithering down a shriveled tree trunk. Seized by fear, she runs away toward her mother who "holds her very tight and strokes her face."[14] When she opens her eyes from reliving this memory, her fear has vanished. She begins to feel a sort of giddiness, as if a gaze was coming "from the sea, from the light in the sky, from the beach."[15] Joseph Campbell sheds light on Lalla's survival mechanism. For Campbell, humanity possesses the power of life, which has shaped us all in our mother's womb. "And this kind of wisdom lives in us, and it represents the force of this power, this energy … But it's a transcendent energy. It's an energy that comes from a realm beyond our powers of knowledge."[16] It becomes obvious that there is a close link between her mother and some other natural or supernatural force.

According to Lalla's friend, wise old Naman the fisherman: "Maybe it is the sea that is always looking on in that way, the deep gaze of the waves of water, the dazzling gaze of the waves of salt and sand … [T]he sea is like a woman … The gaze comes from all sides at once."[17] Even though her mother is physically absent, Lalla constructs an image of her that is connected to the wider natural environment. In short, she relies on her imagination, memory-stories, and songs to discover not only a version of her mother but also a source of energy found in nature and perhaps even cultivate resistance and resilience.

When Lalla ventures alone into the desert, she is assured that the gaze of her ancestor, the Great Blue Warrior al-Ser, will support her: "He is surely going to come, his eyes will look straight into the deepest part of her being and give her the strength to fight against the man in the suit, against the death hovering over Naman, and will transform her into a bird."[18] By communicating with her Berber ancestor, who may very well be traumatized daily by the harsh desert, Lalla assumes "the proportions of a giant who would live for a very long time."[19] Although the term "traumatized daily by the harsh desert" seems to dilute the concept of trauma, the novel does portray the daily life of the Berbers as just that, traumatic. The unrelenting sun, heat, and winds of the desert burn the skin, scorch the head, dry the throat, and make the mind spin relentlessly.

Stories serve as another source of comfort for Lalla. Namen tells her about an emir whose kingdom was plagued by severe drought: A wise man from Egypt informs the king that the drought is the result of a spell cast upon him for having sentenced to death an innocent man. The only way to break the spell would be to send his daughter Princess Leila to the forest to be devoured by wild beasts. Though overwhelmed by a sense of impending doom, the king brings his daughter to the forest and leaves her tied to a tree. Upon hearing the news of the tragic fate awaiting the princess, a prince turns himself into a songbird that soothes the wild beasts, and Leila is spared.

This fairy tale contains a timeless lesson about nature. It reminds Lalla that nature can be soothed, just as Orpheus tamed the wild animals with his lyre. In the absence of real parents, the fairy tale offers guidance to an adolescent who is trying to make sense of the world. Lalla's reaction to the story is kindred to what Cyrulnik wrote about stories: "Unhappiness is supportable as long as stories are made from it."[20] Additionally, the story serves as a mirror image of Lalla's (Leila's) own life. The wild birds, along with the rest of nature, soothe her by chasing away the tormenting beasts of her mind.

> She really does hear, in the whoosh of the sea and the wind, in the sharp cries of the gulls seeking out a beach for the night, she hears the soft voice repeating its lament, the clear, yet somewhat shaky voice, as if it already knew death was coming to silence it, the voice which is

as pure as the water you can't drink enough of after long scorching days. It's a music born of the heavens and of the clouds … It's singing for Lalla, just for Lalla, it envelopes her and cleanses her in its fresh waters, it runs its hand through her hair, over her forehead, across her lips, it declares its love, it descends upon her and gives her its blessing.[21]

In the absence of human love, the adolescent orphan girl communes with Mother Nature. She consumes nature's sounds voraciously. The angelic tune is restorative, as it should be, for it was designed especially for her, according to the narrator. Nature's music embraces her, and she undergoes a cathartic experience. Detractors might argue that this scene is straight from the playbook of Romantic writers and that the argument about Lalla finding solace in nature is unoriginal. However, the narrator is prepared for such a knee-jerk reaction. The use of the terms "really," "already knew death was coming to silence it," and "just for Lalla" are added, lest readers dismiss Lalla's form of therapy as Romantic gibberish. These terms force readers to slow down and to readjust their Western centered judgment. When there is no Prozac to take, no psychotherapist to call, or mother to approach, the birds, the sea, and the wind may indeed provide the solace Lalla so desperately needs and help her to cultivate resistance, resilience, and growth.

The narrator does not entertain an idealized view of nature. The desert is often portrayed in raw form, as evidenced in these lines: "The wind doesn't wait. It does what it wants, and Lalla is happy when it's there, even if it does burn her eyes and ears, even if it does throw handfuls of sand in her face."[22] The narrator reminds us that the "Night has eased the fever of the sun and the dryness. Thirst, hunger, anxiety have all been relieved by the light of the galaxy, and on her skin, like droplets, are the marks of each star in the sky."[23] Lalla transcends her own weakness and vulnerability by uniting herself with the power of nature. Campbell's work illuminates what I shall call Lalla's sources of solace. He writes: "So the psychological problem, the way to keep from becoming blocked, is to make yourself—and here is the phrase—transparent to the transcendent."[24] In Lalla's case, she erases herself and thus links herself with the near infinite and immortal elements of the universe to be filled with their energy and strength.

The man with the gray green suit is a potential threat to this acquired strength. This mysterious character is known precisely as that. He needs no name because he is a dominant man cut from the fabric of "people called to dominate the world."[25] The peculiar title of "the man with the gray green suit" is akin to the term *pied-noir*, which literally translated is "black foot," or a person of European origin who lived in Algeria during the French colonial period. Black foot or the gray-green-suit man wants to take Lalla away and marry her. She flees, knowing that the man is the very embodiment of the cause of her trauma. The wind of ill fortune never strikes people like him. He is the "other" who lives without the trauma associated with the ill consequences of colonization and globalization. The sociologist Albert Memmi sheds light on what could happen to Lalla were she to marry the mysterious man. Memmi writes: "the colonized means little to the colonizer. Far from wanting to understand him [her, in this case] as he really is, the colonizer is preoccupied with making him [her] undergo this urgent change ... It consists, in the first place, of a series of negations."[26] Even if Lalla lives in post-colonial times, the man in the gray green suit still represents a colonizer, an oppressor of the mind. Besides losing her mother, her land, and her culture, Lalla would lose herself completely if she married the man. All the efforts she had made to build herself through memories, stories, and nature would be wiped out by the voracious need of the colonizer who seems to devour everything in his path. The narrator states in fact: "What did these foreigners want? They wanted the entire earth; they wouldn't stop until they had devoured everything, that was certain."[27]

By speaking with her deceased mother and her great ancestor and by listening to Naman's stories, Lalla comprehends at a conscious and/or unconscious level that the man in the gray green suit represents her figurative death. Had she been suffering from anhedonia (the inability to experience pleasure), which is a common symptom of infant trauma, then she might not have been able to revolt against him.[28] Numbed to the core, she would have had the expectation of being neither happy nor unhappy. Lalla does not appear to be vulnerable to anhedonia. She constantly seeks the pleasure of nature's company. The narrator describes her first and last intimate sexual encounter with a shepherd boy in the desert mountains:

> The cold, beautiful night envelops them, holding them in blue darkness. Never has Lalla seen such a beautiful night. Back there in the Project, or on the shores of the sea, there was always something that came between you and the night mist or dust. There was always a veil dulling it, because there were people everywhere, with their fires.[29]

This passage highlights the sharp contrast between Mother Nature's ability to inspire and humanity's tendency to tarnish life with a matte finish. Though readers may be tempted once again to dismiss this as Romantic rhetoric, a dose of caution must temper this reading for other reasons. What must be stressed is the psychological motivation behind her desire to find pleasure in nature. Kindred to Sisyphus, Lalla has chosen to revolt against the traumatic memories that define her. Rather than raising stones in defiance against her fate, she engages in mechanisms, whether it is listening to stories and songs or allowing Mother Nature to envelope her. She is in the right mood for finding solace, as opposed to succumbing to nihilism, as discussed in the chapter on Sisyphus and trauma survivors (Chapter 6).

It should also be underscored that nature not only helps Lalla to create a healthy setting in which she can thrive imaginatively. It also provides the backbone of Naman's stories. (Recall the story about the emir who was constrained to send his daughter Leila to the forest to be devoured by wild beasts to break the drought and that a prince turned himself into a songbird to soothe the wild beasts so Leila would be spared.) The link between stories and nature is welded together in Le Clézio's work. In fact, the author admits that he cannot write a novel without thinking about the earth, fire, air, and water; they are equally as important as societies.[30] What might be going on in Lalla's mind as she listens to stories where Mother Nature centers front and center? And how might stories help her to reach her traumatic experiences?

As pointed out in our discussion of Don Quixote, fairy tales are often used to treat children who have been traumatized.[31] They can be therapeutic to children, because they often take place in dark forests where the mind enters a supernatural world of mystery resembling the unconscious realm. Children are asked to take a magic carpet ride to the underworld, the world of the unconscious, where they can work out their own trauma in the masked forms of big bad wolves.[32] Put in another way, nature's infinite complexity defines itself by the unknown, which mirrors the unknown of the unconscious realm. Whether listening to or constructing fairy tales or stories depicting humans turning into bugs, these exercises are highly creative, especially compared to a Sisyphean task. This may very well encourage Lalla and other trauma survivors to approach their own stories of trauma from a perspective that is as liberating as donning gigantic leather boots to flee ogres.

While there might be a convincing explanation about the therapeutic quality of stories centered on nature, what about stories in general? As reviewed in Chapter 6, stories might help trauma survivors to create healthy mental states by bathing minds in a solution of imaginative language. Metaphors, litotes, oxymora, hyperboles, ironies, analogies, allegories, and allusions all jolt the mind from a state of inertia. These tools have the power not only to cut away (like a scalpel) at encrusted images but also to implant new ones. They can excise outdated images and reveal hidden ones in the tissues of the mind, while constructing others from scratch. Once images have been assigned language, they evoke more words in turn: images cultivate words just as words foster images. The resulting polysemy of words and meaning promotes conscious awareness. Conversely, without words, images have the power to torment like demons trapped in a cerebral labyrinth. When the mind fails to produce words that reflect the intensity of trauma, it wallows in confusion. Stories are a dogged attempt to locate words that somehow mirror the haunting images of a reality, past or present. They attempt to cut through the fog of reality, so that the traumatic memory can be re-imagined and retold anew. If stories loaded with uncanny language and images have the power to stimulate the brain, then it must also stimulate the body, as reviewed in Chapter 6. After all, much of what we think and feel, we think and feel with our body. Tears of sadness and joy, sweating brows and hands are all a part of the body's emotional language.

Finally, listening to stories is a creative process and thus can serve as an aesthetic and pleasurable escapade of the mind. The pleasure of the sonority of words can be therapeutic, like music. This experience appears analogous to what the psychoanalyst Melanie Klein describes in her essay "The Psycho-analytic Play Technique" about her patient Rita.[33] The playground was a therapeutic environment for the young girl. She found the open space a safer place than the psychiatrist's office to act out her trauma. Since storytelling is an aesthetic creation of sounds and images, the reader and writer may find (just as Rita did) a safe and soothing environment in which to thrive.

The Cultural Trauma of Colonialism in the Desert and beyond

Before Lalla flees the man in the gray green suit, the narrator first exposes the yoke of cultural trauma that burdens her. According to Jeffrey Alexander, "Cultural trauma occurs when members of a collectivity feel they have been subjected to a horrendous event that leaves indelible marks upon their group consciousness, marking their memories forever and changing their future identity."[34] Lalla's individual trauma is in fact a reflection of a deeper and wider cultural trauma. Le Clézio weaves together her story with a story of colonization. At the center of this wider story appears a young nomad, Nour, who acts as an icon of colonization. Readers are never told explicitly that he is an orphan, but he is traveling in the desert with other nomads without his immediate family. The Berbers are desperately and futilely searching for a new home, after having been pushed out of their homeland by the colonizing French. What happens to Lalla on an individual scale—losing her mother—has thus happened on a wider cultural scale: her ancestors, the blue people, were orphaned from Mother Nature.

The author uses a particular stylistic device to ensure that readers do not remain indifferent to the blue people's suffering. Intense sensual descriptions guarantee that readers feel their physical pain. Gusts sweep through the pages. Readers see the powerful wind sweep across miles of open desert; feel it burning their face; taste its acridity on their lips; and hear it howling. The desert wind is no gentle breeze. "The blue men had left, one after the other, taking their rags with them. But so many had died on the way! Never would they find the peace they had known before, never would the wind of ill fortune leave them in peace."[35] Except for a few who return to the south where only they can live, the blue people were swept away by the wind of ill-fortune or by the cold night that crushed their limbs. Frantz Fanon states explicitly what Le Clézio conveys metaphorically with the wind: "But the war goes on, and we will have to bind up for years to come the many, sometimes ineffaceable, wounds that the colonialist onslaught has inflicted on our people."[36] This is exactly where Lalla steps in. She unbinds wounds and fosters healing. The blue men are not completely dead or petrified, after all. There is a sense of recovery from the trauma of colonization, and even a particular form of resistance, seen in the next panel.

Global Trauma and "Benevolent Retaliation"

The global trauma described in the final panel of the triptych is like a disease. Its true nature is hidden under layers of protective skin and tissue. On an ostensible level, the third story is about Lalla's escape from the potential trauma of being married to the man in the gray green suit. On a deeper level, it is about overcoming the individual and cultural traumas described in the previous two panels. The traumas are intimately related just as the panels in any triptych. The poet and politician Aimé Césaire reminds us in fact that "no one colonizes innocently, that no one colonizes with impunity either; that a nation which colonizes, that a civilization which justifies colonization—and therefore force—is already a sick civilization, a civilization that is morally diseased."[37] Colonization is only a metastasis of a greater disease found in Europe, which Lalla experiences firsthand.

Even if Lalla's decision to leave for Marseille seems counterintuitive—since it brings her to the very world responsible for her cultural trauma—it is at the heart of an individual and cultural cure. In France, she works as a maid at a hotel where mostly lonely, deracinated, and alienated foreigners live. This new source of trauma appears altogether different from the individual and collective trauma she faced at home. She observes it daily in the hotel and in the streets of Marseille and cannot remain impervious to it. The philosopher Slavoj Žižek describes in theoretical terms what Le Clézio captures in prose: "If the Freudian name for the 'unknown known' is the unconscious, the Freudian name for the 'unknown unknowns' is trauma, the violent intrusion of something radically unexpected, something the subject was absolutely not ready for, and which it cannot integrate in any way."[38] Lalla's experience in Marseille is traumatic precisely because she did not expect it to be so. Naman the fisherman had always conveyed an idealized image of France. Her fairy tale has turned into a nightmare. The narrator paints a dark portrait of European society: "The evil wind is blowing in the street, that is what is creating the void over the city, the fear, the poverty, the hunger: that is what ... makes silence weigh down in lonely rooms where children and old people are suffocating."[39] The voice of the narrator grows so tainted with outrage and disgust that the reader has the impression that it is a first-hand account. Lalla seems to have assumed the role of narrator:

> There is so much despair in this street, as if it kept drifting endlessly down through the different degrees of hell ... There is so much hunger, unsatisfied desire, violence ... Perhaps, there is no love anywhere, no pity, no gentleness. Perhaps, the white veil separating the earth from the

sky has smothered the men, stopped the palpitations of their hearts, made all of their memories, all of their old desires, all of the beauty die.[40]

All too aware of the lamentable state of the European city, Lalla falls into a state of alexithymia. To understand the condition of alexithymia in general terms, it is helpful to consult Krystal's research, again. "To describe people as traumatized is to say that they have withdrawn into a kind of protective envelope, a place of mute, aching loneliness, in which the traumatic experience is treated as a solitary burden that needs to be expunged by acts of denial and resistance."[41] In Marseille, Lalla pushes away emotions, shies away from social attachments, and behaves almost robotically to create a protective wrap from the misery around her. This statement alludes to the fact that alexithymia can be a coping mechanism, albeit a less than ideal one.

She breaks forth from her protective shell when one of the few jovial residents from the hotel dies, and she is forced to bid farewell to his embalmed corpse. This figure of death is completely foreign to her. In her native culture, this is how people die: "Each day, with the same motions, they erased the traces of their fires, they buried their excrement. Turned toward the desert, they carried out their wordless prayer. They drifted away, as if in a dream, disappeared."[42] When Lalla realizes that the dead in the West do not disappear with the wind, but instead are entrapped in a corpse, she snaps. She quits her job at the hotel, collects her pay, and ventures into the metaphorical forest of the city to confront the beasts. Unlike Leila from Naman's fairy tale, Lalla will need no prince to save her, for she can soothe the beasts herself. She purchases new clothes and "Her eyes are sparkling with joy."[43] She walks through the streets of Marseille, as if completely transformed, but not because of her new designer clothes.

The transformation defining Lalla comes into clear focus only gradually. A photographer, who is dining at the same restaurant as Lalla and her gypsy friend Radicz, admires her singular beauty: "He has never seen a more beautiful, more luminous face."[44] Without twisting Lalla's arm too much, he convinces her to pose for him as a model.

At first glance, this might seem perplexing. One would expect Lalla to shun Western society altogether. On closer inspection, it becomes obvious that she must take this step to rework the traumatic events that precipitated her initial trauma. Her choice to become a model makes sense in the same way that writers have embraced the power of paradox. Lalla knows that there is something wrong with Western culture, but she paradoxically becomes a part of it, just as the poet Miguel de Unamuno prays to a nonexistent God in his "The Atheist's Prayer" ("*La oracion del ateo*"). Lalla's choice also makes sense in the way that Richard Wagner's God from his opera *The Ring Cycle* comes up with the idea that he is no longer needed. Lalla participates fully in the Western world to abandon it, as Wagner's God abandons religion. It is precisely from a wounded state that Lalla must make her wound comprehensible. She unwraps the bandages covering her wounds, exposing herself to the very disease (Western culture) that had sickened her, while hoping to develop resistance to it.

A career as a model allows Lalla to purge herself of the overwhelming trauma that has defined her and her people. She reenacts traumatic scenes but reverses the roles. Now she is in a position of power and esteem, while the rest of the Westernized world stagnates in sorrow. In some respects, she can get even with the masterminds of colonization and globalization by outdoing them. Lalla changes the dust upon which the Western Culture walked upon into gold. Cyrulnik refers to this process as a form of mental alchemy, an alchemy of pain.[45] Orpheus calms the beasts with his lyre; Lalla soothes the "beasts" of the West with her dance, which is performed in a nightclub where the guests stand frozen around the dance floor in awe of her beauty. She "retells" her life story amid the culture that had enslaved her people, just as Scheherazade tells stories to save her life from her brutal captor husband. Lalla's career is short-lived, which guarantees that she is never possessed like an object.

Instead of using violence to protest a culture that has traumatized her and her people, she revolts against the West with beauty. She plays the game of the West and then returns to her homeland, a slap in the face to a culture that is otherwise so esteemed. Most importantly, she takes control of her life retaliating against a culture that had controlled her, her culture, and the natural environment. But she retaliates by honoring and projecting her own beauty. This is what I call "benevolent retaliation." It resembles Sisyphus's act of defiance and Roquentin's belief in creative writing. Lalla does not literally raise stones but figuratively does. She crafts herself into a beautiful piece of artwork. This existential and aesthetic act translates into an imaginative mechanism to foster resistance, resilience, and growth.

While Lalla employs "benevolent retaliation," she is not completely cured of her traumatic experiences. "The triumph of resilience is fragile,"[46] writes Catherine Malabou. "The wound is transformed, but it never heals completely. When a subject is severely damaged by existence, he finds himself obliged constantly to uphold the process of resilience to the day of his death."[47] Moreover, the narrator gives us a jolt when it is revealed that Lalla's trip to Marseille could have been a dream. The following lines give us reason to entertain the possibility that Lalla might have left for France only in her mind, "But it's as if nothing had ever happened, as if she'd never left the Projects of planks and tarpaper, or the plateau of stones and the hills where the Hartani live, as if she'd simply fallen asleep for an hour of two."[48] We also have reason to believe that it is only a dream, since it is hard to imagine that Lalla could have been a model while she was in the third trimester of her pregnancy, an important fact to be discussed in greater detail shortly. In addition, the fact that it seems counterintuitive (at first glance) for Lalla to have become a model in Western society suggests that we might not be in "reality," but rather in the unconscious realm.

If Lalla did fall asleep and dream of Marseille, then she found a therapeutic outlet in the unconscious. Campbell writes, "It was Sigmund Freud, Carl Jung, and Jacob Adler who realized that the figures of dreams are really figures of personal mythologization."[49] It makes sense to see Lalla's story in this light, as it is often argued that the only way to understand trauma is for it to be understood unconsciously.[50] This encounter with the self in the unconscious realm ensures that Lalla can move beyond her traumatic past.

When Lalla awakes from her dream (or when she returns to Morocco), she finds herself on the shore where she gives birth to a child with the help of a tree. She wraps a belt around the tree and squats, while the tree supports her during labor. It is at this moment that she can shake herself free from the global, cultural, and individual trauma that has defined her. She comes to life at that moment, as she gives birth to her child in a spot where her mother had given birth to her in the company of Mother Nature. This should not be seen as kitschy or callow. Campbell reminds us again that, "Being the mother, the woman becomes the symbolic counterpart, the personification of the power of the earth."[51] While we witness the destruction of the blue people and the faceless immigrants of European cities, while we watch Radicz and Nour simply disappear, Lalla's imagination blooms and her voice sings the song that soothes the beasts of her mind and the rest of the troubled world. Thus seen, *Desert* is less about depletion from trauma and more about new life.

Conclusions: Connecting Literature and Literary Theory with Reality

Wrapping up our research journey to explore how a Literary Arts Praxis might get at trauma, this chapter has examined how the character Lalla engages in mechanisms designed to cultivate resistance, resilience, and perhaps even growth posttraumatic experiences. She undertakes imaginative escapades consisting of listening to stories and fairy tales; recalling comforting memories and building memory-stories; listening to music; and soothing the body through physical contact with nature. Building on existentialism and aesthetics, I have also developed the term "benevolent retaliation," a form of resistance against perpetrators of trauma. By establishing herself as a beautiful model, Lalla rebels aesthetically against the trauma suffered by her culture and community. Even though it might be tempting for readers to look askance at her treatment (because it is not an exacting science), it makes little sense to rely exclusively on one template (such as the *DSM-5*) to understand the subjective experience of trauma and most importantly, other cultures' methods to foster resistance, resilience, and growth, as so poignantly portrayed in *Desert*.

We might even put forward that Le Clézio creates a healthy environment in which Lalla can craft her own methods. The author or narrator does not simply allow her fate to be determined. That is, she is not simply "touched by the grace of God" or healed by a doctor who prescribes a course of pharmacotherapy. Lalla embarks on her own imaginative escapades and assumes eventually the role of narrator. The author hands a bucket to Lalla who dips it into the deep well of her imagination. Thanks to her example, readers may feel encouraged to learn that the mind is not only a place of pathology and weakness, but also one of strength. With this is in mind, perhaps Le Clézio should have entitled his book *Oasis* rather than *Desert*.

Finally, Edward Said's comment about myopic research perspectives may provide elucidation about how this study on *Desert* might help define future research in trauma studies. In his *Culture and Imperialism* (1994), Said voices concern about professional humanists' inability to make a "connection between the prolonged and sordid cruelty of practices such as slavery, colonialist and racial oppression, and imperial subjection on the one hand, and the poetry, fiction, philosophy of the society that engages in these practices on the other."[52] This is curious for the genealogy of literature in the last century is replete with authors, such as Le Clézio, who have raised their voices against sordid practices and given a voice to victims. Perhaps Said was therefore referring to literary theorists, rather than to literary authors. If so, this leads us to question whether our creative and critical research, especially in cultural trauma studies, might benefit from connecting more with reality and creating somehow healthier environments for trauma survivors to find their own oases.

Notes

1 My comment that neither the tree's prolific blossoming nor the dominance of male characters on its branches is so remarkable should not be misconstrued. I am insinuating that in the nineteenth-century male-dominated society in which the rising bourgeoisie contributed prolifically to writing fiction, it is no small wonder that literature neglected to depict characters who were marginalized members of society, including women, children, and minorities.

2 Levine, "Children," S24.

3 Ibid., S22.

4 Ibid., S28.

5 See NCTSN, "Defining."

6 I am alluding here to Caruth's reliance on the concept of the "unknown" of trauma, a topic discussed in detail in Chapter 4.

7 Nobel Prize, "Nobel."

8 Brown, "Not Outside," 100; this definition stems from the *DSM-III-R*.

9 Erikson, "Notes," 183.

10 Krystal, "Trauma," 79.

11 Le Clézio, *Desert*, 138.

12 Coles writes that, "A memory is, of course, a story, an aspect of experience that lives in a particular mind." Coles, *Call*, 183–184.

13 Coles describes how memory-stories are life sustaining: "Yet Dostoevsky is not advocating memory as a means of clarifying our mental problems or as a distorted representation of what 'really' took place. He is talking instead about what we might consider memory's more 'superficial' sense, a recollected moment

in which someone has tasted of life, a moment forceful enough, charged enough, to survive many other moments." Ibid., 183.

14 Le Clézio, *Desert*, 121.
15 Ibid., 122.
16 Campbell, *Pathways*, 16–17.
17 Le Clézio, *Desert*, 122.
18 Ibid., 162.
19 Ibid., 159.
20 Cyrulnik, *Merveilleux*, 105.
21 Le Clézio, *Desert*, 144.
22 Ibid., 55.
23 Ibid., 177.
24 Campbell, *Pathways*, 11.
25 Deleuze, *Critique*, 14. My translation; the original reads: "*ce n'est pas un peuple appelé à dominer le monde.*"
26 Memmi, *Colonizer*, 83.
27 Le Clézio, *Desert*, 343.
28 See Krystal, "Trauma," 79–80.
29 Le Clézio, *Desert*, 176.
30 See Kéchichian, "Le Clézio."
31 Bruno Bettelheim, Vladimir Propp, Muriel Bloch, and René Diatkine, among others, provide ample evidence in their research of the therapeutic effects of fairy tales; the latter three have studied especially how fairy tales benefit traumatized children.
32 It is curious that Naman's story is a cross between a *1,001 Nights* fairy tale in the Arabic, Indian, and Persian emir tradition and a Perrault and Brothers Grimm fairy tale from a European forest tradition.
33 Klein, "Psycho-analytic," 37–38.
34 Alexander, *Trauma*, 1.
35 Le Clézio, *Desert*, 324.
36 Fanon, *Wretched*, 249.
37 Césaire, *Discourse*, 4.
38 Žižek, *Living*, 292.
39 Le Clézio, *Desert*, 252.
40 Ibid., 253.
41 Ibid., 186.
42 Ibid., 352.
43 Ibid., 268.
44 Ibid., 271.
45 See Cyrulnik, *Merveilleux*, 20.
46 Malabou, *New Wounded*, 183.
47 Ibid.
48 Le Clézio, *Desert*, 332.
49 Campbell, *Myths*, xvii.
50 See Alexander, *Trauma*, 10.
51 Campbell, *Pathways*, 30.
52 Said, *Culture*, xiv.

Conclusion
Summing up and Sailing forward

Where have we have journeyed to in this book? Each chapter was designed to be like an island, while the book itself was a chain of islands, an archipelago. When Charles Darwin traveled to the Galapagos on board the *Beagle* in 1860, he discovered that even though the different islands of the archipelago were geographically close to one another, even though they shared common basic traits, their life forms were distinct.[1] Free from the gales of wind, neither seeds, insects, nor birds could travel easily among the islands, whereas the depths of the waters prevented easy crossing. From these limitations, came unique collections of plants and animals. They underwent metamorphoses to meet the conditions of the islands. Similarly, this book has aimed to present a series of distinct, albeit related, histories and concepts of trauma and traumatism from the perspectives of the sciences, clinical medicine, and the humanities to cultivate metamorphoses. Where have the pages taken us in this archipelago and what metamorphoses have we observed? The direction of the compass needle has pointed in four directions.

We first sailed north in Chapters 1 and 2 and explored embryonic concepts of trauma and traumatism from Cuneiform clay tablets to Enlightenment philosophy, as well as findings from Briquet, Charcot, Janet, Fanon, and, Chodoff, who offered a more contextual and integrated understanding of trauma and traumatism. This more expansive view not only translates into a metamorphosis of the historical narrative of trauma studies but also responds to Herman's and Tallis's concerns about narrowly focused and biologically oriented research on human emotional experiences.

Heading next east, we examined current trauma theories from the perspectives of medicine, the biological sciences, and the humanities. In Chapter 3, I painted a landscape of contemporary scientific trauma theories, while in Chapter 4, I sketched a portrait of cultural trauma studies. These syntheses were designed to offer multidisciplinary investigations to respond to a dearth of such research, according to Tedeschi and Luckhurst, and to the complexity of psychological trauma. At the end of each chapter, I highlighted examples of traumatologists from the fields of science, medicine, and the humanities who have built bridges between distinct domains. I also

DOI: 10.4324/9781003284642-15

attempted to paint a wide horizon where a transdisciplinary project, a metamorphosis of the field of trauma studies, could eventually come to light in the form of new imaginative notions.

We then traveled south in Chapters 5 and 6, providing a synthesis of recognized medical treatments for trauma survivors, while unveiling the main creative concept, a Literary Arts Praxis, and question of this book: how might a Praxis get at trauma? Following Herman's, Tedeschi's, and Calhoun's recommendation for trauma survivors to don a philosopher's hat, following Winnicott's, Rank's, Herman's, Levine's, Cyrulnik's, and Richman's invitation for survivors to make gold out of mud through creative exercises, I proposed a Literary Arts Praxis, an educational training in the literary arts (listening and telling stories; reading and interpreting literature rich in philosophical content from existentialism, phenomenology, and aesthetics; and creative writing, as seen in Camus's *The Plague*). In addition, the Praxis is built on several other research findings. From Janet, I borrow the concepts of a "re-education" and a "psychological evolution"; from Briquet, the notion that traumatic suffering (or hysteria, as he called it) is often caused by social circumstances that can be altered. The Praxis is inspired as well by different versions of Cognitive Behavioral Therapy (from Beck, Tedeschi, Calhoun, Foa, and Cloitre) and its emphasis on exercises that build individual coping skills, including emotional understanding.

We next moved west in Part IV (Chapters 7, 8, and 9) and analyzed World Literature and specifically how characters seemed to undergo metamorphoses. From Cervantes's Don Quixote to Camus's Dr. Rieux and Le Clézio's Lalla, these characters engage in creative mechanisms drawn from the literary arts to overcome traumatic experiences. These mechanisms include, among others: (1) An engagement in creative linguistic and literary acts of resistance, which finds resonance in existentialism; (2) the stimulation of bodily sensations, images, and emotions through the literary arts, so that survivors can readjust the compass of their body and mind, which corresponds with phenomenology; and (3) the transformation of personal identity through an imaginative, unconscious, and creative adventures of self-identity, which is built on aesthetics.

What creative contributions might a Literary Arts Praxis bring to the field of trauma studies? How do I expand on other findings on the connection between trauma and the literary arts? And how do I propose that the Praxis might get at trauma? While I have relied on LaCapra's arguments, I have adjusted them. Though I share his view that literature might provide a haven for trauma survivors, I stress that alliances forged between existential characters and trauma survivors can foster safe settings. Though I echo his argument that the arts can offer imaginative openings to reinterpret reality from odd angles, I do not attribute this to surrealistic situations, but rather to psycho-philosophical content in condensed and clear form. Though I agree with LaCapra that literature can provide piercing commentary on social realities and thus help survivors to understand the bigger picture behind their traumatic experiences, I put forward that existential literature paints universal portraits of the human condition striking a profound chord in many readers. Though my explanations on phenomenological and phenomenologically induced emotional experiences resonate with his position that "writing trauma" spurs readers' emotions and actions, I put forward that the stimulation of emotions and bodily sensations might help survivors to develop emotional "antibodies" needed to confront the memories of their own traumatic experiences.

Beyond amplifying LaCapra's positions, I also develop creative arguments in response to other traumatologists' research. While I do refer to testimonies, I have underscored that they might be seen as precursors to creative stories. Further, the Praxis adjusts the idea that trauma is a wound that is given shape (Laub) or sutured up (Cyrulnik) by words. If trauma is a wound; posttraumatic experiences can be like a spreading cancer. Posttraumatic conditions can be just as harrowing and painful as the original traumatic event. Hence, I propose the idea of excising the cancer of trauma through an exposure to creative words and images. Finally, the Praxis is founded on the idea of revolt, a concept that I have yet to encounter among other scholars, save for Arthur Frank. These revolts do not take place in the streets, but in the imaginative space between our ears. They involve interpretative reading and creative writing exercises. For example, they include first the creation of a testimony (that is more rigid) and then flexible and imaginative stories.

Whereas some might look askance at the concept of a Literary Arts Praxis because it is not founded on the scientific method and while cultural theorists might scoff at it since it appears to unravel the rainbow of the arts, it is important to stress again that several prominent traumatologists point to a relationship between the literary arts and posttraumatic conditions. Even if they uphold this position, they fail to elaborate on it, and hence the reason for this book.

An engagement in the Praxis boils down to a training that promotes a psychological evolution or a metamorphosis of the mind. Creativity and deep thinking obviously do not come easily to everyone, especially during the debilitating consequences of trauma. These skills are like any other from playing tennis to quantizing gravity. They require training and practice. If psychiatrists and psychologists have called for trauma survivors to play the role of philosopher and creative writer as part of their recovery processes, then they may very well consider a training such as a Literary Arts Praxis. And Sisyphus, Roquentin, Don Quixote, Rieux, and Lalla may very well serve as companions to trauma survivors on journeys through posttraumatic continents.

When Darwin and other explorers set sail on vast oceans, the night heavens ironically provided just as much, if not more, navigational information as illuminated skies of the day. On clear nights, the North Star guided seafarers in the northern hemisphere, whereas the astrolabe taught them about constellations to consider as points of directional reference. The North Star argument of this research project has been the importance of the humanities in understanding trauma and traumatism. Through examples, I have argued not only that literature, philosophy, art, and clinical research–enriched by trans-disciplinary perspectives–provide a valuable resource for researchers, clinicians, and trauma survivors, but that the humanities can serve as a driving force to change our understanding of psychological trauma.

Although this statement may seem self-evident, it is more nuanced as it responds to one of Herman's main arguments. She maintains that the history of the field of trauma studies shows that improving scientific knowledge and fostering public awareness are only preliminary steps to ending violence. "Moving from awareness into social action requires," she elaborates, "a political movement strong enough to overcome pervasive denial, the passive resistance of institutional inertia, and the active resistance of those who benefit from the established order."[2] She goes on to lament that "unfortunately, no popular movement has shown this kind of power, whether in the public domain of war and war crimes or in the private domain of crimes against women and children."[3] The Me Too and Black Lives Matter movements are two contemporary political forces that have appeared on the scene since Herman made these remarks in her book's epilogue in 2015. Whereas these political movements have developed to address violence and very often traumatic experiences, they could benefit from a reinforcement. Just as Enlightenment philosophers employed the tool of literature to raise conscious awareness about human suffering caused by injustices, the humanities today are called upon to stimulate political movements to overcome the resistance of the establishment and inspire creative acts of defiance.

Literature, philosophy, and the arts are obviously political in nature. If there is any doubt about this, one need only consider a few literary examples from the nineteenth and twentieth centuries to appreciate their political potency. After visiting Charcot's investigative theater, Émile Zola painted portraits of posttraumatic conditions in his novels. *The Human Beast* (1890) attacks the subject of trauma from both the physiological and psychological sides. If Kardiner treated traumatized war veterans for "shell shock" after the Great War, surrealists Guillaume Apollinaire and André Breton (both war veterans) portrayed in masked form first-hand war experiences in poetry, essays, and prose, as did British poets Robert Graves, Siegfried Sassoon, and Wilfred Owen.[4] And if Niederland, Eitinger, Chodoff, and Krystal investigated the posttraumatic states of Holocaust survivors, authors Elie Wiesel, Aharon Appelfeld, and Primo Levi explored the inexplorable in their autobiographical novels. What is unique about this amplified "story" of trauma studies is how authors of literature gave a voice to voiceless trauma survivors when it was difficult to arouse widespread interest in trauma and posttraumatic conditions.

This conclusion brings us back to this book's port of entry. We return to the humanities classroom to imagine engaging in the literary arts in new ways. As my students exhibited and the research presented in this book suggests raising consciousness on individual and collective levels involves sophisticated cognitive processes that occur in the intercranial darkness of the mind. A pedagogical engagement in literature, philosophy, and the arts seems to offer a trade route to those far-to-reach places. This position is rooted in the notion that while it is the job of neuroscience to study the brain, it is the task of the humanities to demystify the mind.

Where might we go once the final pages of this book have been reached? Embarking on related research projects in the future, a Literary Arts Praxis potentially and unabashedly could join the ranks of Bibliotherapy and Narrative Medicine. The former is a treatment modality involving subjects reading literature, whereas the latter involves practices that provide clinicians with methods to understand stories better because medicine is a "narrative undertaking fortified by learnable skills."[5] The Praxis distinguishes itself from Bibliotherapy in that it centers on literature rich in existential, phenomenological, and aesthetic musings. It comes closer to Narrative Medicine, except that it is designed for trauma survivors (not just clinicians). Perhaps for Bibliotherapy, Narrative Medicine, and a Literary Arts Praxis to gain recognition from evidence-based medicine, they would need to push for interdisciplinary dialogues and collaborative research projects. Such an approach could be grounded in Darwin's concept that all in the world is "netted together" and that a cross-fertilization of distinctly different memes (genes) may elicit a bountiful harvest of ideas.[6]

Whereas my students' stories of trauma and traumatism provided a constant wind to embark on this research journey, gales have propelled this book project forward, too. The staggering reality of a pandemic has projected a dark cloud on humanity's collective horizon, while mass migrations cast an even darker one. Trauma has escaped beyond the walls of counseling centers. Large swaths of the world's population experience it. Refugees board overcrowded planes desperately fleeing tyrants, civil conflicts, and persecution in the Middle East. Others cross the cemetery of the Mediterranean Sea in rubber boats, escaping poverty and natural disasters in Africa. And still others from Central America cling to anything that floats, crossing the Rio Grande River leaving behind cartel violence and droughts. As they travel in search of a brighter future, they carry with them the baggage of traumatic experiences, not to mention stories of resistance, resilience, and growth. Their narratives of traumatic displacement might be echoed by great swaths in the future, as we are displaced from our homes destroyed by violent storms, flooding, and fires. Many of us may very well find ourselves in a lifeboat, searching for beacons to help guide us forward. Today, more than ever, it is important for health professionals, scientists, and scholars from the humanities to understand psychological trauma and posttraumatic treatments, including those from the humanities, as this book has aimed to explore. After all, it may very well be that novelists have discoveries to share about these topics, precisely because they are curious about distant lands that beckon exploration; persistent about doors that must be opened; and passionate about topics that offer resistance.

Notes

1 See Darwin, *Origin*, 378–380.
2 Herman, *Trauma*, 263.
3 Ibid., 264.
4 For an excellent treatise on the history of creative writing written by Anglo-American writers during and after World War I, consult Paul Fussell, *Great*.
5 Charon, "Membranes," 342.
6 Darwin, *Notebook B*.

Bibliography

Abdul-Hamid, Walid Khalid, and Jamie Hacker Hughes. "Nothing New under the Sun: Post-Traumatic Stress Disorders in the Ancient World." *Early Science and Medicine* 19. 6 (2014): 549–557.

Abelard, Peter, and Heloise. *The Letters of Abelard and Heloise*. Translated by Betty Radice and M.T. Clanchy. London: Penguin Books, 2003. Kindle.

Adorno, Theodor. *Aesthetic Theory*, edited by Gretel Adorno and Rolf Tiedemann. Translated by Robert Hullot-Kentor. Minneapolis: University of Minnesota Press, 1997. Kindle.

Adorno, Theodor. *Notes to Literature*, edited by Rolf Tiedemann. Translated by Shierry Weber Nicholson. New York: Columbia University Press, 2019. Kindle.

Agaibi, Christine, and John P. Wilson. "Trauma, PTSD, and Resilience: A Review of the Literature." *Trauma, Violence, and Abuse* 6. 3 (July 2005): 195–216.

Akhtar, Salman, and Glenda Wrenn. "The Biopsychosocial Miracle of Human Resilience: An Overview." In *The Unbroken Soul: Tragedy, Trauma, and Human Resilience*, edited by Henri Parens, Harold P. Blum, and Salman Akhtar, 2–20. Lanham, MD: Jason Aronson, 2008. Kindle.

Alexander, Jeffrey. *The Meanings of Social Life: A Cultural Sociology*. Oxford: Oxford University Press, 2003. Kindle.

Alexander, Jeffrey. *Trauma: A Social Theory*. Malden, MA: Polity Press, 2012. Kindle.

American Psychiatric Association. *Diagnostic and Statistical Manual of Mental Disorders: DSM-III-R*. 3rd rev. edition. Washington, DC: American Psychiatric Association, 1987.

American Psychiatric Association. *Diagnostic and Statistical Manual of Mental Disorders: DSM-IV*. 4th edition. Washington, DC: American Psychiatric Association, 1994.

American Psychiatric Association. *Diagnostic and Statistical Manual of Mental Disorders: DSM-5*. 5th edition. Washington, DC: American Psychiatric Association, 2013.

American Psychiatric Association. "What is Post-traumatic Stress Disorder?" www.psychiatry.org/patients-families/ptsd/what-is-ptsd. Last modified August 2020.

American Psychological Association. "Medications for PTSD." www.apa.org/ptsd-guideline/treatments/medications. Last modified July 21, 2017.

Andermahr, Sonya. "Decolonizing Trauma Studies: Trauma and Postcolonialism-Introduction." *Humanities* 4 (2015): 500–505.

Argenti-Pillen, Alex. *Masking Terror: How Women Contain Violence in Southern Sri Lanka*. Philadelphia, PA: University of Pennsylvania Press, 2003.

Aristotle. *Éthique à Nichomaque*, livre VI. Translated by Philippe Arjakovsky. Paris: Agora Pocket, 2007.

Aristotle. *The Nicomachean Ethics*. Translated by Hugh Tredennick, J.A.K. Thomson, and Johnathan Barnes. London: Penguin Classics, 2004.

Aupperle, Robin L., Carolyn B. Allard, Erin M. Grimes, Alan N. Simmons, Taru Flagan, Michelle Behrooznia, Shadha H. Cissell, et al. "Dorsolateral Prefrontal Cortex Activation During Emotional Anticipation and Neuropsychological Performance in Posttraumatic Stress Disorder." *Archives of General Psychiatry* 69. 4 (2012): 360–371.

Barel, Efrat, Abraham Sagi-Schwartz, Marinus Van IJzendoorn, and Marian Bakermans-Kranenburg. "Surviving the Holocaust: A Meta-Analysis of the Long-Term Sequelae of a Genocide." *Psychological Bulletin* 136. 5 (2010): 677–698.

Barthes, Roland. *Le degré zero de l'écriture*. Paris: Seuil, 1953.

Barthes, Roland. *Mourning Diary*. Translated by Richard Howard. New York: Hill and Wang, 2009.

Barthes, Roland. *S/Z*. Paris: Editions du Seuil, 2015. Kindle.

Baudelaire, Charles. "Épilogue." In *Les Fleurs du mal*. Paris: Garnier, 1961.

Baudelaire, Charles. "The Invitation to the Voyage." In *Paris Spleen*. Translated by James Huneker, Joseph T. Shipley, and Arthur Symons. Digireads, 2015. Kindle.

Beá, Josep, and Victor Hernandez. "Don Quixote: Freud and Cervantes." *The International Journal of Psycho-Analysis* 65 (1984): 141–153.

Beauvoir, Simonede. *The Second Sex*. Translated by Constance Borde and Sheila Malovany-Chevallier. New York: Knopf Doubleday Publishing, 2019. Kindle.

Beck, Aaron T. *Cognitive Therapy and the Emotional Disorders*. New York: Penguin, 1976. Kindle.

Beck, Judith. *Cognitive Behavioral Therapy: Basics and Beyond*. 3rd edition. New York: Guilford, 2021.

Belsher Bradley, Erin Beech, Daniel Evatt, Derek J. Smolenski, M. Tracie Shea, Jean Lin Otto, Craig S. Rosen, et al. "Present-centered Therapy (PCT) for Post-traumatic Stress Disorder (PTSD) in Adults." *Cochrane Database of Systematic Reviews* 11 (2019): 1–3.

Bernardin de St. Pierre, Jacques-Henri. *Oeuvres complètes*, 12 vols., vol. 5. Paris: Mequinon-Mavis, 1818.

Bettelheim, Bruno. *The Uses of Enchantment: The Meaning and Importance of Fairy Tales*. New York: Vintage Books, 2010.

Bisson, Jonathan, Neil P. Roberts, Martin Andrew, Rosalind Cooper, and Catrin Lewis. "Psychological Therapies for Chronic Post-traumatic Stress Disorder (PTSD) in Adults." *Cochrane Database of Systematic Reviews* 12 (2013): 1–163.

Black, Michele C., Kathleen C. Basile, Matthew J. Breiding, Sharon G. Smith, Mikel L. Walters, Melissa T. Merrick, Jieru Chen et al. "*The National Intimate Partner and Sexual Violence Report (NISVS): 2010 Summary Report*." Atlanta: National Center for Injury Prevention and Control, Center for Disease Control and Prevention, 2010.

Blum, Harold. "Resilience and Its Correlates." In *The Unbroken Soul: Tragedy, Trauma, and Human Resilience*, edited by Henri Parens, Harold P. Blum, and Salman Akhtar, 173–191. Lanham, MD: Jason Aronson, 2008. Kindle.

Bonanno, George. "Meaning Making, Adversity, and Regulatory Flexibility." *Memory* 21. 1 (2013): 150–156.

Bonanno, George. "Resilience in the Face of Potential Trauma." *Current Directions in Psychological Science* 14. 3 (2005): 135–138.

Bonanno, George, and Erica D. Diminich. "Annual Research Review: Positive Adjustment to Adversity–Trajectories of Minimal–Impact Resilience and Emergent Resilience." *The Journal of Child Psychology and Psychiatry* 54. 4 (2013): 378–401.

Brenner, Ira. "On Genocidal Persecution and Resilience." In *The Unbroken Soul: Tragedy, Trauma, and Human Resilience*, edited by Henri Parens, Harold P. Blum, and Salman Akhtar, 67–84. Lanham, MD: Jason Aronson, 2008. Kindle.

Breton, André. *Manifesto of Surrealism*. Translated by Richard Seaver and Helen R. Lane. Ann Arbor, MI: University of Michigan Press, 1969.

Breuer, Josef, and Sigmund Freud. *Studies on Hysteria*. New York: Basic Books, 2009.

Briere, John, and Catherine Scott. *Principles of Trauma Therapy: A Guide to Symptoms, Evaluation, and Treatment*. Thousand Oaks, CA: Sage Publishing, 2006.

Briquet, Pierre. *Traité clinique et thérapeutique de l'hystérie*. Paris: J.B. Baillière et fils, 1859.

Bronowski, Jacob. *Origins of Knowledge and Imagination*. New Haven: Yale University Press, 1978. Kindle.

Brown, Laura S. "Not Outside the Range: One Feminist Perspective on Psychic Trauma." In *Trauma: Explorations of Memory*, edited by Cathy Caruth, 100–112. Baltimore: John Hopkins University Press, 1995.

Broyard, Anatole. *Intoxicated by My Illness, and Other Writings on Life and Death*. New York: Ballantine Books, 1992.

Calhoun, Lawrence, and Richard Tedeschi. *Handbook of Posttraumatic Growth: Research and Practice*. Florence: Taylor and Francis Group, 2006.

Calhoun, Lawrence, and Richard Tedeschi. *Posttraumatic Growth in Clinical Practice*. New York: Routledge, 2013. Kindle.

Campbell, Joseph. *Pathways to Bliss: Mythology and Personal Transformation*. Novato, CA: New World Library, 2004.

Campbell, Joseph. *Myths of Light. Eastern Metaphors of the Eternal*. Novato, CA: New World Library, 2003.

Camus, Albert. *Algerian Chronicles*. Translated by Arthur Goldhammer. Cambridge, MA: Belknap Press of Harvard University Press, 2014. Kindle.

Camus, Albert. *The Myth of Sisyphus and Other Essays*. Translated by Justin O'Brien. New York: Vintage International, 1991. Kindle.

Camus, Albert. *Notebooks: May 1935–February 1942*. Translated by Ivan R. Dee. New York: Paragon House Publishing, 1991.

Camus, Albert. *La Peste*. Paris: Gallimard, 1947.

Camus, Albert. *The Plague*. Translated by Stuart Gilbert. New York: Vintage Books, 1991. Kindle.

Camus, Albert. *The Rebel: An Essay on Man in Revolt*. Translated by Anthony Bower. New York: Vintage, 1991. Kindle.

Caruth, Cathy, ed. *Listening to Trauma: Conversations with Leaders in the Theory and Treatment of Catastrophic Experience*. Baltimore: Johns Hopkins University Press, 2014. Kindle.

Caruth, Cathy, ed. *Trauma: Explorations in Memory*. Baltimore: Johns Hopkins University Press, 1995.

Caruth, Cathy, ed. *Unclaimed Experience: Trauma, Narrative and History*. Baltimore: John Hopkins University Press, 1996. Kindle.

Cervantes Saavedra, Miguel de. *Don Quixote*. Translated by John Ormsby. Minneapolis, MN: Lerner Publishing Group, 2014.

Cervantes Saavedra, Miguel de. *El Ingenioso Hidalgo Don Quijote de la Mancha*. Valencia: Editorial Alfredo Ortells, 2004.

Césaire, Aimée. *Discourse on Colonialism*. New York: Monthly Review Press, 2001.

Chadwick, Henry. "Introduction." In SaintAugustine, *Confessions*, ix–xxvi. Oxford: Oxford University Press, 1991. Kindle.

Charcot, Jean-Martin. *La foi qui guérit*. Paris: F. Alcan, 1897.

Charcot, Jean-Martin. *Leçons du mardi à la Salpêtrière de professeur Charcot*, vol. I. Wentworth Press, 2018. Kindle.

Charcot, Jean-Martin. "Sur les divers états nerveux déterminés par l'hypnotisation chez les hystériques." *Comptes rendus hebdomadaires des séances de l'Académie des sciences* 94 (1882): 403–405.

Charcot, Jean-Martin, and Paul Richer. *Les Démoniaques dans l'art: avec 67 figures intercalées dans le texte*. Paris: A. Delahaye et E. Lecrosnier, 1887. Kindle.

Charon, Rita. "At the Membranes of Care: Stories in Narrative Medicine." *Academic Medicine* 87. 3 (March 2012): 342–347.

Charon, Rita. *Narrative Medicine: Honoring the Stories of Illness*. Oxford: Oxford University Press, 2008.

Chartier, Roger. *Les Origines culturelles de la revolutions française*. Paris: Éditions du Seuil, 2000.

Chateaubriand, François-René, de. *Memoirs from Beyond the Tomb*. Translated by Robert Baldick. London: Penguin, 2014. Kindle.

Chelouche, Tessa. "Leo Eitinger MD: Tribute to a Holocaust Survivor, Humane Physician and Friend of Mankind." *Israel Medical Association Journal* 16 (April 2014): 208–211.

Chodoff, Paul. "The Holocaust and Its Effects on Survivors: An Overview." *Political Psychology* 18. 1 (March 1997): 147–157.

Chodoff, Paul. "The Nazi Concentration Camp and the American Poverty Ghetto–A Comparison." *Journal of Contemporary Psychotherapy* 1. 1 (Fall 1968): 27–36.

Cloitre, Marylène, Lisa R. Cohen, Kile M. Ortigo, Christie Jackson, and Karestan C. Koenen. *Treating Survivors of Childhood Abuse and Interpersonal Trauma STAIR Narrative Therapy*. 2nd edition. New York: Guilford Press, 2020. Kindle.

Coles, Robert. *The Call of Stories: Teaching and the Moral Imagination*. New York: Houghton Mifflin Harcourt, 1989. Kindle.

Cramer, Holger, Dennis Anheyer, Felix J. Saha, and Gustav Dobos. "Yoga for Posttraumatic Stress Disorder–a Systematic Review and Meta-analysis." *BMC Psychiatry* 18. 72 (2018): 1–9.

Craps, Stef. *Postcolonial Witnessing: Trauma Out of Bounds*. London: Palgrave Macmillan, 2013. Kindle.

Craps, Stef, and Gert Buelens. "Introduction: Postcolonial Trauma Novels." *Studies in the Novel* 40. 1–2 (Spring–Summer–Spring–Summer 2008): 1–12.

Cusack, Karen, Daniel E. Jonas, Catherine A. Forneris, Candi Wines, Jeffrey Sonis, Jennifer Cook Middleton, Cynthia Feltner, et al. "Psychological Treatments for Adults with Posttraumatic Stress Disorder: A Systematic Review and Meta-analysis." *Clinical Psychology Review* 43 (February 2016): 128–141.

Cyrulnik, Boris. "Children in War and their Resiliences." In *The Unbroken Soul: Tragedy, Trauma, and Human Resilience*, edited by Henri Parens, Harold P. Blum, and Salman Akhtar, 23–36. Lanham, MD: Jason Aronson, 2008. Kindle.

Cyrulnik, Boris. *Un Merveilleux malheur*. Paris: Odile Jacob, 2002.

Cyrulnik, Boris. *La nuit, j'écrirai des soleils*. Paris: Odile Jacob, 2019. Kindle.

Cyrulnik, Boris. *Resilience: How Your Inner Strength Can Set You Free*. Translated by David Macey. New York: Penguin, 2011. Kindle.

Damasio, Antonio. *Descartes' Error: Emotion, Reason, and the Human Brain*. New York: Penguin Books, 2005.

Damrosch, David. *Comparing the Literatures*. Princeton: Princeton University Press, 2020. Kindle.

Damrosch, David. *What is World Literature?* Princeton: Princeton University Press, 2018. Kindle.

Dantzer, Robert, Sheldon Cohen, Scott J. Russo, and Timothy G. Dinan. "Resilience and Immunity." *Brain, Behavior, and Immunity* 74 (2018): 28–42.

Darwin, Charles. "Letter to J. D. Hooker, 13 July 1856." Darwin Correspondence Project, University of Cambridge. www.darwinproject.ac.uk/letter/DCP-LETT-1924.xml.

Darwin, Charles. *Notebook B: Transmutation of Species (1837–1838)*. Transcribed by Kees Rookmaaker. http://darwin-online.org.uk/content/frameset?itemID=CUL-DAR121.-&pageseq=38&viewtype=side. Accessed September 1, 2021.

Darwin, Charles. *The Origin of Species*. New York: Penguin, 1958. Kindle.

Davoine, Françoise. *Fighting Melancholia: Don Quixote's Teaching*. London: Karnac Books, 2016. Kindle.

Davoine, Françoise. "A Quixotic Approach to Trauma and Psychosis." In *Lost in Transmission: Studies of Trauma Across Generations*, edited by M. Gerard Fromm, loc. 2692–2981. London: Karnac Books, 2012. Kindle.

Davoine, Françoise, and Jean-Max Gaudillière. "Mad Witnesses: A Conversation with Françoise Davoine and Jean-Max Gaudillière." Interview with Cathy Caruth. *Listening to Trauma: Conversations with Leaders in the Theory and Treatment of Catastrophic Experience*, edited by Cathy Caruth, 81–110. Baltimore: Johns Hopkins University Press, 2014. Kindle.

De las Casas, Bartolomé. *The Tears of the Indians: Being an Historical and True Account of the Cruel Massacres and Slaughters of above Twenty Millions of Innocent People; Committed by the Spaniards in the Islands of Hispaniola, Cuba, Jamaica, &c. As Also, in the Continent of Mexico, Peru, & Other Places of the West-Indies, to the Total Destruction of Those Countries*. Translated by John Phillips. London: Nath. Brook at the Angel, 1656. https://quod.lib.umich.edu/e/eebo/A35553.0001.001?view=toc.

Deleuze, Gilles. *Critique et Clinique*. Paris: Éditions de Minuit, 1999.

De Man, Paul. "Resistance to Theory." *Yale French Studies* 63 (1982): 3–20.

Derrida, Jacques. *Dissemination*. Translated by Barbara Johnson. Chicago: University of Chicago Press, 2017. Kindle.

Desgenettes, René-Nicolas. *Histoire médicale de l'armée d'Orient par le médecin en chef R. Desgenettes*. Paris: Croullebois, 1802.

Diderot, Denis. "Encyclopedia." *The Encyclopedia of Diderot and d'Alembert Collaborative Translation Project*. Translated by Philip Stewart. Ann Arbor, MI: Michigan Publishing, University of Michigan Library, 2002.

Diderot, Denis. *Supplément au voyage of Bougainville*. Project Gutenberg, 2012. www.gutenberg.org/cache/epub/6501/pg6501.html.

Doidge, Norman. *The Brain That Changes Itself: Stories of Personal Triumph from the Frontiers of Brain Science*. New York: Penguin, 2007.

Eagleton, Terry. *After Theory*. New York: Basic Books, 2003.

Eagleton, Terry. *How to Read Literature*. New Haven: Yale University Press, 2013.

Eagleton, Terry. *Literary Theory: An Introduction*. Minneapolis: University of Minnesota Press, 1996.

Eitinger, Leo. *Concentration Camp Survivors in Norway and Israel*. Dordrecht: Springer Netherlands, 2012. Kindle.

Epstein, Mark. *The Trauma of Everyday Life*. New York: Penguin, 2014.

Erichsen, John Eric. "Mr. Erichsen's Work, 'Railway and Other Injuries of the Nervous System.'" Correspondence. *British Medical Journal* 2. 311 (December 15, 1856): 678–679.

Erichsen, John Eric. *On Concussion of the Spine, Nervous Shock, and Other Obscure Injuries to the Nervous System in Their Clinical and Medico-Legal Aspects*. New York: William Wood, 1883.

Erichsen, John Eric. *On Railway and Other Injuries of the Nervous System*. Philadelphia: Henry C. Lea, 1867.

Erikson, Kai. *Everything in its Path: Destruction of Community in the Buffalo Creek Flood*. New York: Simon and Schuster, 1976.

Erikson, Kai. "Notes on Trauma and Community." In *Trauma: Explorations in Memory*, edited by Cathy Caruth, 183–199. Baltimore: John Hopkins University Press, 1995.

Fanon, Frantz. *Black Skin, White Masks*. Translated by Richard. Philcox. New York: Grove Press, 1967.

Fanon, Frantz. *Toward the African Revolution*. Translated by Hakoun Chevalier. New York: Grove Press, 1967.

Fanon, Frantz. *The Wretched of the Earth*. Translated by Richard Philcox. New York: Grove Press, 2004.

Färber, L., B. Lattrell, A-K. Adloff, T. Welsh, V. Heeschen, and H.P. Hartung. "Hermann Oppenheim. Anmerkungen zu seinem Leben und Wirken." *Nervenarzt* 87 (2016): 1100–1106.

Felman, Shoshana. "Education and Crisis, or the Vicissitudes of Teaching." In *Trauma: Explorations of Memory*, edited by Cathy Caruth, 13–60. Baltimore: John Hopkins University Press, 1995.

Felman, Shoshana, and Dori Laub. *Testimony: Crises of Witnessing in Literature, Psychoanalysis, and History*. New York: Routledge, 1992. Kindle.

Fireman, Gary D., Ted E. McVay, and Owen J. Flanagan. *Narrative and Consciousness Literature, Psychology, and the Brain*. Oxford: Oxford University Press, 2003.

Foa, Edna, Seth J. Gillihan, and Richard A. Bryant. "Challenges and Successes in Dissemination of Evidence-Based Treatments for Posttraumatic Stress: Lessons Learned from Prolonged Exposure Therapy for PTSD." *Psychological Science in the Public Interest* 14. 2 (2013): 65–111.

Foa, Edna, Terrence M. Keane, and Matthew J. Friedman. "Guidelines for Treatment of PTSD." *Journal of Traumatic Stress* 13. 4 (2000): 539–580.

Forsyth, David. "Functional Nerve Disease and the Shock of Battle: A Study of the So-Called Traumatic Neuroses Arising in Connexion with the War." *The Lancet* (December 25, 1915): 1399–1403.

Frank, Arthur. *The Wounded Storyteller: Body, Illness, and Ethics*. 2nd edition. Chicago: University of Chicago Press, 2013.

Frankl, Victor. *Man's Search for Meaning*. Boston: Beacon Press, 1992.

Freud, Sigmund. *Civilization and Its Discontents*. Translated by James Strachey. New York: Norton, 1961.

Freud, Sigmund. *Dream Psychology: Psychoanalysis for Beginners*. Translated by M. D. Eder. Digireads, 2010. Kindle.

Freud, Sigmund. *The Interpretation of Dreams*. 4th edition. Translated by A. A. Brill. Digireads, 2017. Kindle.

Freud, Sigmund. *Introductory Lectures on Psychoanalysis*. Translated by G. Stanley Hall. Digireads, 2013. Kindle.

Friedman, Matthew J. "Finalizing PTSD in *DSM-5*: Getting Here from There and Where to Go Next." *Journal of Traumatic Stress* 26.5 (2013): 548–556.

Fromm, Erich. *Escape from Freedom*. New York: Henry Holt, 1969.

Fulton, Jessica J., Patrick S.Calhoun, H.Ryan Wagner, Amie R. Schry, Lauren P. Hair, Nicole Feeling, Eric Elbogen, et al. "The Prevalence of Posttraumatic Stress Disorder in Operation Enduring Freedom/Operation Iraqi Freedom (OEF/OIF) Veterans: A Meta-analysis." *Journal of Anxiety Disorders* 31 (2015): 98–107.

Fussell, Paul. *The Great War and Modern Memory*. Oxford: Oxford University Press, 2013.

García Márquez, Gabriel. "Interview: The Art of Fiction No. 69." Interview by Peter Stone. *Paris Review* 82 (Winter 1981). www.theparisreview.org/interviews/3196/the-art-of-fiction-no-69-gabriel-garcia-marquez. Last accessed September 11, 2021.

Gawande, Atul. *Being Mortal: Medicine and What Matters in the End*. New York: Metropolitan Books, 2014.

Genette, Gérard. *Figures I*. Paris: Seuil, 2014. Kindle.

Glick, Shimon. "The Empathic Physician: Nature and Nurture." In *Empathy and the Practice of Medicine: Beyond Pills and the Scalpel*, edited by Howard Spiro, Mary G. McCrea Curnen, Enid Peschel, and Deborah St James, 85–102. New Haven: Yale University Press, 1993.

Goethe, Johann Wolfgang, von, and Johann Peter Eckermann. *Conversations of Goethe with Johann Peter Eckermann*. Translated by John Oxenford. Boston, MA: De Capo Press, 2014. Kindle.

Goetter, Elizabeth M., Eric Bui, Rebecca A. Ojserkis, Rebecca J. Zakarian, Rebecca Weintraub Brendel, Naomi M. Simon. "A Systematic Review of Dropout from Psychotherapy for Posttraumatic Stress Disorder Among Iraq and Afghanistan Combat Veterans." *Journal of Traumatic Stress* 28. 5 (2015): 401–409.

Gracia Guillén, Diego. "Discreet Follies: Variations on Don Quixote's Folly." *Anales De La Real Academia Nacional De Medicina* 122. 1 (2005): 105–121.

Halpern, Jodi. *From Detached Concern to Empathy: Humanizing Medical Practice*. Oxford: Oxford University Press, 2011.

Haour, F., and C. de Beaurepaire. "Évaluation Scientifique de la psychothérapie EMDR pour le Traitement des Traumatismes Psychiques." *L'Encéphale* 24. 3 (2016): 284–288.

Harel, Zev, Kahana, Boaz, and Kahana, Eva. "The Effects of the Holocaust: Psychiatric, Behavioral, and Survivor Perspectives." *The Journal of Sociology and Social Welfare* 11. 4 (December 1984): 915–929.

Harnett, Nathaniel G., Adam M. Goodman, and David C. Knight. "PTSD-related Neuroimaging Abnormalities in Brain Function, Structure, and Biochemistry." *Experimental Neurology* 330 (2020): 1–11.

Hartman, Geoffrey. "On Traumatic Knowledge and Literary Studies." *New Literary History* 26. 3 (Summer 1995): 537–563.

Hartman, Geoffrey. "Words and Wounds." In *Listening to Trauma: Conversations with Leaders in the Theory and Treatment of Catastrophic Experience*, edited by Cathy Caruth. Baltimore: Johns Hopkins University Press, 2014. Kindle.

Haury, Gaston. *Les Anormaux et les malades mentaux au régiment. Avec une préface du Dr E. Régis*. Paris: Masson, 1913.

Heidegger, Martin. *Being and Time*. Translated by John Macquarrie and Edward Robinson. New York: Musthavebooks, 2021. Kindle.

Heim, Gerhard and Karl-Ernst Bühler. "Pierre Janet's Views on the Etiology, Pathogenesis, and Therapy of Dissociative Disorder." In *Rediscovering Pierre Janet*, edited by Giuseppe Craparo, Francesca Ortu, and Onno van der Hart, 177–191. New York: Routledge, 2019. Kindle.

Henke, Suzette. *Shattered Subjects: Trauma and Testimony in Women's Life-Writing*. New York: St. Martin's Press, 1998.

Herman, Judith. "Recovery from Psychological Trauma." *Psychiatry and Clinical Neurosciences* 52 (October 1998): S145–S150.

Herman, Judith. *Trauma and Recovery: The Aftermath of Violence, from Domestic Abuse to Political Terror*. New York: Basic Books, 2015. Kindle.

Herodotus. *Histories*. Translated by George Rawlinson. Digireads, 2016. Kindle.

Hippocrate. *Maladies des femmes*, Livre II. Paris: J.B. Baillière, 1841.

Holdorff, Bernd, and Tom Dening. "The Fight for 'Traumatic Neurosis', 1889–1916: Hermann Oppenheim and his Opponents in Berlin." *History of Psychiatry* 22. 4 (2011): 465–476.

Horney, Karen. *Our Inner Conflicts: Constructive Theory of Neurosis*. New York: Norton, 1945.

Hoskins, Matthew, Jennifer Pearce, Andrew Bethell, Liliya Dankova, Corrado Barbui, Wietse A. Tol, Mark van Ommeren et al. "Pharmacotherapy for Post-traumatic Stress Disorder: Systematic Review and Meta-analysis." *The British Journal of Psychiatry: The Journal of Mental Science* 206. 2 (2015): 93–100.

Huizinga, Johan. *The Autumn of the Middle Ages*. Translated by Rodney J. Payton and Ulrich Mammitzsch. Chicago: University of Chicago Press, 1996.

Husserl, Edmund. *Ideas: General Introduction to Pure Phenomenology*. New York: Taylor and Francis, 2013. Kindle.

Iser, Wolfgang. *The Act of Reading: A Theory of Aesthetic Response*. Baltimore: John Hopkins University Press, 1980.

Jakobson, Roman. *Huit questions de poétique*. Paris: Éditions du Seuil, 1977.

Janet, Pierre. *L'automatisme psychologique*. Philaubooks, 2019. Kindle.

Janet, Pierre. *État mental des hystériques: les stigmates mentaux*. Paris: Rueff, 1893.

Janet, Pierre. *L'évolution psychologique de la personnalité*. FV Éditions, n.d. Kindle.

Janet, Pierre. *The Major Symptoms of Hysteria: Fifteen Lectures Given in the Medical School of Harvard University*. 2nd edition. New York: The Macmillan Company, 1924.

Janet, Pierre. *Les médications psychologiques: études historiques, psychologiques et cliniques sur les méthodes de la psychothérapie. Les économies psychologiques II*. Paris: F. Alcan, 1919.

Janet, Pierre. *Les médications psychologiques: études historiques, psychologiques et cliniques sur les méthodes de la psychothérapie. Les acquisitions psychologiques III*. Paris: F. Alcan, 1919.

Janet, Pierre. *Les névroses*. Paris: Flammarion, 1909.

Janet, Pierre. *Principles of Psychotherapy*. Translated by H.M. Guthrie and E.R. Guthrie. MacMillan CAPA, 1924.

Jeffreys, Matt. *Clinician's Guide to Medications for PTSD*. US Department of Veterans Affairs. www.ptsd.va.gov/professional/treat/txessentials/clinician_guide_meds.asp. Accessed September 27, 2021.

Johnson, Carroll. *Madness and Lust: A Psychoanalytical Approach to Don Quixote*. Berkeley, CA: University of California Press, 1983.

Jones, Therese, Felicia Cohn, and Johanna Shapiro. "Minding the Gap(s): Narrativity and Liminality in Medical Student Writing." *Literature and Medicine* 30. 1 (2012): 103–123.

Jung, Carl Gustav. *The Art of C.G. Jung*. New York: Norton and Company, 2018.

Jung, Carl Gustav. *Modern Man in Search of a Soul*. Translated by W.S. Dell and Cary F. Baynes. Christopher Prince, North American eBook, 2011. Kindle.

Kafka, Franz. *The Metamorphosis and Other Stories*. Translated by Willa Muir and Edwin Muir. New York: Schocken Books, 1975. Kindle.

Kardiner, Abram. *Traumatic Neurosis of War*. New York: Paul B. Hoeber, 1941.

Kardiner, Abram, and Herbert Spiegel. *War, Stress, and Neurotic Illness*. New York: Paul B. Hoeber, 1947.

Kéchichian, Patrick. "Le Clézio, Nobel de 'la rupture.'" *Le Monde*, October 10, 2008. www.lemonde.fr/livres/article/2008/10/10/le-clezio-nobel-de-la-rupture_1105439_3260.html.

Kelm, Zak, James Womer, Jennifer K. Walter, and Chris Feudtner. "Interventions to Cultivate Physician Empathy: A Systematic Review." *Medical Education* 14. 219 (2014).

Klein, Melanie. "The Psycho-analytic Play Technique." In *The Selected Melanie Klein*, edited by Juliet Mitchell, 35–54. New York: Free Press, 1986.

Kleinman, Arthur. *The Illness Narratives: Suffering, Healing, and the Human Condition*. New York: Basic Books, 1989.

Kramer, Peter D. *Moments of Engagement: Intimate Psychotherapy in a Technological Age*. New York: Penguin, 1989.

Kristeva, Julia. *Soleil noir: Dépression et mélancolie*. Paris: Éditions Gallimard, 1987.

Krystal, Henry. "Trauma and Aging: A Thirty-Year Follow-up." In *Trauma: Explorations in Memory*, edited by Cathy Caruth, 76–99. Baltimore: John Hopkins University Press, 1995.

Krystal, Henry, and John Krystal. *Integration and Self-healing: Affect, Trauma, Alexithymia*. New York: Routledge, 2015. Kindle.

Kurtz, Roger. "Introduction." In *Trauma and Literature*, edited by Roger Kurtz, 1–17. Cambridge: Cambridge University Press, 2018.

Lacan, Jacques. *Écrits: A Selection*. Translated by Alain Sheridan. London: Routledge, 1989.

LaCapra, Dominick. *History and Reading: Tocqueville, Foucault, French Studies*. Toronto: University of Toronto Press, 2000.

LaCapra, Dominick. *Writing History, Writing Trauma*. Baltimore: Johns Hopkins University Press, 2014. Kindle.

LaLonde, Suzanne. *Paris and Its Revolutionary Ideas*. San Diego: Cognella Academic Press, 2020.

Lancaster, Steven, Benjamin F. Rodriguez, and Rebecca Weston. "Path Analytic Examination of Cognitive Model of PTSD." *Behaviour, Research, and Therapy* 49. 3 (March 2011): 194–201.

Laub, Dori. "A Record that Has Yet to Be Made: An Interview with Dori Laub." Interview with Cathy Caruth. *Listening to Trauma: Conversations with Leaders in the Theory and Treatment of Catastrophic Experience*, edited by Cathy Caruth, 47–77. Baltimore: Johns Hopkins University Press, 2014. Kindle.

Le Clézio, Jean-Marie Gustave. *Desert*. Boston: David Godine Publishing, 2009.

Le Clézio, Jean-Marie Gustave. "Une littérature de l'envahissement." Interview by Gérard de Cortanze. *Magazine Littéraire* 362. 02 (1998): 18–35.

Lejeune, Philippe. *Le Pacte autobiographique*. Paris: Seuil, 1996. Kindle.

Levine, Murray. "Children Come First? A Brief History of Children's Mental Health Services." *American Journal of Orthopsychiatry* 85. 5S (2015): S22–28.

Levine, Peter. *In an Unspoken Voice: How the Body Releases Trauma and Restores Goodness*. Berkeley, CA: North Atlantic Books, 2010. Kindle.

Levine, Peter, and Ann Frederick. *Waking the Tiger: Healing Trauma*. Berkeley, CA: North Atlantic Books, 1997. Kindle.

Lévi-Strauss, Claude. *Myth and Meaning: Cracking the Code of Culture*. New York: Schocken Books, 1995.

Leys, Ruth. "Death Masks: Kardiner and Ferenczi on Psychic Trauma." *Representation* 53 (Winter 1996): 44–73.

Leys, Ruth. *Trauma: A Genealogy*. Chicago: University of Chicago Press, 2000. Kindle.

Liberzon, Israel, and James L. Abelson. "Context Processing and the Neurobiology of Post-Traumatic Stress Disorder." *Neuron* 92. 1 (2016): 14–30.

Lifton, Robert Jay. *Witness to an Extreme Century: A Memoir*. New York: Free Press, 2011. Kindle.

Luckhurst, Roger. *The Trauma Question*. New York: Routledge, 2008.

Lucretius. *Nature of Things*. Translated by Alicia Stallings. New York: Penguin, 2007.

Malabou, Catherine. *The New Wounded: From Neurosis to Brain Damage*. Translated by Steven Miller. New York: Fordham University Press, 2012.

Marbot, Marcellin, de. *Mémoires du général Bon de Marbot*. Paris: Plon, 1891.

Maslow, Abraham. *Toward a Psychology of Being*. Rediscovered Books, 2014. Kindle.

McFarlane, Alexander, and Bessel van der Kolk. "The Long-Term Effect of Psychological Trauma: A Public Health Issue in Kuwait." *Medical Principles and Practice* 5. 2 (1996): 59–75.

McNally, Richard. "Debunking Myths about Trauma and Memory." *Canadian Journal of Psychiatry* 50. 13 (November 2005): 817–822.

Memmi, Albert. *The Colonizer and the Colonized*. Boston: Beacon, 1961.

Mendes Da Costa, Jacob. *Medical Diagnosis: With Special Reference to Practical Medicine*. Miami: Hardpress, 2017. Kindle.

Mengel, Ewald, and Michela Borzaga, eds. *Trauma, Memory, and Narrative in the Contemporary South Africa Novel*. New York: Rodopi, 2012.

Merleau-Ponty, Maurice. *Le Visible et l'invisible*. Paris: Gallimard, 2014.

Michelet, Jules. *Histoire de France au seizième siècle: Renaissance réforme. Œuvres complètes de Jules Michelet*. Edited by Robert Casanova. Paris: Flammarion, 1978.

Montaigne, Michel. *The Complete Essays of Michel de Montaigne*. Translated by Charles Cotton. Digireads, 2017. Kindle.

Mukherjee, Siddhartha. *The Laws of Medicine: Field Notes from an Uncertain Science*. New York: Simon and Schuster, 2015.

Müller, Gesine. *Crossroads of Colonial Cultures: Caribbean Literatures in the Age of Revolution*. Translated by Marie Deer. Berlin: de Gruyter, 2018.

Mutloatse, Mothobi, ed. *Forced Landing: Africa South: Contemporary Writings*. Johannesburg, South Africa: Ravan Press, 1981.

NCBI. "Neurocirculatory Asthenia." www.ncbi.nlm.nih.gov/medgen/14347. Accessed October 23, 2021.

NCTSN. "Defining Child Traumatic Stress." www.nctsn.org/what-is-child-trauma/about-child-trauma.

Nicholson, Andrew, Maria Densmore, Paul A. Frewen, Jean Théberge, Richard W. Neufeld, Margaret C. McKinnon, and Ruth A. Lanius. "The Dissociative Subtype of Posttraumatic Stress Disorder: Unique Resting-State Functional Connectivity of Basolateral and Centromedial Amygdala Complexes." *Neuropsychopharmacology* 40 (2015): 2317–2326.

Niederland, William. "Psychiatric Disorders among Persecution Victims: A Contribution to the Understanding of Concentration Camp Pathology and Its After-Effects." *Journal of Nervous and Mental Disease* 139 (1964): 458–474.

Nobel Prize. "Nobel Prize in Literature 2008." www.nobelprize.org/prizes/literature/2008/press-release. Accessed August 31, 2021.

Nock, Matthew K., Robert Ursano, Steven G. Heeringa, Murray B. Stein, Sonia Jain, Rema Raman, Xiaoying Sun, et al. "Mental Disorders, Comorbidity, and Pre-enlistment Suicidal Behavior Among New Soldiers in the US Army: Results from the Army Study to Assess Risk and Resilience in Servicemembers (Army STARRS)." *Suicide & Life-Threatening Behavior* 45. 5 (2015): 588–599.

North, Carol S., Alina M. Suris, and David E. Pollio. "A Nosological Exploration of PTSD and Trauma in Disaster Mental Health and Implications for the COVID-19 Pandemic." *Behavioral Sciences* 11. 1 (2021): 1–14.

Ogden, Thomas. "Kafka, Borges, and the Creation of Consciousness, Part II: Borges—A Life of Letters Encompassing Everything and Nothing." *The Psychoanalytic Quarterly* 78. 2 (April 2009): 369–396.

Oppenheim, Janet. *"Shattered Nerves": Doctors, Patients and Depression in Victorian England*. New York: Oxford University Press, 1991.

Pai, Anushka, Alina M. Suris, and Carol S. North. "Posttraumatic Stress Disorder in the *DSM-5*: Controversy, Change, and Conceptual Considerations." *Behavioral Sciences* 7. 1 (2017): 7.

Palmab, Jose-Alberto, and Fermin Palmab. "Neurology and Don Quixote." *European Neurology* 68. 4 (2012): 247–257.

Philoof Alexandria. *De Somniis*. Translated by J.H.A. Hart. *The Jewish Quarterly Review* 18 (1906): 330–346. https://archive.org/details/jstor-1451071.

Pinker, Stephen. *The Better Angels of Our Nature: Why Violence Has Declined*. New York: Penguin, 2011. Kindle.

Pitman, Roger K., Ann M. Rasmusson, Karestan C. Koenen, Lisa M. Shin, Scott P. Orr, Mark W. Gliberston, Mohammed R. Milad. "Biological Studies of Posttraumatic Stress Disorder." *Nature Reviews Neuroscience* 13. 11 (2012): 769–787.

Plato. *The Republic*. Translated by G.M.A. Grube. Indianapolis: Hackett Publishing, 1992. Kindle.

Poulet, Georges. "Phenomenon of Reading." *New Literary History* 1. 1 (1969): 53–68.

Rank, Otto. *Art and Artist: Creative Urge and Personality Development*. New York: Alfred Knopf, 1932.

Raynal, Guillaume-Thomas-François. *A History of the Two Indies: A Translated Selection of Writings from Raynal's Histoire philosophique et politique des établissements des Européens dans les Deux Indes.* Edited and translated by Peter Jimack. London: Routledge, 2017. Kindle.

Régis, Emmanuel. *Précis de psychiatrie.* 3rd edition. Paris: Octave. Doin, 1906.

Richman, Sophia. *Mended by the Muse: Creative Transformations of Trauma.* New York: Routledge, 2014. Kindle.

Ricoeur, Paul. "Narrative Identity." *Philosophy Today 35.* 1 (Spring 1991): 73–81.

Riess, Helen, John M. Kelley, Robert W. Bailey, Emily J. Dunn, and Margot Phillips. "Empathy Training for Resident Physicians: A Randomized Controlled Trial of a Neuroscience-Informed Curriculum." *Journal of General Internal Medicine* 27. 10 (2012): 1280–1286.

Rose, Nikolas, and Joelle Abi-Rached. *Neuro: The New Brain Sciences and the Management of the Mind.* Princeton: Princeton University Press, 2013.

Rothberg, Michael. "Decolonizing Trauma Studies: A Response." *Studies in the Novel* 40 (2008): 224–234.

Rousseau, Jean-Jacques. "A Discourse on the Origin of Inequality," in *The Basic Political Writings.* 2nd edition. Translated by Donald A. Cress. Indianapolis, IN: Hackett Publishing, 2011. Kindle.

Rubin, David, Adriel Boals, and Dorthe Bernsten. "Memory in Posttraumatic Stress Disorder: Properties of Voluntary and Involuntary, Traumatic and Non-traumatic Autobiographical Memories in People with and without Posttraumatic Stress Disorder Symptoms." *Journal of Experimental Psychology* 137. 4 (2008): 591–614.

Sacks, Oliver. *An Anthropologist on Mars: Seven Paradoxical Tales.* New York: Vintage, 1995.

Said, Edward. *Culture and Imperialism.* New York: Vintage, 1994.

Sartre, Jean-Paul. *Carnets de la drôle de guerre September 1939-Mars 1940.* Paris: Gallimard, 2018. Kindle.

Sartre, Jean-Paul. *Existentialism is a Humanism.* Translated by Carol Macomber. New Haven: Yale University Press, 2007. Kindle.

Sartre, Jean-Paul. *Nausea.* Translated by Lloyd Alexander. New York: New Directions, 2013. Kindle.

Scaer, Robert C. *The Body Bears the Burden: Trauma, Dissociation, and Disease.* 2nd edition. New York: Haworth Medical Press, 2007.

Scott, Michael. *CBT for Common Trauma Responses.* London: Sage, 2013.

Scurlock, Jo Ann, and Burton Andersen. *Diagnoses in Assyrian and Babylonian Medicine: Ancient Sources, Translations, and Modern Medical Analyses.* Champaign: University of Illinois Press, 2010.

Shapiro, Barbara. "Resilience, Sublimation, and Healing." In *Unbroken Soul: Tragedy, Trauma, and Resilience*, edited by Henri Parens, Harold Blum, and Salman Akhtar, 118–128. Lanham, MD: Jason Aronson, 2008. Kindle.

Shengold, Leonard. "Insight as Metaphor." *The Psychoanalytic Study of the Child* 36. 1 (2017): 289–306.

Showalter, Elaine. *The Female Malady: Women, Madness and English Culture, 1830–1980.* London: Virago, 1987.

Siegal, Daniel J., and Marion F. Solomon. Introduction. In *Healing Trauma: Attachment, Mind, Body and Brain*, edited by Daniel J. Siegal and Marion F. Solomon, loc. 81–257. New York: W.W. Norton and Company, 2003. Kindle.

Sokal, Alan and Bricmont, Jean. *Fashionable Nonsense Postmodern Intellectuals' Abuse of Science*. New York: Picador, 1998.

Sommer, Lauren. "Climate Change Is the Greatest Threat to Public Health, Top Medical Journals Warn." September 7, 2021. www.gpb.org/news/2021/09/07/clima te-change-the-greatest-threat-public-health-top-medical-journals-warn. Accessed September 13, 2021.

Stahnisch, Frank. "William G. Niederland (1904–1993)." *Journal of Neurology* 264 (2017): 2187–2189.

Stein, Dan, Johnathan C. Ipser, and Soraya Seedat. "Pharmacotherapy for Posttraumatic Stress Disorder (PTSD)." *Cochrane Database of Systematic Reviews* 1 (January 2006): 1–97.

Stephanson, Raymond. "The Plague Narratives of Defoe and Camus: Illness as a Metaphor." *Modern Language Quarterly* 48. 3 (1987): 224–241.

Tallis, Raymond. *Aping Mankind: Neuromania, Darwinitis and the Misrepresentation of Humanity*. London: Acumen Press, 2011.

Tansella, Christa. "The Seminal Work of Carlo Zinelli." *Epidemiology and Psychiatric Sciences* 22. 1 (2013): 15–16.

Tedeschi, Richard, Jane Shakespeare-Finch, Kanako Taku, and Lawrence G. Calhoun. *Posttraumatic Growth*. New York: Routledge, 2018. Kindle.

Thomas Jefferson University. "Jacob Mendes Da Costa." https://library.jefferson.ed u/archives/exhibits/notable_alumni/jacob_mendes_dacosta.cfm Accessed October 23, 2021.

Toremans, Tom. "Deconstruction: Trauma Inscribed in Language." In *Trauma and Literature*, edited by Roger Kurtz, 51–65. Cambridge: Cambridge University Press, 2018.

Tsai, Jack, Vanessa Schick, Belinda Hernandez, and Robert H. Piertrzak. "Is Homelessness a Traumatic Event? Results from the 2019–2020 National Health and Resilience in Veterans Study." *Depression and Anxiety* 37. 11 (2020): 1137–1145.

Tyrer, Peter. "A Comparison of DSM and ICD Classifications of Mental Disorders." *Advances in Psychiatric Treatment* 20. 4 (2014): 280–285.

Unamuno, Miguel de. *Analogía Poética*. Madrid: Alianza, Biblioteca Unamuno, 2009.

US Department of Veterans Affairs. "How Common is PTSD in Adults?" www.ptsd. va.gov/understand/common/common_adults.asp. Accessed May 3, 2021.

Van der Hart, Onno, Ellert Nijenhuis, and Kathy Steele. *The Haunted Self: Structural Dissociation and the Treatment of Chronic Traumatization*. New York: W.W. Norton and Company, 2006. Kindle.

Van der Hart, Onno, Ellert Nijenhuis, and Kathy Steele. "Pierre Janet's Treatment of Post-traumatic Stress." In *Rediscovering Pierre Janet*, edited by Giuseppe Craparo, Francesca Ortu, and Onno van der Hart, 163–177. New York: Taylor and Francis, 2019. Kindle.

Van der Kolk, Bessel. *The Body Keeps the Score: Brain, Mind, and Body in the Healing of Trauma*. New York: Viking, 2014. Kindle.

Van der Kolk, Bessel. "Introduction." In *Overcoming Trauma through Yoga: Reclaiming Your Body*, by David Emerson and Elizabeth Hopper, xvii–xxiv. Berkeley, CA: North Atlantic Books, 2011.

Van der Kolk, Bessel. "Posttraumatic Stress Disorder and The Nature of Trauma." In *Healing Trauma: Attachment, Mind, Body and Brain*, edited by Daniel J. Siegal and Marion F. Solomon, 168–195. New York: W.W. Norton and Company, 2003. Kindle.

Van der Kolk, Bessel. "Trauma and Memory." *Psychiatry and Clinical Neurosciences* 52. S1 (1998): S52–S64.

Van Gogh, Vincent. *The Letters of Vincent van Gogh*. Translated by Arnold Pomerans. London: Penguin, 2003. Kindle.

Vissier, Irene. "Decolonizing Trauma Theory: Retrospect." *Humanities* 4 (2015) 250–265.

Vissier, Irene. "Trauma in Non-Western Contexts." In *Trauma and Literature*, edited by Roger Kurtz, 124–139. Cambridge: Cambridge University Press, 2018.

Voltaire. *Age of Louis XIV*. Translated by William F. Fleming. New York: St. Hubert Guild, 1901. Kindle.

Voltaire. *Lettres choisies*. Paris: Garnier, 1963. Kindle.

Voltaire. *Philosophical Dictionary: Unabridged and Unexpurgated*. New York: E.R. DuMont, 1901. Kindle.

Voltaire. *Zadig and L'Ingénu*. Translated by John Butt. London: Penguin Books, 1964. Kindle.

Walker, John I., and James L. Nash. "Group Therapy in the Treatment of Vietnam Combat Veterans." *International Journal of Group Psychotherapy* 31. 1 (January 1981). 379–389.

Wallon, Henri. "Lésions nerveuses et troubles psychiques de guerre." *Journal de psychologie normale et pathologique*, 1920.

Watters. Ethan. *Crazy Like Us: The Globalization of the American Psyche*. New York: Free Press, 2011.

Whitehead, Anne. *Trauma Fiction*. Edinburgh: Edinburgh University Press, 2004.

World Health Organization. *International Statistical Classification of Diseases and Related Health Problems: ICD-10*. Geneva: World Health Organization, 2010. https://icd.who.int/browse10/2019/en. Accessed September 2, 2021.

Wilson, Edward O. *Consilience: The Unity of Knowledge*. New York: Vintage, 1999. Kindle.

Wilson, John, and Rhiannon Brywnn Thomas. *Empathy in the Treatment of Trauma and PTSD*. New York: Brunner-Routledge, 2004.

Winnicott, Donald. *Psycho-Analytic Explorations*. New York: Routledge, 2018. Kindle.

Wood, Michele, Alexander Molassiotis, and Sheila Payne. "What Research Evidence Is There for the Use of Art Therapy in the Management of Symptoms in Adults with Cancer? A Systematic Review." *Psycho-oncology* 20. 2 (2011): 135–145.

Wu, Gang, Adriana Feder, Hagit Cohen, Joanna J. Kim, Solara Calderon, Dennis S. Charney, and Aleksander A. Mathé. "Understanding Resilience." *Frontiers in Behavioral Neurosciences* 7. 10 (February 15, 2013): 1–15.

Yalom, Irvin. *Existential Psychotherapy*. New York: Hachette, 1980.

Young, Allan. *The Harmony of Illusions*. Princeton: Princeton University Press, 1995.

Žižek, Slovaj. *Living in the End of Times*. New York: Verso, 2011.

Zoladz, Phillip R., and David M. Diamond. "Current Status on Behavioral and Biological Markers of PTSD: A Search for Clarity in a Conflicting Literature." *Neuroscience and Biobehavioral Reviews* 37. 5 (2013): 860–895.

Index

Page numbers followed by 'n' refer to notes.

For Product Safety Concerns and Information please contact our EU
representative GPSR@taylorandfrancis.com
Taylor & Francis Verlag GmbH, Kaufingerstraße 24, 80331 München, Germany

www.ingramcontent.com/pod-product-compliance
Lightning Source LLC
Chambersburg PA
CBHW060252220326
41598CB00027B/4070